Nanobiomaterials Science, Development and Evaluation

Related titles

Nanomaterials in Tissue Engineering,
(ISBN: 978-0-85709-596-1)

Nanotechnology and Nanomaterials in the Treatment of Life-threatening Diseases
(ISBN: 978-0-323-26433-4)

Nanotechnology Applications for Tissue Engineering
(ISBN: 978-0-323-32889-0)

Woodhead Publishing Series in Biomaterials

Nanobiomaterials Science, Development and Evaluation

Edited by

Mehdi Razavi

Avnesh Thakor

ELSEVIER

WP
WOODHEAD PUBLISHING
An imprint of Elsevier

Woodhead Publishing is an imprint of Elsevier
The Officers' Mess Business Centre, Royston Road, Duxford, CB22 4QH, United Kingdom
50 Hampshire Street, 5th Floor, Cambridge, MA 02139, United States
The Boulevard, Langford Lane, Kidlington, OX5 1GB, United Kingdom

British Library Cataloguing-in-Publication Data
A catalogue record for this book is available from the British Library

Library of Congress Cataloging-in-Publication Data
A catalog record for this book is available from the Library of Congress

ISBN: 978-0-08-100963-5 (print)
ISBN: 978-0-08-100968-0 (online)

For information on all Woodhead Publishing publications
visit our website at https://www.elsevier.com/books-and-journals

Publisher: Matthew Deans
Acquisitions Editor: Laura Overend
Editorial Project Manager: Natasha Welford
Production Project Manager: Poulouse Joseph
Cover Designer: Greg Harris

Typeset by MPS Limited, Chennai, India

Contents

List of Contributors

Farzaneh Aavani Amirkabir University of Technology, Tehran, Iran

Samad Ahadian University of Toronto, Toronto, ON, Canada

Ebru Altuntaş Istanbul University, Istanbul, Turkey

Yasemin Budama-Kilinc Yildiz Technical University, Istanbul, Turkey

Rabia Cakir-Koc Yildiz Technical University, Istanbul, Turkey

Ayse Candayan Bogazici University, Istanbul, Turkey

Sefa Celik Istanbul University, Istanbul, Turkey

Kyriakos Dalamagkas Harvard Medical School, Boston, MA, United States; University College of London, London, United Kingdom; Weiss Memorial Hospital, Chicago, IL, United States

Kubra Gozutok Yildiz Technical University, Istanbul, Turkey

Madalina Elena Grigore University Politehnica of Bucharest, Bucharest, Romania

Alexandru Mihai Grumezescu University Politehnica of Bucharest, Bucharest, Romania

Alina Maria Holban Department of Microbiology and Immunology, Faculty of Biology and Research Institute of the University of Bucharest, University of Bucharest, Bucharest, Romania

Mohammed Inayathullah Biomaterials and Advanced Drug Delivery Laboratory, Stanford University School of Medicine, Palo Alto, CA, United States; Cardiovascular Pharmacology Division, Cardiovascular Institute, Stanford University School of Medicine, Stanford, CA, United States

Serda Kecel-Gunduz Istanbul University, Istanbul, Turkey

Amirsalar Khandan Islamic Azad University, Isfahan, Iran

Nasim Kiaie Amirkabir University of Technology, Tehran, Iran

M. Miraftab University of Bolton, Bolton, Lancashire, United Kingdom

M. Rezaa Mohammadi Biomaterials and Advanced Drug Delivery Laboratory, Stanford University School of Medicine, Palo Alto, CA, United States

Fatemeh Mohandes Sharif University of Technology, Tehran, Iran

Parisa Nazemi Isfahan University of Technology, Isfahan, Iran

Wanting Niu Harvard Medical School, Boston, MA, United States; VA Boston Healthcare System, Boston, MA, United States

Farideh Ordikhani Sharif University of Technology, Tehran, Iran

Burak Ozdemir Yildiz Technical University, Istanbul, Turkey

Aysen E. Ozel Istanbul University, Istanbul, Turkey

Burcu Özkan Yildiz Technical University, Istanbul, Turkey

Olga N. Oztel Liv Hospital Center for Regenerative Medicine and Stem Cell Manufacturing (LivMedCell), Istanbul, Turkey

Milica Radisic University of Toronto, Toronto, ON, Canada

Jayakumar Rajadas Biomaterials and Advanced Drug Delivery Laboratory, Stanford University School of Medicine, Palo Alto, CA, United States; Cardiovascular Pharmacology Division, Cardiovascular Institute, Stanford University School of Medicine, Stanford, CA, United States

Mehdi Razavi Stanford University, Palo Alto, CA, United States

Anzelika Schreiber Charité – Universitätsmedizin, Berlin, Germany

Abdolreza Simchi Sharif University of Technology, Tehran, Iran

Wenchao Sun Biomaterials and Advanced Drug Delivery Laboratory, Stanford University School of Medicine, Palo Alto, CA, United States; Cardiovascular Pharmacology Division, Cardiovascular Institute, Stanford University School of Medicine, Stanford, CA, United States

Magdalini Tsintou Harvard Medical School, Boston, MA, United States; University College of London, London, United Kingdom

Cang Wang Zhejiang University, Hangzhou, China

Ding Weng Tsinghua University, Beijing, China

Frank Witte Charité – Universitätsmedizin, Berlin, Germany

Gülgün Yener Istanbul University, Istanbul, Turkey

Serap Yesilkir-Baydar Yildiz Technical University, Istanbul, Turkey

Yi-Nan Zhang University of Toronto, Toronto, ON, Canada

Yu S. Zhang Harvard Medical School, Cambridge, MA, United States

Kai Zhu Harvard Medical School, Cambridge, MA, United States; Fudan University, Shanghai, China; Shanghai Institute of Cardiovascular Disease, Shanghai, China

Introduction

1

Mehdi Razavi
Stanford University, Palo Alto, CA, United States

Researches on nanobiomaterials over the past decades have inspired innovation in novel materials, processing techniques, performance evaluation, and applications. Significant progress has been made toward scaffold materials for structural support. Degradable bioscaffolds with controlled porosity and tailored properties are possible today because of innovation in bioscaffold production by advanced technologies. Different research groups have tried to manipulate the mechanical properties such as stiffness, strength, and toughness of bioscaffolds by the design of nanostructures including the inclusion of nanoparticles or nanofiber reinforcements in polymer matrices to mimic tissue's natural nano architecture [1].

Within the stem cell niche, micro-/nanoscale interactions with extracellular matrix (ECM) components constitute another source of passive mechanical forces that can affect stem cell behaviors. The ECM is composed of a wide spectrum of structural proteins and polysaccharides that span over different length scales, with strands of collagen fibrils dominating at the nanometer level, with a diameter between 35 nm and 60 nm and a length that can extend over the micron range [3]. It is via such well-choreographed spatiotemporal dialog between stem cells and their micro-/nanoenvironment that long-term maintenance and control of stem cell behavior are achieved. The advent of sophisticated small-scale technologies has now made it possible for researchers to produce a platform that is able to be utilized to gain valuable insights into stem cell biomechanics [4]. Besides, bioinspired and mimicking substrates with micro-/nanofeatures have been used to recognize and control stem cell differentiation. However, despite the importance of stem cell mechanobiology, how mechanical stimuli regulates the stem cells behaviors both in vivo and ex vivo have yet to be fully understood [5]. To better mimic the nanostructure in natural ECM, over the past decade, bioscaffolds manufactured from nanoparticles, nanofibers, nanotubes, and hydrogel have newly emerged as promising selections in fabrication of bioscaffolds that resemble the ECM and efficiently replace defective tissues [5]. Since natural tissues or organs are nanometer in dimension and cells directly interact with (and create) nanostructured ECMs, the biomimetic features and outstanding physiochemical behaviors of nanomaterials play a key role in stimulating cell growth and guiding tissue regeneration [6]. Stem cells are able to differentiate into different cell types, proposing opportunities and alternatives not only for the treatment of diseases but also for the tissues and organs regeneration beyond complex surgical treatments or tissue/organ transplantation. The construction of synthetic ECMs inspired by tissue-specific niches for programmed stem cell fate and response, including proliferation and differentiation, is a topic of interest in the field of tissue regeneration. By nanogrooved matrices mimicking the native tissues, Kim et al. [7] understood that the body and nucleus of human mesenchymal stem cells (hMSCs) with the sparser nanogrooved

Nanobiomaterials Science, Development and Evaluation. DOI: http://dx.doi.org/10.1016/B978-0-08-100963-5.00001-X

pattern elongated and orientated more along the direction of nanogrooves than those with the quite denser nanogroove patterns [1].

The current developments in the field of nanotechnology extremely enhanced the area of nanomedicine. There are numerous profits of nanotechnology-based methods to therapy, personalized medicine, targeted drug delivery, and intelligent drug design. Personalized or individual-based medicine, aims to develop drugs based on the patient's genotype by making use of nanoarrays for molecular diagnostics, whereas conventional method tries to match the existing drugs with the patients in the most appropriate way [8]. Intelligent drugs are being made to respond to stimuli and particularly react with the target and existing drugs are being modified so that their side effects, immunogenicity, or toxicity might be reduced. Nanotechnology approaches can also be utilized to increase the efficiency of the molecule as a therapeutic agent. For instance, the poor aqueous solubility of drug candidates confines their bioavailability and the drug-discovery process. This solubility restriction can be addressed by decreasing the particle size of drug to nanometer scale [9]. One of the most promising applications of nanotechnology include design and fabrication of intelligent delivery systems that are capable of indicating responsive behavior upon a certain environmental signal including temperature, pH, ionic strength, electric and magnetic field. Nanoscale responsive delivery systems are very favorable, since they offer numerous advantages including specific targeting, stimuli-dependent release behavior, and increased ability of escaping from phagocytotic uptake and, therefore, prolonged circulation times because of their nanoscale sizes [10]. Numerous investigations have been carried out on delivery of protein-peptide drugs, genes, and antisense oligonucleotides by such intelligent nanosystems [1,11].

Tissue engineering is the use of a scaffolding material to either induce formation of tissue from the surrounding tissue or to act as a carrier or template for implanted cells or other agents. Materials utilized as tissue-engineered bioscaffolds may be rigid or injectable, with the latter necessitating an operative implantation procedure. Conventional tissue engineering bioscaffolds have utilized different pore-forming approaches to recreate the macroscale and microscale properties of native tissues, but the nanoscale structures and properties were neglected. But, the nanoscale structures are vital to regulating cell functions, including proliferation, migration, differentiation, and the formation of ECM. To simulate the hierarchical organization of natural ECM, one important strategy is to build nanoscale and microscale features in the three-dimensional (3D) scaffolds design. The normally accepted definition of nanomaterials refers to materials with well-defined features between 1 nm and 100 nm, including nanopattern, nanofibers, nanotubers, nanopores, nanospheres, and nanocomposites [12,13] (Fig. 1.1a–f) [1].

There are various techniques to improve the surfaces and provide patterns to reach to cells organization. These patterns could be two-dimensional (2D) or 3D, although the resulting cell organization is usually in 2D. The dimension of the patterns could be at the micro- or nanometer level. Achieving nanopatterns is a more challenging procedure than micropatterns since low micron level is what can be reached with most of the recent methods employed. Investigations on the effect of micropatterns on cell

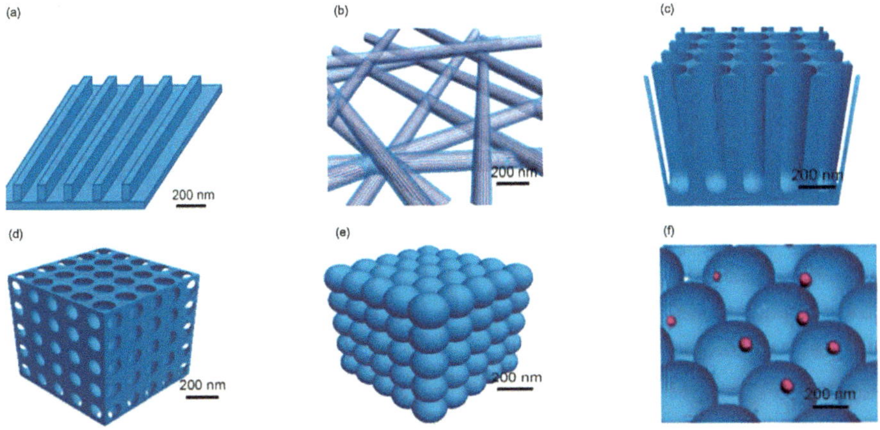

Figure 1.1 Nanostructures with features of nanopattern (a), nanofibers (b), nanotubers (c), nanopores (d), nanospheres (e), and nanocomposites (f) with structural components with a feature size in the nanoscale.
With permission from Nature Publishing Group [1].

guidance are displaying an enhance and the data accumulated show that cells could be responsive to nanolevel chemical and physical cues [2].

As is known, synthetically nanofabricated topography can also effect cell morphology, alignment, adhesion, migration, proliferation, and cytoskeleton organization [14]. The symmetry and order of the nanopits was found to considerably influence the expression of osteopontin and osteocalcin, two bone-specific ECM proteins, in both cell types (Fig. 1.2a–c) [15]. While hMSCs cultured on entirely ordered or completely random nanopits did not result in the expression of these two proteins, hMSCs cultured on slightly irregular substrates did show considerable amounts of these proteins of interest. Enhanced bone nodule formation was also evident in hMSCs cultured on these substrates in relation to substrates with either completely ordered or completely random features. The results from the researches indicated the potential of nanotopography to direct cell fate. Together, a few common observations can be drawn from the aforementioned studies of the mechanosensitivity of stem cells. All the studies possess explicitly or implicitly suggested the involvement of cytoskeleton contractility in regulating the mechanosensitivity of stem cells, suggesting the significance of the force balance along the mechanical axis of the ECM–integrin–cytoskeleton linkage and their regulation by the mechanical signals in the stem cell niche (Fig. 1.2d) [16]. Furthermore, strong evidence recommended that the differentiation potentials of stem cells toward distinct lineages could be maximized if the cells were cultured in the mechanical microenvironment mimicking their tissue elasticity in vivo [17]. Moreover, nanoscale manipulation of surface features including surface texture, geometry, spatial position, and height might potentially change clustering of the integrins, the development of focal adhesions, and cytoskeletal structure, therefore effecting the osteogenic differentiation to the surface [1,18].

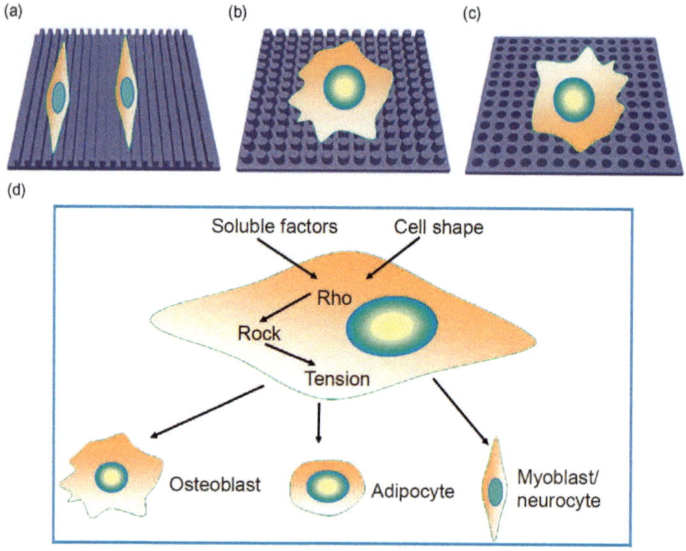

Figure 1.2 Schematic depictions of representative nanotopography geometries. Three basic nanotopography geometries include nanogrooves (a), nanopost array (b), and nanopit array (c). The speculative pathways (d) for cell-shape-directed osteogenic and adipogenic differentiations of MSCs were examined in growth medium. RhoA, Ras homolog gene family member A; ROCK, Rho-associated protein kinase.
With permission from Nature Publishing Group [1].

Tissue engineering and regenerative medicine using nanobiomaterials is still in its infancy but upward strides are being made to advance and enhance protocols for clinical applications. In this book, we focused on reviewing the classification and design of nanostructured materials and nanocarrier materials, their cell interaction properties, and their application in tissue engineering and regeneration. Additionally, some new challenges about the future research on the application of nanomaterials are described in the conclusion and future parts. Sometimes nanoparticle interactions with biomolecules in vivo or their aggregation states may alter their toxicity to humans. But the often contradictory results of recent researches are obviously not sufficient to provide the final answer concerning nanomaterial toxicity. In-depth examinations of nanomaterials on human health and the environment are essential to fully elucidate whether nanoparticles should be utilized in biomedical applications. New frontiers of research should be directed toward better biomimicking the natural process of tissue regeneration. Although it is difficult to mimic nature, current scientific and technological results display potential to achieve bioscaffolds that would encourage local and systemic biological functions. Proper selection of bioscaffold materials, their geometry, pore size, and size distribution, and ability to release biomolecules at an anticipated rate will play critical roles in the future development of bioscaffolds. Nonetheless, nanotechnology alone may not be the answer to improving the mechanical properties of bioscaffolds. The restrictions in processing techniques, in part, have hampered the progress in the development of new bioscaffolds to form structures with a multidimensional architecture. The challenge is to use these technologies in combination with nanomaterials. It is possible that at the end an optimum bioscaffold combining several materials and techniques (e.g., a complex polymer structure can be created by ice-templating or computer-assisted production that can later be mineralized to reach to the desired mechanical and biodegradation responses) will become reality.

References

[1] Gong T, Xie J, Liao J, Zhang T, Lin S, Lin Y. Nanomaterials and bone regeneration. Bone Res 2015;3(August):15029.

[2] Hasirci V, Vrana E, Zorlutuna P, Ndreu A, Yilgor P, Basmanav FB, et al. Nanobiomaterials: a review of the existing science and technology, and new approaches. J Biomater Sci Polym Ed 2006;17(11):1241–68.

[3] Li X, Wang L, Fan Y, Feng Q, Cui FZ, Watari F. Nanostructured scaffolds for bone tissue engineering. Journal of Biomedical Materials Research - Part A 2013:2424–35.

[4] Stevens MM. Biomaterials for bone tissue engineering. Materials Today 2008:18–25.

[5] Stevens MM, George JH. Exploring and engineering the cell surface interface. Science 2005;310(November):1135–8.

[6] Chen CS, Mrksich M, Huang S, Whitesides GM, Ingber DE. Geometric control of cell life and death. Science 1997;276(5317):1425–8.

[7] Kim J, Kim HN, Lim K-T, Kim Y, Seonwoo H, Park SH, et al. Designing nanotopographical density of extracellular matrix for controlled morphology and function of human mesenchymal stem cells. Sci Rep 2013;3:3552.

[8] Jain KK. The role of nanobiotechnology in drug discovery. Adv Exp Med Biol 2009;655:37–43.

[9] Pathak P, Meziani MJ, Desai T, Sun YP. Nanosizing drug particles in supercritical fluid processing. J Am Chem Soc 2004;126(35):10842–3.

[10] Wang CH, Wang CH, Hsiue GH. Polymeric micelles with a pH-responsive structure as intracellular drug carriers. J Control Release 2005;108(1):140–9.

[11] Hu Y, Chen Y, Chen Q, Zhang L, Jiang X, Yang C. Synthesis and stimuli-responsive properties of chitosan/poly(acrylic acid) hollow nanospheres. Polymer (Guildf) 2005;46(26):12703–10.

[12] Kotela I, Podporska J, Soltysiak E, Konsztowicz KJ, Blazewicz M. Polymer nanocomposites for bone tissue substitutes. Ceram Int 2009;35(6):2475–80.

[13] Rogel MR, Qiu H, Ameer GA. The role of nanocomposites in bone regeneration. J Mater Chem 2008;18(36):4233.

[14] Li X, van Blitterswijk CA, Feng Q, Cui F, Watari F. The effect of calcium phosphate microstructure on bone-related cells in vitro. Biomaterials 2008;29(23):3306–16.

[15] Dalby MJ, Gadegaard N, Tare R, Andar A, Riehle MO, Herzyk P, et al. The control of human mesenchymal cell differentiation using nanoscale symmetry and disorder. Nat Mater 2007;6(12):997–1003.

[16] Yao X, Peng R, Ding J. Effects of aspect ratios of stem cells on lineage commitments with and without induction media. Biomaterials 2013;34(4):930–9.

[17] Engler AJ, Sen S, Sweeney HL, Discher DE. Matrix Elasticity Directs Stem Cell Lineage Specification. Cell 2006;126(4):677–89.

[18] Guilak F, Cohen DM, Estes BT, Gimble JM, Liedtke W, Chen CS. Control of Stem Cell Fate by Physical Interactions with the Extracellular Matrix. Cell Stem Cell 2009:17–26.

Particles/Fibers/Bulk

2

Nasim Kiaie[1], *Farzaneh Aavani*[1] *and Mehdi Razavi*[2]
[1]Amirkabir University of Technology, Tehran, Iran
[2]Stanford University, Palo Alto, CA, United States

2.1 Introduction

The approach of science and techniques for regeneration of tissues and systems of drug delivery has attracted the attention of researchers to biomaterials. Biomaterials are defined as "any substance or combination of substances, other than drugs, synthetic or natural in origin, which can be used for any period of time, which augments or replaces partially or totally any tissue, organ or function of the body, in order to maintain or improve the quality of life of the individuals," based on American National Institute of Health. Hence the focus of this chapter is on the classification of biomaterials in different forms.

In general, all materials are classified as organic or inorganic materials. Organic materials are carbon-containing chemical compounds existing in living organisms. Carbohydrates, lipids, proteins, and nucleic acids are four major types of organic materials. All of these materials are composed of carbon, hydrogen, and oxygen atoms, but the ratio of atoms is different among categories. In contrast, inorganic biomaterials are not consisting of or deriving from living sources and molecular structure of most of them lacks carbon element except carbon monoxide, carbondioxide, carbonates, cyanides, cyanates, and carbides.

Previously, biomaterials were classified as bioceramics, biometals, biopolymers, and biocomposites. Bioceramics and biometals are always inorganic materials but it is different in the case of biopolymers. They might be organic or inorganic based on the presence and percentage of carbon atoms in their backbone chain. Biocomposites are a little more complicated. We put them in inorganic sub-category in acondition that all components of which to be inorganic. But in some cases,an organic material combines with an inorganic one for specific purposes. We put these types in organic–inorganic materials. If the phases of the composite are in molecular level it is not a composite anymore, it is named biohybrid.

In this chapter, we tried to classify organic and inorganic biomaterials based on the above explanations and mention some examples for each type. As nanotechnology is a promising tool for the betterment of characteristics of biomaterials, examples presented in this chapter contain various shapes of biomaterials especially in the nano dimensions.

Nanobiomaterials Science, Development and Evaluation. DOI: http://dx.doi.org/10.1016/B978-0-08-100963-5.00002-1

2.2 Organic biomaterials

If organic materials have some properties such as biocompatibility, nontoxicity and noncarcinogenicity could replace or restore function to a body tissue and to replace hard or soft tissues, they are regarded as organic biomaterials [1]. Some of the biopolymers fall into this category.

2.2.1 Organic biopolymers

The biopolymer is a polymer generated by living organisms. In other words, biopolymers are organic biomaterials that are formed of a number of monomers. Their backbone chains are made entirely or mostly of carbon atoms. Another factor distinguishing biopolymer from other polymers is their structure. In fact, most of the biopolymers tend to fold into secondary and tertiary structures while other polymers have much simpler and more random structures. The other difference between biopolymers and other polymers is in the molecular mass distribution. In other words, monodispersity is the characteristic of biopolymers while other polymers have high polydispersity values. The reason behind this phenomenon is that the control of molecular mass in the synthesis of the polymer is difficult but this is controlled by nature in the case of natural biopolymers.

The polynucleotide (with 13 or a lot more nucleotide monomers), polypeptides, and polysaccharides (such as cellulose, hemicelluloses, lignin, silk, and starch) are three main types of biopolymers. Plus, some types of synthetic polymers with determined carbon percentage fall into the category of biopolymers according to European standard CEN/TS 16295:2012.

Biopolymers have the widest range of applications in biomedical field. Because of their properties, ease of fabrication, and low price, they are advantageous over inorganic biomaterials. They could be produced in various forms including bulk (such as film, sheet, etc.), particles, and fibers. Organic biopolymers gathered in Table 2.1 could be categorized as bioinert and bioresorbable.

2.2.1.1 Different types of biopolymers based on tissue interactions

Organic biopolymers use as biomaterials are either bioinert or bioresorbable based on interactions with the tissues. In cases where a biopolymer is used to replace the functions of a hard tissue or it is to be used for long-term applications, it would be necessary to elicit minimum interactions with the human body. It means that they should be bioinert. Being inertness in some organic biopolymers makes them suitable for use in orthopedic devices or hard tissues substitute [2–4]. These biopolymers are presented in Table 2.1.

On the other side, bioresorbable biopolymers are ideal for tissue engineering scaffolds. In fact, what determines the success of scaffolds in replacing tissues is the rate of biodegradation of them. Scaffolds made of bioresorbable biopolymers have the ability to degrade via hydrolytic (when a hydrolysable bond exists) or enzymatic

Table 2.1 Organic biopolymer classification based on degradation and origin

Bioinert	Biopolymer	Origin
	Thermoplastic polyurethane (TPU)	Synthetic
	Polyamide (PA) (such as nylon)	Synthetic
	Poly(ethylene terephthalate) (PET)	Synthetic
	Polypropylene (PP)	Synthetic
	Polyethylene (PE), low-density polyethylene (LDPE), high-density polyethylene (HDPE), PTFE (Teflon)	Synthetic
Bioresorbable	Poly-3-hydroxybutyrate (PHB), polyhydroxyvalerate (PHV), polyhydroxyalkanoate (PHH)	Natural
	Polyamides (PA) (such as protein, silk, wool, collagen)	Natural
	Nucleic acid	Natural
	Starch, chitosan, and cellulose	Natural
	Polylactic acid	Renewable Resource
	Polycaprolactone	Synthetic
	Polyvinyl chloride (PVC)	Synthetic
	Polystyrene (PS)	Synthetic
	Polybutylene succinate	Synthetic
	Polyvinyl alcohol	Synthetic
	Polyanhydrides	Synthetic

processes. After breaking down, the residues of the biopolymer is gradually absorbed by the body and do not initiate an intense immune response. As it is shown in Table 2.1, all natural biopolymers are bioresorbable [5–10].

2.2.1.2 Different forms of biopolymers as nanobiomaterials

Biopolymers in biomedical applications adopt different shapes based on expected properties and application. In almost all of medical instruments, the bulk of the material is usable. For example, blood storage and urine bags, blood tubing, heart and lung bypass sets, endotracheal tubes, intravenous solution dispensing sets all are made of an organic biopolymer, PVC, because of flexibility, strength, and durability of this polymer, which is a bulk feature [11]. Another organic biopolymer, whose bulk properties makes it interesting for medical devices, is PP used for hollow fiber membranes of oxygenators [12].

In spite of medical devices, bulk properties of organic biopolymers in the reconstruction of tissues become important. Two examples are high-density polyethylene used for facial skeleton reconstruction [13] and polyethylene terephthalate (PET) used for ligament and tendon reconstruction [14].

Polytetrafluoroethylene (PTFE), another organic biopolymer, is used as wound dressing membranes. This membrane prevents blood clotting, adhesion of tissue, and attachment of bacteria [15]. This polymer is also used for replacement of the rabbit abdominal aortic artery [16]. Both applications are based on bulk properties of this polymer.

Although the bulk of the material is important, surface properties should be considered. The surface of biomaterials determine bio and blood compatibility, adsorption phenomenon, wettability, surface erosion, roughness, surface oxidation, and so on, in some cases it is needed to modify the surface of biomaterials without changing bulk properties. As a case, in order to improve blood compatibility of hydrophobic polymers such as PVC, the surface could become hydrophilic via grafting of water-soluble moieties such as polyethylene glycol (PEG) [7]. Another example is immobilizing heparin on PET grafts to prevent platelet deposition and thrombogenesis. As a result, surface properties improved while needed flexibility of bulk of biopolymer is saved [17].

Biopolymers might be used in the nanoparticle state, especially in applications such as drug and gene delivery and imaging probes. Drug-loading capacity is an important factor in drug delivery systems, which could be achieved in nanoparticles because of their high surface area. Additionally, nanoparticles facilitate endosomal uptake and drug delivery into the cells.

Examples of using organic biopolymers as drug delivery vehicles are too numerous to list. The particle itself or the coating on it could be made from biopolymers. For example, PVC is used to coat nanoparticles to improve the antiinfection ability of them [18]. Polystyrene nanoparticles have also applications as drug delivery, biosensors, and as an imaging probe for early cancer detection [19]. These particles could be used for targeted delivery of chemotherapeutic drugs to ovarian cancer cells [20]. Chitosan is another biopolymer that is used frequently as drug vehicle and the impact of different factors on its final characteristics simulated and predicted by some authors [21–23].

Biopolymers in fiber state are fabricated routinely via electrospinning apparatus as woven or nonwoven forms. The most important field of utilization of such fibrous structures is in building tissue scaffold, because fibers imitate the natural extra cellular matrix (ECM) structure as cell niche. A good example is a synthetic small diameter vascular prosthesis made from nonwoven fibers of PET. In this study, a tubular structure similar to arteries was produced with suitable mechanical compliance and nonthrombogenicity [24]. A nanofibrous scaffold made of organic biopolymers enables us to load therapeutics into fibers as well. Antibacterial wound dressing made of polyurethane (PU) fibers is a good case of a nanofibrous structure releasing an antibiotic such as mupirocin (Mu) [25].

2.2.2 Organic lipid-based biomaterials

Beside biopolymers, there is a small group of organic materials that are based on lipids. Liposomes and niosomes are two subtypes of these materials. Both these materials are biocompatible and their nontoxicity is reported. Extensive efforts have been done by researchers to prepare liposome and niosome nanoparticles owing to the fact that these materials are suitable for drug and gene delivery applications and their structures have made loading of both hydrophilic and hydrophobic drugs possible. Vesicle of the liposome is made from one or more phospholipid bilayers, therefore exist as unilamellar or multilamellar liposomes. Phospholipids are present abundantly in the cell membrane. Through changing the composition of lipid, charge of the liposome and its characteristic may change. Some liposome formulations for anticancer drug delivery have acquired food and drug administration (FDA) and entered the market successfully. Niosomes are rather newer than liposomes. They have a similar structure to liposomes and are made of self-association of nonionic surfactants in an aqueous phase. Chemical stability of niosomes is higher than liposomes, plus their surface modification is easier. For further reading, there are valuable reviews on the applications of these two nanoparticles in drug delivery [26,27].

2.3 Inorganic biomaterials

Inorganic biomaterials are those lacking carbon element except a few combinations named in the introduction section. Inorganic materials could have crystalline or glass structures. As in the case of organic biomaterials, if these materials are used to replace or restore function to a body tissue and to replace human tissues they could be named inorganic biomaterials. Here we discussed four major types of inorganic biomaterials including bioceramics, biometals, inorganic biopolymers, and biocomposites made from two or more inorganic components.

2.3.1 Bioceramics

Bioceramics are biocompatible ceramics. They are regarded as the hardest biomaterials with high toughness and elastic modulus. They are brittle, heat- and corrosion-resistant, and therefore used in musculoskeletal system applications. In fact, bioceramics have many applications in biomedicine from eye contact lenses to ear implants; they can be used for orthopedic purposes to replace hips, knees, joints, tendons, and ligaments. They can be used in bone tumor surgeries as filler and spinal fusion surgeries. They can repair cranial or iliac crest. Plus, they have applications in dentistry as dental implants, augmentation of the jaw bone, periodontal pockets, maxillofacial reconstruction, gold porcelain crowns, glass-filled ionomer cement and dentures [28].

2.3.1.1 Different types of bioceramics based on tissue interactions

We can put them into three groups based on their interaction with the tissues: bioinert, bioactive, or surface reactive (semi-inert), and biodegradable or resorbable bioceramics (noninert).

Inert bioceramics are those with wear resistance and minimal biological response, it means they can be stable in terms of stiffness, strength, and toughness for a long period of time. Although, besides inertness, processing, size, and shape of bioceramics are determinants for their mechanical integrity. Hence, as inert bioceramics are used in long-term applications, failure probability, and crack growth behavior at different load levels should be predicted via tools such as fracture mechanics and statistical distributions. Biocompatibility would not be a concern as in the case of long-term application of bioinert ceramics. Inert bioceramics adopt different forms in biomedical applications, they can be used as a dense structure attaching to the tissue via tissue outgrowth or a grouting agent or they can have a porous shape in which a mechanical attachment is created between bioceramic and tissue via ingrowths of tissue. Some examples of inert bioceramic are ceramic oxides such as alumina and zirconia, silicon nitrides, and carbons.

Bioactive bioceramics are regarded as bulk reactive ceramics. They can form a chemical bond with the tissues. Owing to the brittleness of this category, they found applications for periodontal anomalies and filling of small bone defects. Important uses of bioactive ceramics are mimicking biomineralization of bone and coatings on metallic substrates and porous scaffolds for bone tissue engineering. Glass ceramics, bioactive glasses, and hydroxyapatites (HAs) are some examples of bioactive bioceramics.

Resorbable bioceramics can integrate with the tissues and could be completely degraded to be replaced with host tissue. In fact, grain boundaries cannot tolerate chemical attacks and the whole structure disintegrates physically. Additionally, they may solve in body fluids or be desorbed by cells such as osteoclasts. With attention to their resorption, the utility of them as tissue engineering scaffolds or drug delivery systems is rational. Additionally, they are used to fabricate resorbable screws for anterior cruciate ligament (ACL) reconstruction surgeries. In this category, stability before replacement by the host tissue and adjusting desorption rates to the repair rates are problematic. Two familiar groups of this material are calcium phosphates and calcium aluminates [29].

2.3.1.2 Different forms of bioceramics as nanobiomaterials

Bioceramics could be used as solid pieces or as nanobiomaterials in different states such as bulk (including hollow fiber membrane, coatings), particle, nanotubes, and fiber.

Typically, usage of bioceramics as bulk materials is in tissue engineering scaffolds and graft substitution. As it is expected, resorbable bioceramics are common in such applications because of their degradation ability. For example, HA bioceramic scaffolds were selected for culturing adipose-derived stem cells and the effect of different nano and microtopographies on attachment, proliferation, and osteogenic differentiation of these cells investigated [30]. Calcium silicate scaffolds are also a good substrate for osteogenic differentiation of mesenchymal stem cells (MSCs) because silicon (Si) ions releasing from these structures stimulate osteogenesis and angiogenesis [31]. The bulk properties of this scaffold vary after strontium substitution into the structure. This strategy adds properties such as inhibition of bone resorption to the scaffold, which makes it more preferable for bone defect treatment [32]. Another example of bulk usage of bioceramics, calcium phosphate scaffolds made through 3D printing could be pointed, which are used customarily as synthetic bone graft substitutes [33,34].

Bioceramic used as coatings in numerous studies. The aim of coating medical devices and tissue engineering constructs is an improvement of biocompatibility, osteoconductivity, and the long-term stability [35]. Calcium phosphate, hydroxylapatite, and carbon are some bioceramics with wide applications as a coating of structures such as artificial heart valves [36].

Beside bulk, bioceramic in particle state is a source of interest as a biomaterial. Similar to particulate biopolymers, bioceramics could be used as drug delivery vehicles. In this respect, porous and insoluble glass beads are a good carrier for therapeutic agents such as radioactive isotopes and chemotherapeutics for cancer treatment, enzymes, antibodies, and antigens. Graphene oxide nanoparticles are new interesting bioceramics suitable for drug delivery applications [37]. Another example is a study of the binding of Risedronate (a drug for osteoporosis treatment) to the surface of HA nanoparticles and targeting bone defects [38].

Another form that bioceramics can adopt is hallowed micro- and nanotube. Carbon nanotubes are among the first-known nanotubes, which exist as multiwall or single wall hollow cylinders with the diameter of 0.7–2 nm and very high aspect ratios. Electrical and thermal conductivity and high surface area make this type of bioceramic interesting for drug and gene delivery and tissue regeneration applications. The efficiency of them for hyperthermia therapy is also proved [39]. Graphene oxide nanotubes are analogous to carbon nanotubes with different wall numbers and diameters. They are used predominantly in biosensors and as cell growth and differentiation mediators [37]. One novel material with nanotube structure, which occurs in nature is Halloysite ($Al_2Si_2O_5(OH)_4$-$2H_2O$). This material is an aluminosilicate with a two-layered hollow tubular structure with 15–100 nm diameters. This hollow space could be used as a nanoreactor, for loading of poorly soluble drugs and for cell attachment and proliferation substrate [40]. Titanium dioxide (TiO_2) nanotubes are also new structures with many potential applications in biomedical field. These tubular structures are prepared via anodization on Ti substrate and found applications in drug delivery, biosensors, antibacterial substrates, modulating deposition of HA and orthopedic implants [41].

Bioceramic in fiber form shows interesting features such as emitting far infrared waves. Therefore, woven fibers of bioceramics are a good candidate for fabrication of magnetotherapeutic devices [42]. Moreover, bioceramics such as zirconium dioxide (ZrO_2) in the form of hollow fibers are used as selectively permeable membranes with the aim of immune-isolation of transplanted cell [43]. Fibrous scaffolds that best mimic the natural ECM can be made from nanofibers of bioceramics such as zirconia, alumina, titania, carbon, and calcium phosphate. Electrospinning is the versatile method of producing such nanofibrous bioceramics [44].

2.3.2 Biometals

Some properties of metals including electrical and thermal conductivity make them an interesting material for use in biomedical applications. Deformability of metals is another important feature enabling engineers to form them into desired shapes. This is because metallic bond in the atomic structure of metals is not directional and the location of metal ions could change without breaking down the crystal structure. Metals or their alloys as biomaterials are used mostly in bone fracture plates (Sherman plates) and screws [45,46]. Different metallic elements such as iron (Fe), chromium (Cr), cobalt (Co), nickel (Ni), titanium (Ti), tantalum (Ta), niobium (Nb), molybdenum (Mo), and tungsten (W) and their alloys such as 316L stainless steel (as the first biometal used in surgeries), titanium-base alloys such as [Ti 6% Al 4%V] and [55% Ni and 45% Ti], cobalt- chromium alloys such as [Cr (27–30%), Mo (5–7%), Ni (2.5%)] and [Cr (19–21%), Ni (33–37%), and [Mo (9–11%)], shape memory alloys such as [Ti 45%–55%Ni] are used frequently for biomedical applications. The biggest concern regarding the use of metals in the body is their corrosion and degradation leading to a decrease of toughness and wear strength and consequently disintegration and weakening of the implanted device. This event also reduces biocompatibility and may cause toxicity [47,48]. The physiological fluid contains organic acids, proteins, enzymes, macromolecules, electrolytes and dissolved oxygen, nitrogen, and soluble carbonates. Plus, some compounds secreted by inflammatory and fibrotic cells and the existence of stress, strain, and frictional forces may cause progression of degradation of metals.

Although some metals exist naturally in the body such as iron in red blood cells or cobalt taking part in the synthesis of vitamin B-12, the large amount of them is intolerable by the body because of the fact that the corroded metals released into the body might initiate adverse reactions. Being corrosion-resistant not only keeps the mechanical properties but maintains the biocompatibility of the biometal. Albeit, upon exposure to air or fluids, an oxide layer grows on the surface of some biometals, which makes them corrosion-resistant and then biocompatible, such as titanium oxide layer with a thickness of a few nanometers forming on the surface of titanium alloys spontaneously when exposed to air. Another point affecting the success of metallic biomaterials is being lightweight [49,50].

Biometals have biomedical applications mainly as hard tissue substitution. They can interact with the human tissues or only be used in passive forms. Some of the applications of biometals as biomaterials include bone plates and screws, hip and knee artificial joints, dental implants, and products such as crowns, bridges, and dentures, and root-forming analogs, spinal or blood vessels fixation devices, vascular stents, and occlusion coils, catheter guide wires, artificial heart valves, and pacemakers [51].

2.3.2.1 Different forms of biometals as nanobiomaterials

Different forms of biometals used in biomedical applications are fiber, bulk, or nanotubes. In the form of bulk, biometals are used mostly as bone scaffolds on the growth or differentiation of cells is facilitated. As an example, five different biometals with 12 mm in diameter, 3 mm in height, and with a central hole of 2 mm in diameter, were studied as osteoclast activator and osteoblast promoter in vitro (DePuyOrthopädie GmbH, Johnson & Johnson, Germany). Temporary implants made of stainless steel 316L and titanium alloy Ti6Al4V used as screws or plates for osteosynthesis are also in bulk forms [52]. Ti6Al4V scaffolds are also fabricated with a porous structure for bone tissue engineering [53]. In the bulk shapes, as the surface of biometal exposed to the body is high, surface treatment with the help of laser is required to improve biocompatibility and corrosion of metals [54].

There have been little studies on metallic biomaterials in the form of fibers. Albeit, Toki Corporation (Tokyo, Japan) is leading the utilization of metallic fibers for fabrication of artificial heart muscles. A sophisticated shape memory alloy fiber made of Ni–Ti with 100-micron diameter was used as an actuator attached on the surface of ePTFE conduit (http://www.toki.co.jp).

The most known metallic biomaterials in the particle state are iron and gold nanoparticles. Iron nanoparticles are valuable tools for magnetic separation of different materials and magnetically guided drug delivery. Iron nanoparticle response to the magnetic field and produce heat under changing magnetic field. They could destroy tumor cells as a result of locally heating the tumor. As the oxide state of iron nanoparticles have a lower magnetic moment, usually a shell of gold is applied on the particles to prevent oxidation [55]. Gold nanoparticles alone are an interesting option for drug and gene delivery, hyperthermia, and contrast agents. Gold nanoparticles exhibit properties such as surface plasmon resonance (SPR) and ability to surface modification and functionalization [56].

2.3.3 Inorganic biopolymers

Inorganic biopolymers are relatively a small group rather than organic biopolymers. Inorganic biopolymers against organic polymers have a backbone chain, which is composed primarily of noncarbon atoms. Inorganic biopolymers fall into four categories based on the backbone atoms: silicones or polysiloxanes, polysilanes, polygermanes, and polystannanes, and polyphosphazene. While polysilanes, polygermanes, and polystannanes, and polyphosphazene are nearly new and are waiting for being developed in biomedical field because of their conductivity properties, silicones are the most common inorganic polymers. They are bioinert and are composed of silicon (Si) and oxygen (O_2). It is found abundantly on the earth (59% of crust) and in the human body in nails, hair, and skin, connective tissues and bone in the form of silanate or silicic acid. It has physical forms of crystalline, amorphous, and synthetic amorphous. Deficiency of Si in the body causes diseases and it could be contained in the daily diet. Si could be blended with a verity of substances in the lab. Polysilanes are composed of chains of Si atoms. Two important features of them are heat-resistance and electrical conductivity. If the main chain is made of germanium and tin atoms, polygermanes and polystannanes are produced respectively. Being electric conductor is worth mentioning in these polymers. Polyphosphazenes are made of alternating phosphorus and nitrogen atoms. They are electrical insulators and highly flexible.

Most of the inorganic biopolymers are crystalline, insoluble, and unstable in water. Hence, in the past, it was thought that they couldn't be biologically active. But today they found many applications in biomedical engineering as drug delivery vehicles, antimicrobial substrates, modulator of gene expression, bone tissue engineering, and blood coagulation [57].

2.3.3.1 Different forms of inorganic biopolymers as nanobiomaterials

Among inorganic biopolymers mentioned above, silicone has the most applications in biomedicine. Silicone material is used as grafting and scaffolding material in biomedical applications. It is used in the form of thin films or nanoparticles. Ultra-thin films of silicone are used to cover the electrodes of a glucose biosensor [58]. They can be used as a secondary phase of a biocomposite to stiffen it and attach to polymeric matrix owing to their high specific surface area. Silica is also used as a coating for implants. In bulk state, silicone has been used for decades as pacemaker leads and urinary catheter components. For years, contact lenses industry used the advantage of high oxygen permeability of silicone hydrogels [59,60]. Another field in which bulk of silicone is used is porous cell scaffolds. Elastic porous polydimethyl-siloxane (PDMS) cell scaffolds are suitable for the growth of osteoblasts. The existence of high pores makes them suitable for water adsorption and then cell viability [61]. In some studies, it was shown that changing topography could improve scaffold. For example, patterning surface of PDMS scaffolds with different sizes of channels promoted orientation and migration of Schwann cells [62]. For tissue engineering applications for which bulk of materials is very important, attention has been directed toward polyphosphazene as biodegradable biopolymers. Polyphosphazene has applications in bulk state as stimuli-responsive hydrogels, shape memory polymers and bone, nerve, tendon, and ligament tissue engineering scaffolds [63].

Similar to organic polymers, inorganic biopolymers in nanoparticle state have applications in biomedicine, especially drug delivery systems. Silica nanoparticles are used as drug and gene delivery platforms and therapeutic agent is loaded into their pores. Additionally, it is possible to form core-shell structures based on silica nanoparticles. Hollow nanoparticles are another possible shape with the ability to load a high amount of payload. Their biocompatibility, low toxicity, durability, and versatility, good biodegradability as nanocarriers is comparable to organic nanocarriers. Additionally, silica-based nanosystems are open to modification and functionalizing and have shown good results in vivo. One important advantage of these carriers is easy production and simple purification process, which helps in manufacturability at low cost. One of the applications of silica in the nanoparticle state is contrast enhancer in ultrasound imaging. As well, silica could be used as the coating of iron oxide nanoparticles (SPION) as MRI contrast agent. Silica nanoparticle can carry sensitizing agents, amplifying agents, and guidance agents for ablative therapy [64]. Interestingly, silicon particles of only several nanometers are called Quantum Dots. These semiconductor materials exhibit special optical and electronic properties, which make them favorable for some biomedical applications including real-time tracking of single molecules and cells to study intracellular processes such as cell trafficking, high-resolution cellular imaging, tumor targeting, and utilization as organic dyes [65]. Polyphosphazene is another type of inorganic biopolymer, which has a wide range of applications as drug and gene delivery vehicle, owing to their biodegradation property [66].

2.3.4 Inorganic biocomposites

As mentioned earlier, biocomposites are made to improve the properties of the whole structure. Inorganic biocomposites are those structures which have been composed of phases such as bioceramics, biometals, or biopolymers. The second phase might have different shapes such as a particle, fiber, and so on, and be made of different materials. This second phase could be even air; in this case, the resulted biocomposite is called foam. Bone, dentin, cartilage, and skin are some composites present in the body naturally. Therefore, applications of biocomposite as hard tissue replacement or orthopedic devices are much extended. Biocomposites found applications in tissue engineering as well, such as bone, vascular, and neural scaffolds. In biocomposites, the biocompatibility of each substitute should be noticed. In addition, the interface between phases is very important to have enough resistance to keep the whole composite structure intact. Two common problems regarding these biocomposites are stress shielding and need for a second surgery for the removal of implanted biomaterial. The second problem, which is due to nondegradation of most ceramics, could be prevented with the help of resorbable bioceramics as a primary phase.

As pointed above, the first reason behind creating biocomposite is altering the rate of degradation. An example of such structure is a biocomposite made of iron and a resorbable bioceramic as bone-healing implant. The addition of degradable phase to Fe increased degradation and decreased yield and compressive strength [67].

The second reason could be an improvement of cellular interactions. Consider the case of a porous scaffold of PDMS) for culturing rat bone marrow-derived mesenchymal stem cells. After integrating HA crystals into pores of this scaffold, cell attachment improved dramatically [68]. Another example is a ZrO_2/HA biocomposite. Zirconia alone is not suitable as bone restorative material because of inertness and lack of bone affinity. Mixing of active HA with zirconia increased cell adhesion and bone integration [69].

The third reason for creating biocomposites is combining properties of different materials. For example, ZnO/Ag core-shell nanoparticles are inorganic biocomposites. The presence of silver cause inhibition of the growth of *Staphylococcus aureus* [18]. Another example is hyperthermia treatment of bone cancer with the help of nanocomposites. In a study, a magnetic phase was entered within the glass–ceramic formulation. Glass matrix enabled osteointegration with bone while incorporated Fe_3O_4 induced magnetic properties into the structure. Under a magnetic field, this power was heated and tumor cells were killed [70]. In another case, iron particles were embedded into the walls of carbon nanotubes improving electrical and magnetic properties of the template [71].

The fourth and the most significant reason of creating biocomposites is the improvement of mechanical properties of the structure. For example, composites in which matrix is a ceramic like Al_2O_3 reinforced with carbon fiber to increase toughness, strength, modulus, and thermal stability, which make them suitable for orthopedic applications. The carbon fibers could be loaded with drugs simultaneously [72]. Another example is biocomposites of iron–bioceramic as a degradable bone implant. Not only yield and compressive strength decreased rather than pure Fe but cell viability and proliferation improved, and due to the biodegradability of the ceramic phase bone healing improved [67].

2.4 Organic–inorganic biomaterials

In nature, most of the human tissues are a composite of organic and inorganic materials. A clear example is bone tissue, which is composed of an organic phase (collagen) and inorganic (nanocrystalline HA) components. Therefore, in order to recapitulate the natural tissues, it is necessary to develop a combination of organic and inorganic biomaterials. They could be prepared as composites or hybrids to mimic the natural structures. Different components could bind together via hydrogen or other weak interactions in composites or via cross-linking in hybrids. The other difference between hybrids and composites is that the dimension of dispersion is in the molecular levels in the case of hybrids. Creative hybrid or composite scaffolds could have improved cell responses due to changes in signaling pathways following changes of nanostructures.

2.4.1 Organic–inorganic hybrids

Hybrid organic–inorganic polymers made through adding organic side groups to an inorganic backbone chain. Such hybrid materials have many biomedical applications [73]. For example, coating of implantable glucose sensors is made through blending silica with organic biopolymers in order to prevent fibrous encapsulation and warrant adequate glucose diffusion and to prevent denaturation of the enzyme glucose oxidase [74]. Another example is chitosan–epoxysilane films, which are used to coat zinc substrates and decrease the rate of cathodic delamination by eliminating ion transport [75].

Another strategy to create hybrids is functionalization of the surface of an inorganic substance, such as silicate particles, with organic biopolymers [76]. Therefore, it is a creative way to attach an organic group covalently to inorganic substrates such as siloxane. In fact, it is possible to pattern an inorganic network with organic molecules and present them new functionalities. In a study, such patterned surfaces created for microfluidic devices fabrication [77].

2.4.2 Organic–inorganic composites

Composites are materials in which different phases exist heterogeneously while the phases are bigger than molecular levels (as in the case of copolymers and hybrids). Mainly, the goal of producing a composite with a polymeric matrix is to improve mechanical properties such as strength, stiffness, toughness, and fatigue resistance while other reasons exist, for example creating a biocomposite with two distinct phases in which each phase play a specific role (for more explanation, imagine one component support cell attachment and at the same time the other component play antibacterial role or even release a therapeutic).

Composites in which one phase is polymeric, whether organic or inorganic, have priorities over ceramic biocomposites such as avoiding the problem of stress shielding and preventing a second surgery for removal of implanted biomaterials because of biodegradation of most polymers. Introducing the second phase into the polymer matrix can help to improve properties based on application. Mechanical properties and degradation kinetics could be controlled by the shape and amount of the second phase.

Interfacial bonding strength becomes important in achieving the desired mechanical stability of biocomposite, because it is the site in which fractures take place routinely. Additionally, after placing biocomposite in vivo condition, the interface of fiber and polymer is more prone to deterioration than the matrix and interfacial bonding strength between matrix and fiber weaken after exposure to water and biological fluids.

Mainly, the second phase has two shapes: fibers and particle. Use of particles as fillers to reinforce biocomposite with polymeric matrixes has had successful results in the clinic. Dental restorative resins and bone cement are two examples. Introducing bioactive fillers such as HA in bone cement induces bioactivity and bone-bonding properties in polymeric biocomposite. In addition, with the help of fillers justifying biodegradation rate of the polymeric matrix becomes possible. Another filler material is graphene oxide nanosheets. The nanofillers incorporate into silane coating to promote corrosion [78].

Biocomposites in which the second phase is particle are of immense interest. Incorporation of particles into composites may take place in two ways: they could be incorporated into the polymeric matrix during polymerization or they may introduce into matrix after polymerization and via dispersion. As an example, we could point out silicate particles, which are studied frequently as the second phase of composites. Silicate particles could be incorporated into an organic polymer matrix during the synthesis procedure. Nanoparticles mix with monomers and, after polymerization, they entangle into the final structure [79]. Nanoparticles could also be dispersed into a polymeric matrix through intensive mixing. The dispersion of silica nanoparticles into silane coatings could improve corrosion of the underlying carbon steel [80,81]. In a study, a composite of silica microsphere (as inorganic biopolymers) and collagen (an organic biopolymer) as a wound-healing support was produced. Collagen as the matrix of biocomposite facilitates cell proliferation at the same time the particles of silica are carriers for sustained delivery of an antimicrobial drug. In a study, gold nanoparticles incorporated into PP mesh to mediate degradation of the mesh by foreign body reactions and to improve cellular response [82]. The addition of gold nanoparticles is shown to have beneficial effects on the biocompatibility of biocomposites. Whelove's team improved the biocompatibility of PET patch, designed for the purpose of a hernia (a condition in which fascia, connective tissue over the abdominal muscles, breaks down) repair, via immobilizing gold nanoparticles [83]. In another work, an antimicrobial PP suture is fabricated through immobilization of nanosilver on these sutures [84].

One interesting biocomposite is a hollow-fiber membrane oxygenator made from PP, which is coated with silicone. After creating this coating onto the microporous membrane, leakage of plasma was prevented, which is translated to higher biocompatibility [85].

An artificial vascular graft made from poly(tetrafluoroethylene) (ePTFE) and mesoporous silica was synthesized on it in situ. Because of this mesoporous coating of silica, hydrophobicity and biocompatibility increased the controlled release of heparin from silica particles achieved [86].

2.5 Concluding remarks

In a nutshell, three main types of biomaterials including organic, inorganic, and their combination was reviewed here. These materials could be used as a biomaterials in a condition that they provide satisfactory biocompatibility and nontoxicity. In applications as a biomaterial, these materials could be in different states including bulk, particles, fiber, and tubes. These structures could be prepared in nanodimensions as nanoparticles, nanofiber, and nanotubes depending on the applications. A few examples of each type are presented. While organic biomaterials are limited to organic biopolymers, inorganic biomaterials have the widest range as bioceramics, biometals, inorganic biopolymers, and inorganic biocomposites. Surprisingly, application of these materials in the biomedical field is less than organic biopolymers. Finally, a combination of organic and inorganic biomaterials is discussed. This strategy is favorable to biomimetic and enables us to imitate the normal human tissues.

2.6 Future research

New frontiers of studies should be directed toward finding new hybrids and composites, which can best mimic the natural processes of the human body. In this regard, the first step is having a thorough understanding of biomaterials and their classifications are necessary, which enables us a suitable selection of biomaterials. The second step is finding and inventing new technologies to combine and assembly biomaterials and form different structures with varying properties. It seems that special attention must be paid to silica nanoparticles for a wide variety of applications as drug and gene delivery vehicles. In the case of bioinert or nonresorbable nanobiomaterials, some issues such as toxicity and fate of particles should be studied.

2.7 Conflict of interest

There is no conflict of interest.

References

[1] Fattahi P, Yang G, Kim G, Abidian MR. Biomaterials: a review of organic and inorganic biomaterials for neural interfaces (Adv. Mater. 12/2014). Adv Mater 2014;26:1793.

[2] Navarro M, Michiardi A, Castaño O, Planell JA. Biomaterials in orthopaedics. J Royal Soc Interf 2008;5:1137–58.

[3] Yazdimamaghani M, Razavi M, Vashaee D, Pothineni VR, Rajadas J, Tayebi L. Significant degradability enhancement in multilayer coating of polycaprolactone-bioactive glass/gelatin-bioactive glass on magnesium scaffold for tissue engineering applications. Appl Surf Sci 2015;338:137–45.

[4] Yazdimamaghani M, Razavi M, Vashaee D, Tayebi L. Microstructural and mechanical study of PCL coated Mg scaffolds. Surf Eng 2014;30:920–6.

[5] Casalini T. 3 - Bioresorbability of polymers: chemistry, mechanisms, and modeling. Bioresorbable polymers for biomedical applications. Woodhead Publishing; 2017. p. 65–83.

[6] Chew SA, Hinojosa VA, Arriaga MA. 11 - Bioresorbable polymer microparticles in the medical and pharmaceutical fields Bioresorbable Polymers for Biomedical Applications. Woodhead Publishing; 2017. p. 229–64.
[7] Garbayo E, Pascual-Gil S, Prosper F, Blanco-Prieto MJ. 19 - Bioresorbable polymers for next-generation cardiac scaffolds Bioresorbable polymers for biomedical applications. Woodhead Publishing; 2017. p. 445–67.
[8] Pertici G. 1 - Introduction to bioresorbable polymers for biomedical applications Bioresorbable polymers for biomedical applications. Woodhead Publishing; 2017. p. 3–29.
[9] Heidari F, Razavi M, Bahrololoom ME, Bazargan-Lari R, Vashaee D, Kotturi H, et al. Mechanical properties of natural chitosan/hydroxyapatite/magnetite nanocomposites for tissue engineering applications. Mater Sci Eng C 2016;65:338–44.
[10] Jazayeri HE, Fahmy MD, Razavi M, Stein BE, Nowman A, Masri RM, et al. Dental applications of natural-origin polymers in hard and soft tissue engineering. J Prosthodontics 2016.
[11] Jayakrishnan Lakshmi. Migration resistant, blood-compatible plasticized polyvinyl chloride for medical and related applications. Artif Organs 1998;22:222–9.
[12] Wang Y-B, Gong M, Yang S, Nakashima K, Gong Y-K. Hemocompatibility and film stability improvement of crosslinkable MPC copolymer coated polypropylene hollow fiber membrane. J Membr Sci 2014;452:29–36.
[13] Niechajev I. Facial reconstruction using porous high-density polyethylene (medpor): long-term results. Aesthetic Plast Surg 2012;36:917–27.
[14] Sara A, Sandro M, Paolo P, Simone P, Marina M, Andrea P, et al. Human mesenchymal stromal cell-enhanced osteogenic differentiation by contact interaction with polyethylene terephthalate nanogratings. Biomed Mater 2016;11:045003.
[15] Jhong JF, Venault A, Hou CC, Chen SH, Wei TC, Zheng J, et al. Surface zwitterionization of expanded poly(tetrafluoroethylene) membranes via atmospheric plasma-induced polymerization for enhanced skin wound healing. ACS Appl Mater Interf 2013;5:6732–42.
[16] Zhang J, Huang H, Ju R, Chen K, Li S, Wang W, et al. In vivo biocompatibility and hemocompatibility of a polytetrafluoroethylene small diameter vascular graft modified with sulfonated silk fibroin. Am J Surg 2017;213:87–93.
[17] Al Meslmani B, Mahmoud G, Strehlow B, Mohr E, Leichtweiss T, Bakowsky U. Development of thrombus-resistant and cell compatible crimped polyethylene terephthalate cardiovascular grafts using surface co-immobilized heparin and collagen. Mater Sci Eng C Mater Biol Appl 2014;43:538–46.
[18] Sadeghi B. Preparation of ZnO/Ag nanocomposite and coating on polymers for anti-infection biomaterial application. Spectrochim Acta Part A 2014;118:787–92.
[19] Lunov O, Syrovets T, Loos C, Beil J, Delacher M, Tron K, et al. Differential uptake of functionalized polystyrene nanoparticles by human macrophages and a monocytic cell line. ACS Nano 2011;5:1657–69.
[20] Ekkapongpisit M, Giovia A, Follo C, Caputo G, Isidoro C. Biocompatibility, endocytosis, and intracellular trafficking of mesoporous silica and polystyrene nanoparticles in ovarian cancer cells: effects of size and surface charge groups. Int J Nanomed 2012;7:4147–58.
[21] Kiaie N, Aghdam RM, Tafti SH, Emami SH. Statistical optimization of chitosan nanoparticles as protein vehicles, using response surface methodology. J Appl Biomater Funct Mater 2016;14:e413–22.
[22] Heidari F, Razavi M, Bahrololoom ME, Tahriri M, Rasoulianboroujeni M, Koturi H, et al. Preparation of natural chitosan from shrimp shell with different deacetylation degree. Mater Res Innovations 2016:1–5.

[23] Heidari F, Razavi M, Ghaedi M, Forooghi M, Tahriri M, Tayebi L. Investigation of mechanical properties of natural hydroxyapatite samples prepared by cold isostatic pressing method. J Alloys Compd 2017;693:1150–6.
[24] Dimitrievska S, Petit A, Doillon CJ, Epure L, Ajji A, Yahia L, et al. Effect of sterilization on non-woven polyethylene terephthalate fiber structures for vascular grafts. Macromol Biosci 2011;11:13–21.
[25] Chen X, Zhao R, Wang X, Li X, Peng F, Jin Z, et al. Electrospun mupirocin loaded polyurethane fiber mats for anti-infection burn wound dressing application. J Biomat Sci Polym Ed 2017;28:162–76.
[26] Akbarzadeh A, Rezaei-Sadabady R, Davaran S, Joo SW, Zarghami N, Hanifehpour Y, et al. Liposome: classification, preparation, and applications. Nanoscale Res Lett 2013;8:102.
[27] Moghassemi S, Hadjizadeh A. Nano-niosomes as nanoscale drug delivery systems: an illustrated review. J Controlled Release 2014;185:22–36.
[28] Vallet-Regí M. Evolution of bioceramics within the field of biomaterials. Comptes Rendus Chimie 2010;13:174–85.
[29] Baino F, Novajra G, Vitale-Brovarone C. Bioceramics and scaffolds: a winning combination for tissue engineering. Front Bioeng Biotechnol 2015;3:202.
[30] Xia L, Lin K, Jiang X, Fang B, Xu Y, Liu J, et al. Effect of nano-structured bioceramic surface on osteogenic differentiation of adipose derived stem cells. Biomaterials 2014;35:8514–27.
[31] Razavi M, Fathi MH, Savabi O, Vashaee D, Tayebi L. Biodegradation, bioactivity and in vivo biocompatibility analysis of plasma electrolytic oxidized (PEO) biodegradable Mg implants. Phys Sci Int J 2014;4:708.
[32] Lin K, Xia L, Li H, Jiang X, Pan H, Xu Y, et al. Enhanced osteoporotic bone regeneration by strontium-substituted calcium silicate bioactive ceramics. Biomaterials 2013;34:10028–42.
[33] Inzana JA, Olvera D, Fuller SM, Kelly JP, Graeve OA, Schwarz EM, et al. 3D printing of composite calcium phosphate and collagen scaffolds for bone regeneration. Biomaterials 2014;35:4026–34.
[34] Fahmy MD, Jazayeri HE, Razavi M, Masri R, Tayebi L. Three-dimensional bioprinting materials with potential application in preprosthetic surgery. J Prosthodontics 2016.
[35] Razavi M, Fathi M, Savabi O, Boroni M. A review of degradation properties of Mg based biodegradable implants. Res Rev Mater Sci Chem 2012;1:15–58.
[36] Surmenev RA, Surmeneva MA, Ivanova AA. Significance of calcium phosphate coatings for the enhancement of new bone osteogenesis – a review. Acta Biomaterialia 2014;10:557–79.
[37] Liu J, Cui L, Losic D. Graphene and graphene oxide as new nanocarriers for drug delivery applications. Acta Biomaterialia 2013;9:9243–57.
[38] Rawat P, Manglani K, Gupta S, Kalam A, Vohora D, Ahmad FJ, et al. Design and development of bioceramic based functionalized plga nanoparticles of risedronate for bone targeting: in-vitro characterization and pharmacodynamic evaluation. Pharm Res 2015;32:3149–58.
[39] He H, Pham-Huy LA, Dramou P, Xiao D, Zuo P, Pham-Huy C. Carbon nanotubes: applications in pharmacy and medicine. BioMed Res Int 2013;2013:12.
[40] Yuan P, Tan D, Annabi-Bergaya F. Properties and applications of halloysite nanotubes: recent research advances and future prospects. Appl Clay Sci 2015;112–113:75–93.
[41] Cipriano AF, Miller C, Liu H. Anodic growth and biomedical applications of TiO_2 nanotubes. J Biomed Nanotechnol 2014;10:2977–3003.

[42] Ardizzone V, Bove A. Magnetotherapeutic device with bio-ceramic fibers. Google Patents; 2002.
[43] Liu L, Gao S, Yu Y, Wang R, Liang DT, Liu S. Bio-ceramic hollow fiber membranes for immunoisolation and gene delivery: I: Membrane development. J Membr Sci 2006;280:375–82.
[44] Balu R, Singaravelu S, Nagiah N. Bioceramic nanofibres by electrospinning. Fibers 2014;2:221.
[45] Razavi M, Fathi M, Savabi O, Vashaee D, Tayebi L. Micro-arc oxidation and electrophoretic deposition of nano-grain merwinite ($Ca_3MgSi_2O_8$) surface coating on magnesium alloy as biodegradable metallic implant. Surf Interface Anal 2014;46:387–92.
[46] Kheirkhah M, Fathi M, Salimijazi HR, Razavi M. Surface modification of stainless steel implants using nanostructured forsterite (Mg_2 SiO_4) coating for biomaterial applications. Surf Coat Technol 2015;276:580–6.
[47] Burugapalli K, Razavi M, Zhou L, Huang Y. In vitro cytocompatibility study of a medical β-type Ti-35.5 Nb-5.7 Ta titanium alloy. J Biomater Tissue Eng 2016;6:141–8.
[48] Khodaei M, Meratian M, Savabi O, Razavi M. The effect of pore structure on the mechanical properties of titanium scaffolds. Mater Lett 2016;171:308–11.
[49] Chen Q, Thouas GA. Metallic implant biomaterials. Mater Sci Eng R Rep 2015; 87:1–57.
[50] Khodaei M, Meratian M, Shaltooki M, Hashemibeni B, Savabi O, Razavi M. Surface modification of Ti_6Al_4V implants by heat, H_2O_2 and alkali treatments. Surf Eng 2016;32:786–93.
[51] Jazayeri HE, Tahriri M, Razavi M, Khoshroo K, Fahimipour F, Dashtimoghadam E, et al. A current overview of materials and strategies for potential use in maxillofacial tissue regeneration. Mater Sci Eng C 2017;70:913–29.
[52] Popovich A, Sufiiarov V, Polozov I, Borisov E, Masaylo D. Producing hip implants of titanium alloys by additive manufacturing 2016;2016:2.
[53] Weißmann V, Wieding J, Hansmann H, Laufer N, Wolf A, Bader R. Specific yielding of selective laser-melted Ti_6Al_4V open-porous scaffolds as a function of unit cell design and dimensions. Metals 2016;6:166.
[54] Mahmoudi B, Torkamany MJ, Aghdam ARSR, Sabbaghzade J. Laser surface hardening of AISI 420 stainless steel treated by pulsed Nd:YAG laser. Mater Design (1980–2015) 2010;31:2553–60.
[55] Huber DL. Synthesis, properties, and applications of iron nanoparticles. Small 2005;1:482–501.
[56] Jain S, Hirst DG, O'Sullivan JM. Gold nanoparticles as novel agents for cancer therapy. Brit J Radiol 2012;85:101–13.
[57] Bharti C, Nagaich U, Pal AK, Gulati N. Mesoporous silica nanoparticles in target drug delivery system: a review. Int J Pharm Invest 2015;5:124–33.
[58] Myler S, Collyer SD, Bridge KA, Higson SPJ. Ultra-thin-polysiloxane-film-composite membranes for the optimisation of amperometric oxidase enzyme electrodes. Biosens Bioelectron 2002;17:35–43.
[59] Whitford MJ. The chemistry of silicone materials for biomedical devices and contact lenses. Biomaterials 1984;5:298–300.
[60] Lambert JM. The nature of platinum in silicones for biomedical and healthcare use. J Biomed Mater Res B Appl Biomater 2006;78B:167–80.
[61] Si J, Cui Z, Xie P, Song L, Wang Q, Liu Q, et al. Characterization of 3D elastic porous polydimethylsiloxane (PDMS) cell scaffolds fabricated by VARTM and particle leaching. J Appl Polym Sci 2016:133. n/a-n/a.

[62] Liu C, Kray J, Toomajian V, Chan C. Schwann cells migration on patterned polydimethylsiloxane microgrooved surface. Tissue Eng Part C 2016;22:644–51.
[63] Baillargeon AL, Mequanint K. Biodegradable polyphosphazene biomaterials for tissue engineering and delivery of therapeutics. BioMed Res Int 2014;2014:16.
[64] Liberman A, Mendez N, Trogler WC, Kummel AC. Synthesis and surface functionalization of silica nanoparticles for nanomedicine. Surf Sci Rep 2014;69:132–58.
[65] Cheng X, Lowe SB, Reece PJ, Gooding JJ. Colloidal silicon quantum dots: from preparation to the modification of self-assembled monolayers (SAMs) for bio-applications. Chem Soc Rev 2014;43:2680–700.
[66] Lakshmi S, Katti DS, Laurencin CT. Biodegradable polyphosphazenes for drug delivery applications. Adv Drug Delivery Rev 2003;55:467–82.
[67] Ulum MF, Arafat A, Noviana D, Yusop AH, Nasution AK, Abdul Kadir MR, et al. In vitro and in vivo degradation evaluation of novel iron-bioceramic composites for bone implant applications. Mater Sci Eng C 2014;36:336–44.
[68] Yang Y, Lan D, Huang Y, Li Y, Wang Y, Sun L, et al. Preparation of elastic porous cell scaffold fabricated with combined polydimethylsiloxane (PDMS) and hydroxyapatite (HA). Sheng Wu Yi Xue Gong Cheng Xue Za Zhi 2014;31:625–31.
[69] Matsumoto TJ, An S-H, Ishimoto T, Nakano T, Matsumoto T, Imazato S. Zirconia–hydroxyapatite composite material with micro porous structure. Dental Mater 2011;27:e205–12.
[70] Baeza A, Arcos D, Vallet-Regí M. Thermoseeds for interstitial magnetic hyperthermia: from bioceramics to nanoparticles. J Phys Condens Matter 2013;25:484003.
[71] Liu S, Wehmschulte RJ. A novel hybrid of carbon nanotubes/iron nanoparticles: iron-filled nodule-containing carbon nanotubes. Carbon 2005;43:1550–5.
[72] Cao JJ, Chen HH, Du F, Zhao HC, Fan L. Preliminary study of in situ transformed carbon fibers/Al2O3 ceramic matrix composites. Ceram Int 2013;39:7037–42.
[73] Allcock HR. Inorganic—organic polymers. Adv Mater 1994;6:106–15.
[74] Kros A, Jansen JA, Holder SJ, Nolte RJM, Sommerdijk NAJM. Silane-based hybrids for biomedical applications. J Adhes Sci Technol 2002;16:143–55.
[75] Fernandez-Solis C, Erbe A. Waterborne chitosan-epoxysilane hybrid pretreatments for corrosion protection of zinc. Biointerphases 2016;11:021001.
[76] Xu Q, Sardon H, Chan JMW, Hedrick JL, Yang YY. Polyurethane-coated silica particles with broad-spectrum antibacterial properties. Polym Chem 2015;6:2011–22.
[77] Wang G, Yang J, Shi Q. Preparation of transparent ultrahydrophobic silica film by sol–gel process. J Coat Technol Res 2011;8:53–60.
[78] Ahmadi A, Ramezanzadeh B, Mahdavian M. Hybrid silane coating reinforced with silanized graphene oxide nanosheets with improved corrosion protective performance. RSC Adv 2016;6:54102–12.
[79] Rothe B, Elas A, Michaeli W. In situ polymerisation of polyamide-6 nanocompounds from caprolactam and layered silicates. Macromol Mater Eng 2009;294:54–8.
[80] Tanahashi M, Takeda K. Dispersion of nano-sized hydrophilic silica particles into various hydrophobic polymer networks. J Nanosci Nanotechnol 2014;14:3123–36.
[81] Balan P, Chan ES, Harun MK, Swamy V, Singh Raman RK. Effect of lanthanide activated nano-SiO_2 on the corrosion behavior of silane-based hybrid coatings on low carbon steel. Mater Corros 2015;66:1223–31.
[82] Grant DN, Benson J, Cozad MJ, Whelove OE, Bachman SL, Ramshaw BJ, et al. Conjugation of gold nanoparticles to polypropylene mesh for enhanced biocompatibility. J Mater Sci Mater Med 2011;22:2803–12.

[83] Whelove OE, Cozad MJ, Lee BD, Sengupta S, Bachman SL, Ramshaw BJ, et al. Development and in vitro studies of a polyethylene terephthalate-gold nanoparticle scaffold for improved biocompatibility. J Biomed Mater Res B Appl Biomater 2011;99:142–9.

[84] Saxena S, Ray AR, Kapil A, Pavon-Djavid G, Letourneur D, Gupta B, et al. Development of a new polypropylene-based suture: plasma grafting, surface treatment, characterization, and biocompatibility studies. Macromol Biosci 2011;11:373–82.

[85] Watanabe H, Hayashi J-i, Ohzeki H, Moro H, Sugawara M, Eguchi S. Biocompatibility of a silicone-coated polypropylene hollow fiber oxygenator in an in vitro model. Ann Thorac Surg 1999;67:1315–9.

[86] Li K, Zhou Y, Yang Jy, Zhu Jh, Liu Cj. In vitro biocompatibility evaluation of ePTFE graft with controlled release of heparin from mesoporous material. Appl Surf Sci 2012;258:4041–7.

Porous scaffolds

3

Ebru Altuntaş[1], *Burcu Özkan*[2] *and Gülgün Yener*[1]
[1]Istanbul University, Istanbul, Turkey
[2]Yildiz Technical University, Istanbul, Turkey

3.1 Tissue engineering

Tissue engineering (TE) is a multidisciplinary field that aims to develop artificial tissues for the regeneration of damaged tissues, which are difficult to be treated by conventional drug administration, artificial prostheses, and organ transplantation, or incurable [1]. The basis of the design artificial organs and the development of TE strategies is to understand the structure and function of normal biological tissues in detail. Generally, biological tissues are formed from cells and extracellular matrix (ECM), which is noncellular part. ECM is a heterogeneous component of signaling molecules, functional proteins, proteoglycans, and is arranged in a three-dimensional (3D) shape, and is enriched with various growth factors, cellular components, water, cytokines, and ions to provide structural support to cells [2,3].

ECM functions can be summarized as follows:

- Establishment of hierarchical structured micro/nano environment;
- To provide mechanical and structural support to the cells;
- Regulation of cell shape and polarity;
- Storage of regulatory molecules (gas foaming (GF), multidomain proteins, enzymes);
- Regulation of cell function through biomechanic interactions and mechanical signs (e.g., cell survival, proliferation, migration, differentiation, and growth).

Considering the primary role of cell environment and ECM in determining cell response and behavior, it is quite clear that biochemists and biologists need to deeply understand biological event that govern cell–ECM and cell–cell interactions. Cells must be supported with a scaffold having suitable mechanical and biological properties that allow cell adhesion, proliferation, and spontaneous formation of ECM by cells. For this purpose, materials science plays a role in the production of ECM-substitute scaffold with proper 3D structure, chemical and physical properties [4].

3.2 Scaffolds

Scaffolds are defined as 3D porous biomaterials that are designed to perform some or all of the following functions: (1) contribute cell–biomaterial interactions, cell adhesion, and the accumulation of ECM; (2) enable sufficient transport of gases, regulatory factors, and nutrients to allow proliferation, cell survival, and differentiation; (3) to obtain biodegradation rate that is close to the rate of tissue regeneration at certain culture conditions, and (4) to minimize inflammation or toxicity in vivo [5].

Nanobiomaterials Science, Development and Evaluation. DOI: http://dx.doi.org/10.1016/B978-0-08-100963-5.00003-3

3.3 The critical structural and chemical requirements of scaffolds

For TE applications, scaffolds that are produced from a biodegradable polymer should be porous and 3D structures that function to support tissue mechanics and provide cell survival. These 3D, porous scaffolds including gel, sponge, sphere, and fiber-based structures manufactured by different production methods have a variety of characteristics due to their significant structural architecture [6]. Ideally, a functional scaffold must meet the following challenging requirements [7–9]:

- Be biocompatible to prevent undesired host tissue responses to implants;
- Have a degradation rate that matches the formation rate of new tissue;
- Have adequate surface properties that provide bimolecular signals to cells for cell growth, proliferation, differentiation, and adhesion;
- Have optimum structural features in terms of porosity, pore size, permeability, and pore interconnectivity in order to provide effective nutrient transmission and the removal of wastes;
- Be bioresorbable;
- Show mechanical properties similar to the host tissue;
- Have a production process that allows the scaffold to be structured to fit a range of defective geometries;
- Be up-scalable for mass production;
- Meet the regulatory requirements and can be sterilized for clinical usage.

Biocompatibility is a necessary characteristic for scaffolds. Because of the scaffold works in contact with the tissues and cells in vitro, when the scaffold is implanted in vivo it should not lead to harmful bioresponse [10]. Biocompatibility of the scaffold is affected by important factors such as the scaffold's chemistry, structure, and morphology [11].

Scaffold is intended to be a temporary support that is displaced to regenerated tissue in the organism over time. Therefore scaffold must be biodegradable in human body by molecular degradation mechanisms that result in the gradual disappearance of scaffold and the formation of degradation by-products [12]. In addition, the degradation rate of the scaffold should reflect the rate of tissue formation. It is quite difficult to reach this criteria but it is particularly important in terms of structural supporting role of the scaffold [10,13].

Scaffold surface is the first and primary area that interacts with its surrounding cells and tissues. Even though biodegradable porous scaffolds have good enough interconnected pores that allow cell infiltration and growth also have surface properties such as hydrophilicity/hydrophobicity that originate from the chemical composition may not be sufficient to induce selective cell adhesion, migration, and proliferation. In many cases, specific cellular interactions are required for the desired tissue formation. In general, the surface properties of the biomaterials that are implanted describe the behavior of the protein adsorption with determination of simultaneous cellular interactions. Many studies have been made to mimic the natural ECM by immobilizing biomolecules on the surface of the polymer scaffold [14]. Surface properties can be selectively functionalized through physical adsorption or chemical modification to improve the performance of biomaterials. Cell adhesion proteins such as poly(L-lysine), collagen, and fibronectin, laminin, vitronectin were adsorbed onto a polymeric matrix surface to support cell attachment [15,16]. In addition to this, covalent binding of functional biomolecules is required to provide more stable adhesive layer for the cells. Naturally derived macromolecules such as collagen, gelatin, heparin, hyaluronic acid, Arg-Gly-Asp (RGD), or Tyr-Ile-Gly-Ser-Arg (YIGS) short peptide sequences obtained from cell adhesive proteins and sugar moieties such as galactose or lactose were grafted onto the polymer surface to regulate cell–matrix interactions [14,17].

Pore structure and porosity of the scaffold play an important role in implant placement and 3D tissue formation. Pores are required for tissue formation because it allows cell migration and growth, vascularization, and diffusion of nutrients for cell viability [18,19]. The amount of porosity is related inversely with mechanical properties. High degree of porosity is desirable for cell colonization and provide an opportunity for more rapid tissue formation. However, a high degree of porosity indicates that the scaffold has lower mechanical properties. Therefore, optimized balance should be achieved between these conflicting requirements in each specific application [20]. Cellular growth and penetration in the 3D scaffold structure is greatly influenced by the average pore size of biomaterial scaffolds. Optimum pore size ranges for the different types of cells and tissues are shown in Table 3.1. Generally, the scaffold with a large pore size while allowing effective nutrient supply, gas diffusion, and the removal of metabolic wastes also may lead to low cell adhesion and intracellular signal [21]. If the pore size used is too small, occlusion of pores that prevents ECM production and neovascularization in the inner area of the scaffold will occur by cells [25]. Consequently, structure of scaffold should contain both macropores (pore size >50 μm) and micropores (pore size <10 μm) in order to provide the necessary physical support during the regeneration process [26].

Table 3.1 Optimum pore size ranges for different kinds of cells and tissues [21–24]

Type of cells and tissues	Optimum pore size ranges
Neovascularization	5 μm
Fibroblast	5–15 μm
Adult mammalian skin	20–125 μm
Chondrocyte	70–120 μm
Bone	100–350 μm
Osteoid	40–100 μm
Hepatocyte	20 μm
Liver tissue	45–150 μm
Vascular smooth muscle	60–150 μm
Bladder smooth muscle	100–300 μm
Fibrovascular tissue	>500 μm

The interconnectivity of pores is a critical issue for cell migration, further colonization of the scaffold surface, and the maintenance of cell viability by providing the diffusion of essential nutrients and removal of metabolic wastes [27]. The lack of pore interconnectivity results in insufficient nutrients and oxygen transport as well as limited removal of wastes from the scaffold [28]. This situation may inhibit cell migration and growth even if the biomaterial is highly porous [29]. As a result, production of scaffolds with improved pore interconnectivity is useful for TE applications [30].

The appropriate mechanical properties for a biomaterial that are used in TE applications are critical to the success of the implant. Hence, many tissues undergo mechanical stresses and strains, and it is important that mechanical properties of the scaffold match, as much as possible, those of the regenerated tissue. Thus, the formation of new ECM is not limited due to mechanical weakness [10]. TE scaffolds are applicable clinically and commercially; it should be affordable and possible to scale-up [31]. The development of scalable production process for GMP (good manufacturing practice) has great importance in order to ensure the successful transformation of TE strategies to clinical applications [32].

The above mentioned scaffold features are related to two main factors that play an important role in controlling scaffold properties: (1) the type of polymer material and (2) scaffold production technology. For example, toxic wastes can cause harmful effects when they are released out from the scaffold. Such substances may be monomers, impurities in the initial material, or substances from the material process (degradation products, organic solvents, etc.). Mechanical properties are related to raw materials at first; however, these properties vary considerably depending on the scaffold structure that is determined by the technique used in the production of the scaffold. Another example is bioresorbability and especially the degradation rate is related not only to polymer characteristics (i.e., microstructure of copolymers and molecular weight, chemical composition, and the monomer distribution), but it is also related to scaffold structure (i.e., pore walls and scaffold dimension).

When designing scaffold for a specific application, it must be known which properties the scaffold should exhibit to successfully perform its function. After the necessary scaffolding features are clearly defined, materials science is involved in selecting the appropriate polymer material, production method, and suitable treatments [33].

3.4 Scaffolding biomaterials

Biomaterials are defined as any substance or combination of substances other than drugs that can treat, strengthen, or replace any tissue, organ, or body function, and they can be used as a whole or as a part of a system to maintain or improve the individual's quality of life [34,35]. Previous biomaterial research was carried out on systems that has appropriate physical properties and minimal toxicity to the host tissue and that aim successfully and permanently to replace damaged tissues. Metals, ceramics, and nondegradable polymers are the best examples of conventional systems. Inertness and inadequacy to adapt growth are common features. Today, the concept of an ideal biomaterial has changed with the development of bioactive materials. These bioactive substances have the ability to interact with the biological environment to support the material–host tissue integration and to enhance biological response [36].

Generally a bioactive material is designed to induce specific biological activity [37]. More functional and measurable bioactivity can be defined as the possibility of making feature to create bond with living tissue [38]. In this case, nonbioactive materials leads to the formation of nonadherent tissue layers at the implant interface. Therefore, metals and other nonbiodegradable materials cannot be used in this context; it is clear that biomaterials are suitable to produce bioresorbable scaffolds that degrade in the human body by hydrolitic and/or enzymatic degradation [33].

Biomaterial scaffolding should be selected according to the requirements of the TE application. Some biomaterials are more appropriate than others depending on which tissue is being engineered. TE scaffolds are produced using a variety of organic and inorganic biomaterials including biopolymers, bioceramics, metals, and their composites. Bioceramics, metals, and composites are mostly used in the regeneration of hard tissues due to their high mechanical properties. Furthermore, polymers are used for the reconstruction of soft tissues [39].

3.4.1 *Organic biomaterials (biopolymeric scaffolds)*

Various porous scaffolds have been developed from natural and synthetic polymers that can mimic in vivo extracellular microenvironment to control the functions of the implanted cells. While synthetic polymers are synthesized by the human-directed polymerization process, natural polymers are obtained from the growth and metabolism of microorganism, plants, and animals. Recently, new hybrid polymeric scaffolds that mimic the ECM of a natural tissue have been developed by a combination of natural and synthetic polymers [14,40].

3.5 Naturally derived biopolymers

Natural polymers are described as the first biodegradable biomaterials that are suitable for TE applications and used clinically because they are biocompatible and can be resorbed by the host tissue during implantation [41]. Natural polymers are advantageous compared to synthetic polymers for TE because they are similar to the protein and polysaccharide components of the ECM structure. Cells recognize amino acid and saccharide sequences and have the necessary binding site for them. The good interactions with cells provide the possibility of enhancing cell performance in a biological system [42]. In addition, scaffold materials should have reproducible and controllable properties considering the strict medical regulatory standards for consistent quality and material purity. The structure and chemical components of natural polymers can vary significantly among natural sources [43,44]. As a result, material properties may not be reproducible from batch to batch and makes it difficult to apply the quality assurance/quality control (QA/QC) manufacturing practices in the current situation. In contrast, the synthetic polymer material properties are reproducible from batch to batch because QA/QC practices are well established and their properties are determined by the adjustable process parameters [45].

Natural polymers can be classified as polysaccharides (chitosan, cellulose, dextran, alginate, glycosaminoglycans, and amylose), proteins (collagen, keratin, elastin, silk, gelatin, fibrin, actin, and myosin) or polynucleotides (DNA, RNA) [42].

While type I collagen is the most abundant and main component of bone, skin, ligaments, and tendons, type II collagen is the main component of cartilage. Collagen does not only provide structural support to cells and tissues but it also plays an important role in cellular behavior, chemokine storage, and release [46]. Collagen and denatured form of collagen, gelatin, can form a porous gel matrix. It is also used in the functionalization of the surfaces of synthetic polymers to allow cell adhesion [47]. Collagen scaffolds are widely used clinically in the regeneration of dermal, vascular, orthopedic, and ophthalmic tissues [48].

One of the most common types of natural fibrous protein is silk. Silkworm silk is used in textile production for centuries and has been used as sutures for decades due to superior tensile mechanical and nondegradable properties [49]. This natural macromolecular material has been introduced as a scaffold material in the usage field of TE owing to good biocompability, slow degradation, and good mechanical properties [50,51].

Fibrin has important functions in wound healing such as creating a hemostatic barrier to prevent bleeding and support the natural scaffold for fibroblasts. The polymerization is induced by fibrin monomer conversion to fibrinogen via thrombin [52]. Mostly fibrin has been used to produce hydrogel scaffold formation for cardiovascular tissue [53], neural TE [54], and microvascular networks [55]. Fibrin also can be mixed with calcium phosphate granules to form a porous scaffold [56]. Fibrin is suitable for clinical use as hemostatic agent, tissue adhesive, and significantly improves hemostasis when it is used to strengthen skin graft, as well as develops host tissue graft integration [57].

Elastin, an ECM protein in mammals, plays a supportive role in endothelial cell growth and in controlling of vascular smooth muscle proliferation [58]. Elastic also provides elasticity to tissues and it is found in ligaments, arteries, lungs, and skin. Elastin types that are used for scaffold fabrication contains sequences such as solubilized elastin derived from animal sources, recombinant tropoelast, and elastin [59,60]. Elastin is mainly used in cardiovascular tissue, dermal tissue, and the engineering of vascular channels [61]. Commonly, elastin is incorporated into scaffolds as a mixture with other natural biomaterials especially such as collagen [62] and silk [63].

Polysaccharides are another class of natural polymers. Glycosaminoglycans (GAGs), the basic components of the ECM tissue, are included in the group of polysaccharides and they have many functions for example the preservation of tissue structure and directing the cell function. GAGs that are found in cartilage tissue play a significant role in lubricating articular joints, resisting compressive forces, and cell binding in basal membrane. Hyaluronic acid, dermatan sulfate, chondroitin sulfate, keratan sulfate, and heparin sulfate species that are mainly found in the body; chondroitin sulfate and hyaluronic acid are primarily used for scaffolding in TE. GAG usage in the engineering of dermal [64], brain [65], and adipose tissue [66] has been reported; however, it has been widely produced in the form of hydrogel for cartilage TE.

Alginate is an anionic polysaccharide commonly derived from brown algae cell wall. It is capable of forming gels with high swelling degree in the presence of divalent cations such as Ca^{2+} [67]. Alginate has been studied primarily as a hydrogel scaffold for cartilage in TE. In addition to the alginate hydrogels, alginate can also be electrospun [68] and porous sponges can be produced by adding divalent cations (Ca^{2+}, Mg^{2+}, Ba^{2+}, Sr^{2+}) in the alginate solution [69].

Chitosan is a cationic polysaccharide with hydrophilic properties that is used as scaffold material to support cell adhesion and differentiation [10,11]. Chitosan can generate different material forms including hydrogels [70], electrospun mats [71], microspheres [72], and porous scaffolds [73]. Implanted chitosan causes a minimum level of foreign body response and it has natural antimicrobial and thrombogenic properties [74]. Chitosan bandages are clinically used as wound dressings [75].

3.6 Synthetic biopolymers

The properties of synthetic polymers (e.g., degradation time, porosity, and mechanical characteristics) are very useful in the biomedical field since they are adjusted according to the specific application. One of the most important problems of natural polymers is that they are generally expensive, show differences from batch to batch, and have the possibility of cross-contamination from unwanted diseases or unknown viruses due to isolation from animal, plant, and human tissue. On the other hand, synthetic polymers are usually cheaper than natural polymers; they can be produced uniformly in large quantities, have no immunogenicity, their physicochemical properties can be controlled easily, and they have a long shelf life. Molecular structure and molecular weight can be tunable during synthetic procedures, and the mechanical and physical properties of scaffold that is made from synthetic polymers can be adjusted to the desired location in the human body [76]. Synthetic polymers are divided into two broad categories as (i) biodegradable and (ii) nonbiodegradable. Some nondegradable polymers are poly(hydroxyethylmethacrylate), poly(N-isopropylacryamide), and polyvinyl alcohol (PVA). Some synthetic biodegradable polymers such as polylactide (PLA), polyglycolide (PGA) and their copolymer poly(lactide-co glycolide) (PLGA), poly(hydroxy butyrate) (PHB), poly(ε-caprolactone) (PCL), polyanhydride, polyphosphazene, poly(glycerol sebacate) (PGS), poly(propylene fumarate) (PPF), and biodegradable polyurethanes (PUs) are included in the group of poly(α-hydroxy ester)s. Among these two categories of polymers, synthetic biodegradable polymers have been preferred in TE applications to minimize chronic foreign body reaction and to provide a completely natural tissue formation [77].

Aliphatic polyesters

These polymers can form stable porous 3D scaffold that is insoluble or does not melt in vitro tissue culture conditions [78]. These polymers generally degrade by hydrolysis of ester groups in their structure; degradation rate and degradation products can be adjusted according to the composition, structure, and molecular weight [79].

PLA, PGA, and their copolymer PLGA are synthesized by ring-opening polymerization of monomers (lactide and/or glycolide) and are generally expressed as poly-α-hydroxyacids [80]. In addition to biodegradability and biocompatibility of these polymers, they are among the few synthetic polymers that are approved by US Food and Drug Administration (FDA) for surgical sutures and clinical applications such as some implantable devices. These polymers degrade the products that can be absorbed by the organism (lactic acid that is normally produced by muscular contraction) as a result of exposure to water [81]. PGA has many advantageous properties and it is one of the most widely used polymers for scaffolding. It degrades in vivo or in aqueous solutions and loses its mechanical integrity within two or four weeks depending on the physical structure and molecular weight of material and degradation conditions. Nonwoven fibrous fabrics are made with this polymer and are most commonly used as a scaffold [78,82].

PLA is another biodegradable polymer that is widely used for the manufacture of scaffolds [83]. Extra methyl group in the repeating unit of PLA (compared with PGA) reduces the molecular affinity for water and makes it more hydrophobic leading to slower hydrolysis. Thus, the loss of mechanical integrity of the PLA scaffold or implant takes several months or even years [84,85]. PLGAs were synthesized using various ratios of lactic and glycolic acid to obtain a degradation rate between the rate of PGA and PLA [86]. Also other linear aliphatic polyesters such as PCL [86] and PHB [87] are used in TE. PCL degrades significantly slower when compared to PLA, PGA, and PLGA [87].

Even though slow degradation of PCL makes it less preferable for TE applications, this property of PCL makes it more suitable for long-term implants and controlled release applications. PCL-based copolymers have been synthesized recently to improve the degradation properties [88]. PHB is produced by fermentation of microorganisms [89]. PHB and PHB-based copolymers are less popular for TE applications when compared with PGA, PLA, and PLGA because they degrade very slowly due to their hydrophobic nature. Other important synthetic biodegradable polymer PFF can be degraded by hydrolysis of the ester bond similar to lactide and glycolide polymers [90].

Polyanhydrides

Polyanhydrides can be synthesized easily from appropriate, low-cost sources, and can be adjusted to meet the desired specifications [91]. Polyanhydrides are biocompatible and they degrade into diacid by-products that can be eliminated from the body as metabolites in vivo and are nontoxic. These polymers are essentially designed for drug release applications because they are very hydrophobic and degrade by surface erosion [92]. Drugs, when loaded into such polymers, are better protected because they have almost no penetration of water before polymer erosion [93]. Also these polymers have been searched for the TE scaffolds.

Polyphosphazenes

Polyphosphazenes is a relatively new class of biodegradable polymer by comparison with poly(α-hydroxy acids) and poly(anhydrides) [94]. These polymers contain phosphorus and nitrogen atom sequences in their backbone at the interface between inorganic and organic polymers. Biodegradable polyphosphazenes can be synthesized with the opportunity to adjust the degradation rate over hours, days, months, or years by combining side groups on phosphorus atom, controlling their nature and side substitutes composition [95,96]. They are good candidates of a variety of soft and hard tissue TE applications, thanks to good biocompatibility, synthetic flexibility, nontoxic degradation products, and designed mechanical properties [97–99].

Polyurethanes

PU, which is one of the most popular groups of biomaterials, can be used for a wide range of biomedical applications [100]. They are popular recently due to their segmented-block structural characters that provide adjustable mechanical properties, biological properties, physical properties, blood and tissue compatibility, and versatility in a wide range in terms of biocompatibility [100]. PUs are used as biostable and inert materials in catheters, heart valves, prostheses, and vascular grafts owing to improved durability, biocompatibility, hardness, and stability [101].

Poly(glycerol sebacate)

PGS is a relatively new synthetic, biodegradable, and biocompatible polymer used increasingly in various biomedical applications [102]. PGS has thermoset elastomeric properties and it is relatively inexpensive to produce. In addition, its degradation rate and mechanical properties can be adjusted for a particular application by controlling curing temperature, curing time, reactant concentration, and the acylation degree of acrylated PGS [103]. PGS has mostly been used for soft TE such as cardiac muscle, nerve, blood, retina, and cartilage due to its elastomeric nature. Also applications of PGS has been extended as tissue adhesive, drug delivery, and hard tissue regeneration [104–106].

3.6.1 Inorganic biomaterials (bioceramic scaffolds)

Bioceramics are a class of inorganic nonmetallic materials defined as components or ceramic products of implant and replacements, which are used in medical and dental applications [107]. Considering the inorganic nature and mechanical stiffness of bioceramics, they are generally used for the regeneration of hard tissues such as bone and teeth. However, some studies have shown the potential of bioceramics as an innovative way to regenerate a variety of damaged soft tissues [108,109].

Another development that has been receiving interest is the use of bioactive ceramics, bioglasses, and glass–ceramics as a delivery system for inorganic ions that have a positive effect on tissue regeneration and angiogenesis [110–112].

They can be categorized as bioactive (bioglass, glass–ceramics, and hydroxyapatite (HA)), biosoluble (calcium phosphates), and bioinert (alumina (Al_2O_3), zirconia (ZrO_2), and pyrolytic carbon) according to the types of bioceramic and host tissue interactions. In addition, bioceramics are generally classified as crystalline, semicrystalline, or amorphous in nature [113].

Bioinert ceramics are used as acetabular cups and femoral heads for hip prosthesis as well as used for manufacturing dental implants; however, these materials are inert, and for this reason they are not used as scaffolds. The ability to form a stable bond with the host tissue has major importance in the selection of bioceramic for the production of scaffold. In this context, bioactive and bioresorbable ceramics consisting of the same ions in bone offer a valuable solution. These bioactive ceramics are biocompatible; they bind directly to bone and do not cause any systemic toxicity or immunological reactions. Furthermore, they degrade gradually during the regeneration of natural host tissue and disappear when they have completed their task of acting as templates for new tissue [114–116]. Bioactive ceramics have several major groups including calcium glass–ceramics, phosphate ceramics, and bioactive glasses.

3.7 Calcium phosphate bioceramics

Calcium phosphate is the main mineral component of bones. Only certain calcium phosphates are useful for implantation in the body. Calcium phosphates that have Ca/P ratio less than 1 are not suitable for biological implantation because of their high solubility, but this ratio is greater than 1.67 resorption rate that significantly reduces [117]. Synthetic calcium phosphate bioceramics that are generally named "biphasic calcium phosphate" (BCP), they are a series of combination of HA $Ca_{10}(PO_4)_6(OH)_2$, beta-tricalcium phosphate (β-TCP) ($Ca_3(PO_4)_2$), and HA ve β-TCP (ratio of HA to β-TCP), and they have attracted attention recently [36].

Calcium phosphate bioceramics are generally osteoconductive for TE applications but are not osteoinductive [118,119]. However, several calcium phosphate bioceramics including HA, BCP ve β-TCP have been reported that they have bone-forming capabilities in nonbone areas without additional osteogenic factors [120,121]. Some calcium phosphate bioceramics are defined as having intrinsic osteoinductivity because they have shown osteoinductive properties [119]. These osteoinductive properties are thought to be dependent on various factors such as surface topography, geometry, and pore characteristics of biomaterial and chemical compositions [122].

Calcium phosphate bioceramics HA, BCP, and β-TCP are used as coating in the treatment of craniofacial defects, as femoral stem in hip implants and maxillary floor augmentation [118]. Despite β-TCP scaffolds having the same porosity of HA scaffolds, they have lower resistance. Therefore, the use of these bioceramics porous scaffolds are not recommended in the regeneration of major damage in the load-bearing region because of inadequate strength of β-TCP, weak mechanical response, and limited mechanical reliability [36].

3.8 Bioactive glasses

The first bioactive glass (SiO_2 45 wt.%—Na_2O 24.5 wt.%—CaO 24.5 wt.%—P_2O_5 6 wt. % system) (45S5 Bioglass), which was developed in the late 1960s by Larry

Hench et al., has been the most studied glass in biomedical applications [123]. This glass is a silicate glass based on 3D glass-forming SiO_2. Since that time, many other borate, silicate, glass–ceramics, and phosphate glasses that were shown to be bioactive are recommended for biomedical applications [115,124,125]. These bioactive materials release ions to the cells in their regional physiological environments when they are degraded. During the process of degradation these materials form a carbonate-substituted HA layer on the glass surface. This carbonate-substituted HA layer can bind firmly to the soft tissues and bone similarly phosphate glass fibers for muscle and ligament replacements due to it is similar to the mineral component of the bone [36]. Generally, the ability to change the chemical composition and surface reactivity rate, which provide to bind a wide variety of tissues, are the advantages of bioactive glass. They are disadvantageous in terms of mechanical properties because these materials have a relatively low flexural strength in comparison with other ceramic materials [36].

3.9 Glass–ceramics

Glass–ceramics are crystallized glass that are produced as a result of the controlled thermal process of parent glass or thermal treatment during production. Glass–ceramic, which is produced by casting and melting methods, has better physical and mechanical properties (e.g., fracture toughness, strength) than the parent glass. However, the common challenge of the glass–ceramic scaffolds for TE applications is an unexpected and slow degradation that is formed in the presence of crystalline phases [125].

3.9.1 Biocomposites

Composites that consist of an organic matrix (generally a biodegradable polymer) and an inorganic phase (bioactive material particles such as HA and bioactive glass) draw attention for TE applications, since natural bone tissue consists of collagen fiber matrix (50–500 nm diameter) and HA crystals (70 nm long and 2–5 nm wide) [126–128]. In general, the purpose of forming such composites is combining the osteoconductive properties, power, and hardness of bioceramics with durability, flexibility, and resorbability of polymers. Thus, polymer phase can gain bioactive function as well as its strengthcan be improved. In addition, issues with the fragility and mechanical reliability of bioceramics can be controlled [129].

First-studied composites include TCP or HA as inorganic phases, poly(L-lactic acid) (PLLA), poly(D/L-lactic acid) (PDLLA), PGA, and PLGA as organic phase [130–132]. HA/polyethylene porous composites that were introduced in the market with a commercial name "Hapex" are frequently used for the regeneration of orbital floor fractures in clinical treatment [133]. Bioactive glass that is dispersed in a biodegradable polymer matrix, which has the potential to improve the host tissue/cell interaction or nanocomposites that consist of HA nanoparticles discreetly have been paid

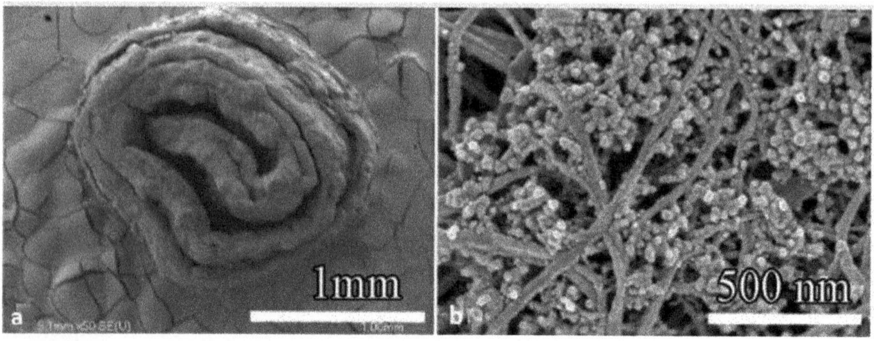

Figure 3.1 (a) Top view low-magnification SEM micrograph of a hybrid roll. (b) High magnification SEM micrographs of DC-nBG gels.
Reprinted from [135], Copyright (2011), with permission from Elsevier.

attention recently [134]. Bioactive glass nanoparticles are incorporated into intensive collagen matrix to mimic microstructure, biological, and mechanical properties of natural bone (Fig. 3.1) [135].

A problem with the above-described nanocomposites is the difficulty of preparing nanoparticles, especially bioactive glass nanoparticles. Another problem is the tendency of nanoparticles to agglomerate, which makes it difficult to disperse homogeneously throughout the matrix. The production of inorganic–organic hybrid for bone and tissue regeneration applications is an alternative approach that draws attention recently [136,137]. Hybrids essentially behave like a single phase causing controlled degradation and designed mechanical properties due to interactions at the molecular level [136].

3.10 Scaffold fabrication techniques

Various techniques are used, which allow the processing of materials into 3D porous scaffolds in order to facilitate cell distribution and to lead the growth of cells into 3D structures. Traditional methods include GF, phase separation, fiber meshes/fiber bonding, self-assembly, freeze-drying, and solvent casting/particle leaching. Other techniques are electrospinning for the production of nanofibrous scaffolds and solid freeform fabrication (SFF; rapid prototyping) for the production of scaffolds from a computer-aided design model. Table 3.2 describes the basic advantages and disadvantages of these techniques. The selection of scaffold production techniques should be done by considering potential and disadvantages of each technique and manufacturing techniques should match the needs of specific tissue to be regenerated. Besides improving the production methods of scaffold with controlled structural and mechanical properties, attention should be paid to improve the properties of scaffolds by modifying biochemical properties of the surface with cell adhesive peptides or leading to cell growth, cell migration, proliferation, or differentiation with growth factors [146].

Table 3.2 Scaffold fabrication techniques for TE applications [29,138–145]

Methods	Advantages	Disadvantages
Fiber meshes	High porosity, high pore interconnectivity, and high surface area to volume ratio	Lack of structural stability
Fiber bonding	High porosity, high pore interconnectivity, and high surface area to volume ratio	Poor mechanical property, high processing temperature, limited control over porosity, residual solvents and porogens
Solvent casting/ particle leaching	Control over porosity and pore geometry, highly porous structures, crystallinity can be tailored, large range of pore sizes	Poor control over the orientation and the degree of pore interconnectivity, limited to the fabrication of thin membranes, limited mechanical property, residual solvents and porogens
Gas foaming	No organic solvents, control over porosity and pore size, suitable for the incorporation of heat sensitive biological agents inside the scaffold	Inadequate pore interconnectivity, limited pore sizes, formation of a nonporous surface
Phase separation	Easily combine with other fabrication technology, allows incorporation of bioactive agents, highly porous structures	Difficult to control precisely scaffold morphology, problems with residual solvent, limited range of pore sizes
Self-assembly	The level of porosity, pore size and the diameter of the fibers are well-controlled, various cell behaviors can be promoted	Designing process is complex, expensive materials required, limited scaffold size
Freeze-drying	Leaching steps are not required, high temperature are not applied	Long processing time, small pore size
Electrospinning	The simplicity of the process, easily scaled-up for mass production, high aspect ratio, surface area, permeability, porosity, and tunable mechanical reliability, suitable for the surface modification of bioactive agents	Limited mechanical property, pore size decrease with fiber thickness, inability to fabricate complex 3D structures
Rapid prototyping	Excellent control over geometry, porosity, no supporting material required	The required equipments are expensive, limited types of polymers can be used.

3.10.1 Fiber meshes/Fiber bonding

Fiber-based scaffolds produced by textile technology are used for the production of nonwoven scaffolds, which is one of the first porous structures for TE and they are made from PGA and PLLA [147]. Despite these fibrous structures having a high degree of porosity (up to 95%) with interconnected pores and high surface area/volume ratio, fiber diameter range is limited to 10–15 μm. The lack of structural strength of this nonwoven scaffolds usually results in significant deformation because of the contractile forces of the cells. This situation has led to the development of fibers binding techniques based on the heat treatment to bind random fiber bundles in order to improve the mechanical properties of the scaffold [138]. The fibers can bind to each other with two different techniques. First technique is developed by Mikos et al. [148]. In this technique, PGA fibers are immersed in PLLA solution. When the solvent evaporates, PGA fibers are embedded in PLLA. After that, composite is heated above the melting temperature of both polymers. PLLA melts in the first place and fills all gaps. This helps in protecting the spatial arrangement of fibers. Then PLLA is removed by performing the dissolution with methylene chloride. Second method for binding PGA fibers uses the atomization of PLLA and PLGA to coat fibers. Chloroform that is dissolved in PLLA or PLGA is sprayed onto PGA fibers [149].

Eventhough fiber bonding techniques produce highly porous scaffolds with interconnected pores, which is suitable for tissue regeneration [148–150], both methods can be toxic to cells if the solvent is not completely removed.

3.10.2 Solvent casting and particulate leaching

This technique was first described in 1994 by Mikos et al. and it uses a water-soluble porogen for the production of pores in a polymer matrix [151]. Briefly, the polymer solution is poured into a mold containing the particles with desired size. After evaporating the solvent, the particles are leached by immersion into water. PLLA and PLGA scaffolds are mainly obtained for this approach. Salt is commonly used as a porogen [151,152]. Also sugar [153], paraffin, and gelatin microspheres are used for this purpose [154].

The pore properties of the obtained scaffold such as the average pore size, pore interconnectivity, and porosity can be controlled by porogen geometry, size, and concentration, and this an important advantage of this method [154]. Highly porous biomaterial with a pore size up to 500 μm and 93% porosity can be produced by using solvent casting/particle leaching method [151]. However, this technique requires the use of large amount of organic solvent, which denatures bioactive molecules, and it affects the time needed for solvent evaporation (days-to-weeks). Also, this method that is used to generate porosity has low control over the orientation and degree of pore interconnectivity [139]. In addition, the production of thin membranes (typically less than 500 μm) is limited because of difficulties relating to the removal of particles from the scaffold. Afterward, these membranes should be assembled within the larger 3D structures [155].

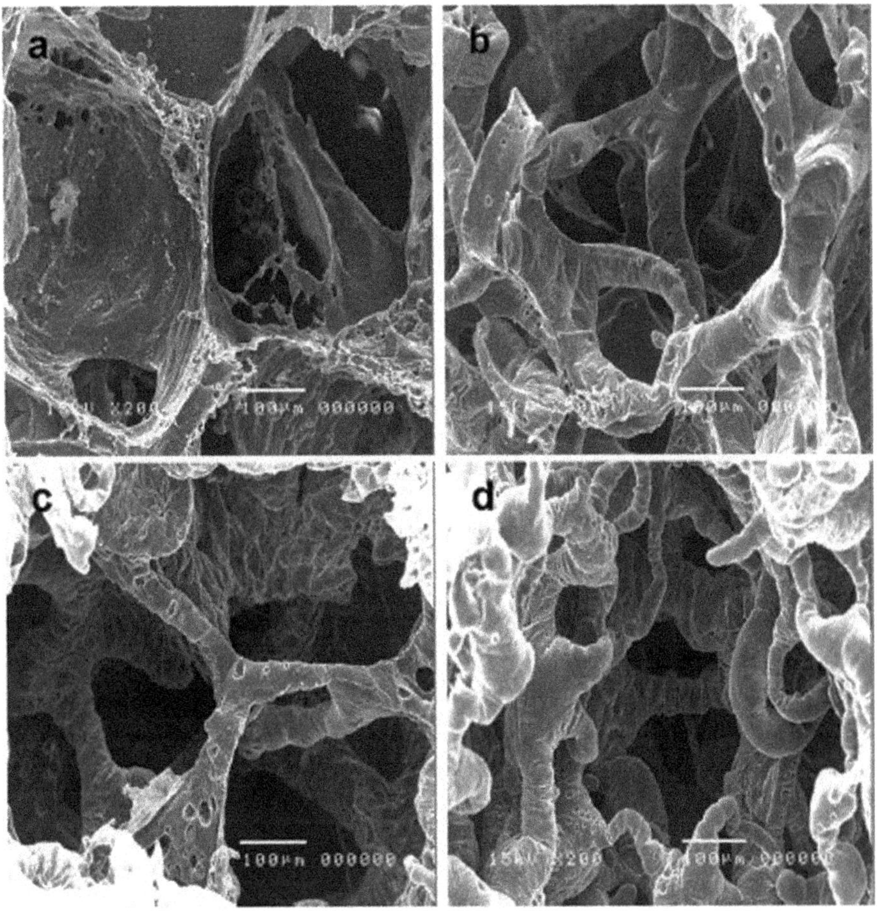

Figure 3.2 SEM images at 2003 magnification illustrating the microstructures of the (a) salt leached, (b) salt-PEG 200 leached, (c) salt-PEG 600 leached, and (d) salt-PEG 1000 leached PCL scaffolds.
Reprinted from [156], Copyright (2013), with permission from John Wiley and Sons.

3D, PCL porous scaffolds with interconnected networks can be produced by using particulate, polymer leaching techniques and modified solvent casting technique that uses sodium chloride and polyethylene glycol (PEG) as porogens (Fig. 3.2). The pores in the scaffold, which is formed by PEG leaching, is larger than the pores formed without PEG leaching and these large pores are more interconnected to each other and they distributed uniformly in the scaffold. As a result, the cells that were cultured on these new PCL scaffolds have a maximum value of mineral accumulation and it was clearly observed to provide much better support to the proliferation of cultured bone cells and differentiation [156].

3.10.3 Gas foaming

GF is widely used to produce microcellular foams of thermoplastic polymers such as poly(methylmethacrylate) and polystyrene [157–160]. However, Mooney et al. used this technique to produce $PLA_{50}GA_{50}$ scaffolds for TE in 1994 [161]. Since then, GF has become a preferable technique for the production of microporous scaffolds [162,163]. High pressure (800 psi) carbon dioxide (CO_2) gas is used for the manufacture of highly porous scaffold in GF technique. Biodegradable polymer such as PLGA is saturated with high pressure CO_2 [161]. The solubility of the gas in polymer decreases rapidly when CO_2 pressure is set to atmospheric levels. This results in nucleation and growth of gas bubbles or cells with sizes ranging between 100 μm and 500 μm in the polymer [161].

The amount of CO_2 dissolved in the polymer solution determines the porosity and pore structure of the scaffold. The main advantage of using CO_2 foaming for the production of scaffolds is to reduce the problems associated with residual solvents, which can be toxic to mammalian cells. However, it is well documented that the formation of nonporous layer in foamed scaffolds, because of the fast diffusion of CO_2, when pressure is released, they can exhibit insufficient pore interconnectivity especially on the scaffold surface [164]. This problem has been overcome by combining GF and particulate leaching techniques [28, 165].

Disks formed from the polymer (e.g., PLGA) and NaCl particles were compression molded at room temperature in GF and particulate leaching techniques, and then it was allowed to reach equilibrium with the high pressure CO_2 (800 psi). Creating a thermodynamic instability led to nucleation and growth of gas pores in polymer particles, resulting in the expansion of the polymer particles. Polymer particles were combined with salt particles to form a continuous matrix. After that salt particles were leached to obtain macroporous in the polymer matrix (Fig. 3.3) [165].

This new process provides to obtain a matrix with well-controlled porosity and a pore structure by combining high pressure GF and particulate leaching techniques. This process prevents potential issues that are related to the use of high temperatures and/or organic solvents in the process of biomaterials [165].

3.10.4 Phase separation

The phase separation (PS) scaffold fabrication technique includes demixing in a homogeneous polymer solution by using another solvent or lowering the temperature to a temperature that is below the bimodal solubility curve [166]. This technique separates the polymer solution to polymer-lean and polymer-rich phases. Polymer is dissolved in a solvent with low melting point and that is easy to sublime such as phenol, naphthalene, and 1,4 dioxane. After the dispersion of a bioactive molecule such as alkali phosphatase is performed [167,168], liquid–liquid phase is separated by decreasing the temperature and quenching the mixture below the freezing point of the solvent forms solid with two phases. Then, the solvent of the polymer-lean phase is removed by means of evaporation, extraction, or sublimation, and it forms a porous polymeric scaffold with bioactive molecules that are integrated into structure and the

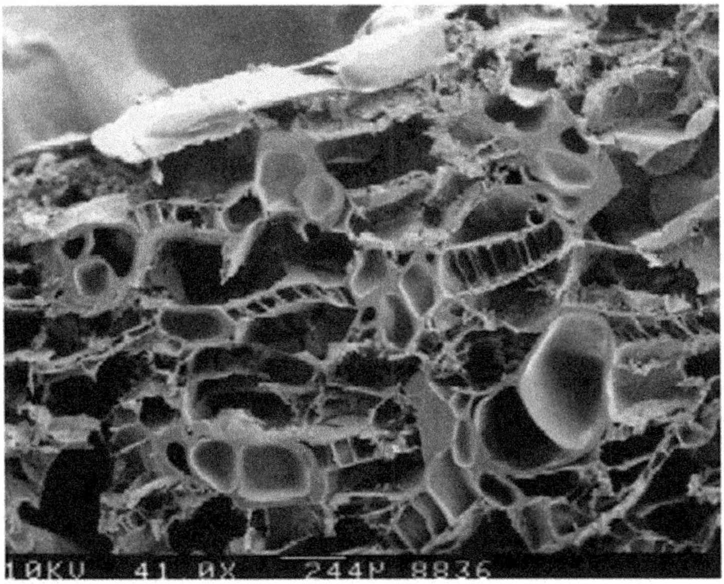

Figure 3.3 High magnification scanning electron photomicrograph of gas foaming and particulate leaching matrix demonstrating macropores, formed by leaching of NaCl particles, and smaller pores formed by the gas pores within the polymer particles.
Reprinted from [165], Copyright (1998), with permission from John Wiley and Sons.

polymer-rich phase [167,168]. It can be combined with particulate leaching technique in designing 3D structures with controlled pore morphology and it is an advantage of the PS technique. However, the use of organic solvents and poor pore interconnectivity of 3D scaffolds are the disadvantages of PS technique [169,170]. The use of surfactants and the coarsening process can be applied to improve pore morphology and the homogeneity of the pore size of the scaffold [166].

Various synthetic polymeric nanofibers are produced by using PS method for TE applications [171,172]. For example, PLLA scaffolds with the diameter ranging from 50 nm to 500 nm, 98% porosity, and continuous 3D nanofibrous network are produced by using liquid–liquid PS method [173]. PLLA/HA porous scaffolds are also prepared by using solid–liquid phase separation method and it has shown better enhancement of the growth and proliferation of osteoblasts in bone TE when comparing with pure PLLA scaffolds (Fig. 3.4) [174].

3.10.5 Self-assembly

Molecules are spontaneously arranged to form an aggregate with a well-defined structure in self-assembly process. Recently, self-assembly principle has been applied to manufacture nanometer-sized fibers with the well-defined chemistry by using the synthesized molecules for 3D cultures or TE applications [175].

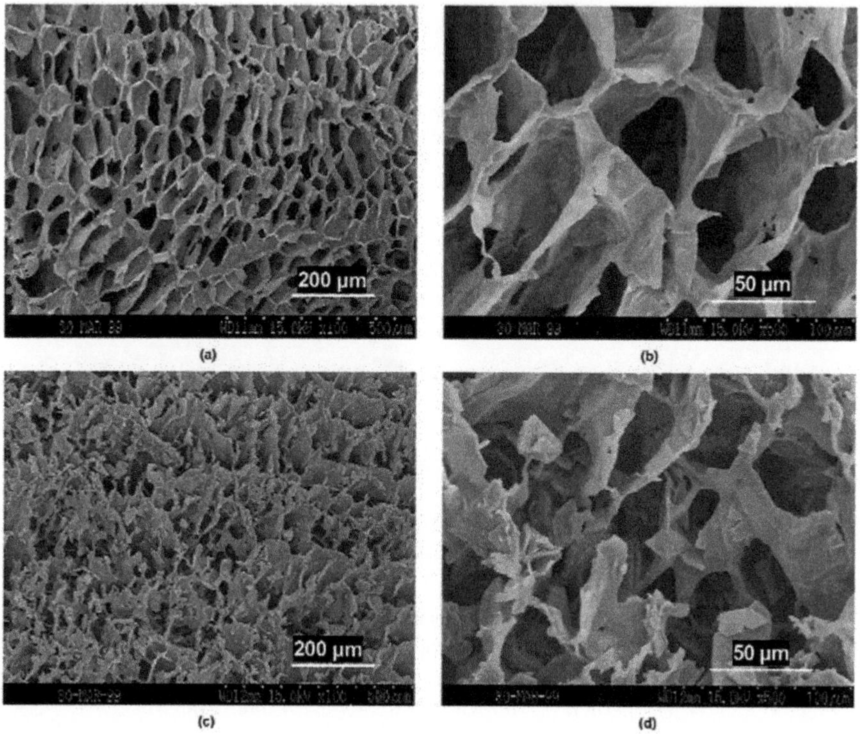

Figure 3.4 Scanning electron micrographs of PLLA and PLLA/HAP (PLLA/HAP: 50:50) foams prepared from a 5% (w/v) PLLA/dioxane solution: (a) PLLA, × 100; (b) PLLA, × 500; (c) PLLA/HAP, × 100; (d) PLLA/HAP, × 500.

Self-assembly process that forms nanofibers can be defined as a process similar to putting pieces of legos together into a large assembly. In the assembly process, molecular legos spontaneously come together with weak, noncovalent bond (i.e., hydrophobic interactions, van der Waals interactions, water-mediated hydrogen bonds, and ionic bonds) [175]. Peptide amphiphiles (PAs) with carbon chain have been developed for the production 3D nanofibrous TE scaffolds [176]. PA is manufactured by alkylation of the NH_2 terminus of the hydrophilic peptide to create a new amphiphilic compound and give hydrophobicity that affects the aggregation of peptide molecules in water and secondary structure. Hydrophobic and hydrophilic regions in PAs form weak noncovalent bonds that exhibit a very stable structure to stabilize the assembly process [177,178]. Changes in PA design provide various self-assemblies including layered and lamellar structures that give flexibility to the system due to its reversible nature. The advantage of self-assembly is the production of finer nanofibers with thin diameter compared to electrospinning [140]. Amino acid residues can be chemically modified by grafting bioactive parts to increase biological activity. RGD peptides include amphiphilic peptides [176] and they increase significant proliferation, functionalized nanofibers attachment, and osteogenesis of the mesenchymal stem cells [179]. Another advantage of self-assembly is the self-assembled nanofibrous scaffold specially suitable for in vivo use due to self-assembly can be carried out in a physiological environment. Therefore avoiding the use of organic solvents in this method reduces cytotoxicity [180].

3.10.6 Freeze-drying

Freeze-drying technique is used in the manufacture of porous scaffolds [181]. This principle is based on the sublimation technique. The polymer is dissolved in a solvent to form a solution with the desired concentration. The polymer solution may contain water (i.e., emulsion-based freeze-drying) or may not contain water (i.e., nonemulsion-based freeze-drying). The solution is frozen and the solvent is removed by freeze-drying under high vacuum. In this way, scaffolds with high porosity and interconnectivity can be produced [182,183]. The main advantages of this technique are providing evaporation of organic solvent completely from scaffold and elimination of the salt-leaching step that negatively affects the purity of scaffold when the trace amount of salt remains in scaffold [184]. However, the control of the average pore size is low when the porous structures are produced by this method and this method is extremely sensitive to the kinetics of the thermal quenching process. Also, freeze-drying is an inefficient technique and is economically uncompetitive because this method is time- and energy-consuming. Low structural stability and generally poor mechanical properties of the produced scaffolds are the other limitations [185].

3.10.7 Electrospinning

Electrospinning (ES) is a low-cost method for the production of fibrous scaffold that has a highly specific surface area with a diameter between the micro- and nanometer scale [186,187]. Polymer solution, which is dissolved in a suitable solvent and prepared from a selected polymer, is loaded into the polymer reservoir to initiate the fiber formation in ES and then a high voltage that eliminates the surface tension and forms a fine-charged jet is applied to a polymer solution. Charged polymer is ejected, dried, and solidified onto the oppositely charged collector plates. The ejected polymer solutions that form nonwoven fibers with a large surface area to volume ratio and having quite a porous structure after solvent evaporation repel each other while travel along the collector (Fig. 3.5) [189].

ES technique can be adjusted as desired by changing several parameters based on this basic procedure [190]. These parameters include the system setup factors (flow rate, distance between the needle, the collector, and applied voltage), properties of the polymer solution (polymer molecular weight, elasticity, concentration, conductivity, surface tension, viscosity), and environmental factors (humidity and temperature).

The use of electrospun fibers has attracted great attention in the last decade in the regeneration of damaged tissue due to the relative simplicity of the production of fibrous morphology that mimics natural ECM structure [140,191]. For example, in the design of bone tissue [192], wound dressing [193,194], artificial blood vessels

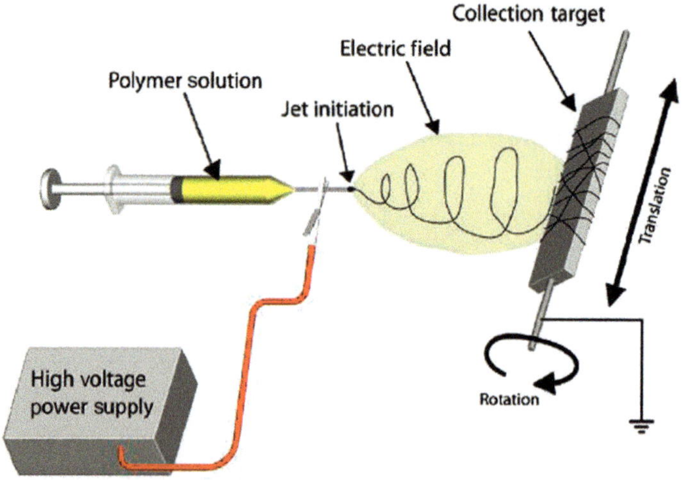

Figure 3.5 Scheme of the electrospinning system with major components.
Reprinted from [188], Copyright (2007), with permission from Elsevier.

[195], nerve tissue [196], and drug delivery vehicles [190,197] has been studied with nanofibrous scaffolds as suitable substrates. Also, ES thin fibers with nanosized diameters provide a potential system with a large surface area for effective transportation of biomolecules [198]. Highly interconnected porosity of nanofibers is useful for cell migration and regenerative tissue growth [141].

The simplicity of this process is that it does not require any complicated and expensive equipment and it can be easily scaled-up for the mass production are the main advantages of this technique. It can be adapted to mimic natural ECM by exhibiting properties such as surface area, porosity, high aspect ratio, mechanical strength that can be adjusted, and permeability for efficient cell growth is another advantage of this technique [140,142,199]. In addition, it can be optimized during production to match the functional properties of regenerated tissue [200,201]. Further, nanofibers are suitable for surface modification of bioactive agent where the biomolecules are adsorbed or immobilized to improve specific cellular functions [191]. However, this technique still has some issues in the production of complex 3D scaffold. Besides, its potential is limited for many TE applications because the control of porosity and the average pore size of electrospun scaffolds is low.

3.10.8 Solid freeform fabrication (rapid prototyping)

Despite many conventional production methods found for the fabrication of TE scaffold, these manual-based methods may not be appropriate for achieving customized production because of their characteristics. In these scaffold production methods, accurate control over interconnectivity and internal structure is also very difficult [202,203]. Therefore, SFF has been prefered recently to produce porous and fully interconnected scaffolds for TE applications and it is referred as rapid prototyping (RP). The SFF method generates controlled 3D structures by stacking computer-aided design (CAD)/computer-assisted manufacturing (CAM) based on two-dimensional (2D) forms.

SFF techniques including fused deposition modeling (FDM), 3D printing (3DP), stereolithography (SL), selective laser sintering (SLS), and various other approaches are practicable for TE. Researchers can control the scaffold parameters in these techniques [204].

One of the main drawbacks of this technique is achieving low resolution by current systems and limitation in the choice of polymeric materials that can be applied for this technique [205].

3.10.8.1 Stereolithography (SL)

SL fabricate 3D scaffolds through selective photocuring of a photopolymer. Solidification occurs because of ultraviolet (UV) laser irradiation on the surface of photopolymer. UV laser scans create 2D patterns and then the desired 3D structure is produced by stacking the solidified 2D patterns together. Nanostereolithography and microstereolithography have been developed based on SL that uses a specific laser system to form 3D structures on micrometer in order to improve resolution. Despite the highest resolution that can be achieved by this technique among SFF technologies, photocurable materials that are limited in supply and costly are necessary [204,206,207].

3.10.8.2 Fused deposition modeling (FDM)

FDM is a production method used for fabrication, production applications, and mechanical system modeling [208]. The technique produces a tissue scaffold by the melt extrusion method that is making use of a layer-by-layer thermoplastic polymer [209]. FDM uses a moving nozzle to extrude a fiber of polymeric material (x- and y-axis control) from which the physical model is built layer-by-layer [167]. FDM technique has some advantages such as there is no unbound loose powder and there is no solvent removal required in FDM differently 3D printing, it provides flexibility to the material in processing and handling [210,211]. FDM technique requires preformed fibers that have a consistent size and material properties for feed through the rollers and nozzle, and it is the main difficulty of this technique [202,210]. PCL is generally used in FDM for TE scaffold production [212]. PCL is preferred due to its high decomposition temperature and low glass transition. Therefore the application of this method to biodegradable polymers except PCL can be limited. Besides, the incorporation of cells or biological factors in the procedure is prevented because of the high temperature.

3.10.8.3 Selective laser sintering (SLS)

The SLS uses a high-power laser, such as a carbon dioxide laser to selectively heat and sinter various materials just below their melting points [213]. The laser selectively fuses powders following the cross-sectional information carried by the predefined CAD data while SLS operation [203]. Since the powders are maintained with low compaction forces after the sintering process in order to generate new layers, structures have an internally porous structure convenient for a bone scaffold [214]. SLS can generate complex structures such as anatomically shaped scaffolds that have controlled porosity, topology, pore sizes, and more conveniently in comparison with other SFF techniques [215,216]. In addition, large numbers of scaffolds can be produced within the powder bed which provide an opportunity to mass production. However, this technique may be limited in the production of biopolymers because of the high operating temperature [202,203,217].

3.10.8.4 Three-dimensional printing (3DP)

3DP method uses ink jet printing technology to eject a binder from a jet head that moves in accordance to the CAD cross-sectional data onto a polymer powder surface. The binder joins adjacent powder particles by dissolving. The unbound powder acts to promote unconnected or overhanging properties and needs to be removed after component completion [167]. 3DP is usually more affordable, faster, and easier to use than other SFF techniques. The versatility and simplicity of 3DP allows the processing of a wide variety of powder materials including polymers, metals, and ceramics. In addition, bioprinting technology can be improved for performing computer-assisted deposition of biomolecules, natural polymers, and viable cells [218,219]. However, if the scaffold is designed to be porous, one problem with powder-supported and powder-filled structures is the difficulty removing the internal unbound powder. Further, scaffold architecture may be limited by the low positional accuracy of the inkjet printer and the nozzle size [202,203,217].

3.11 Conclusion

TE is an interdisciplinary field trying to take advantage of a variety of processing methods with natural and synthetic biomaterials in scaffold production for the regeneration of tissues and organs. Ideally, scaffolds should be designed to be biocompatible to support cell–scaffold interactions with functionalized surface and suitable pore properties conveniently and they can be arranged according to need. Also, they should have the capacity to release biomolecules in a controlled way to facilitate tissue regeneration by mimicking the ECM environment and to provide optimum cell adhesion, proliferation, and differentiation. In this context, engineers should develop new strategies for production techniques using less harmful processes, materials, and new techniques that meet the needs of tissue they want to design and further researches should be carried out associated with the clinical significance of scaffolds that enable long-term in vivo activity. Consequently, the scaffold performance will be able to improve and more sustainable processing routes will be developed in the near future. We think of a bright future for porous scaffolds in the TE area, which will provide an increasing contribution in improving the quality of life of mankind.

References

[1] Ratcliffe A. The translation of product concept to bone products: a partnership of therapeutic effectiveness and commercialization. Tissue Engineering Part B: Reviews 2011;17(6):443–7.

[2] The extracellular matrix as a scaffold for tissue reconstructionBadylak SF, editor. Seminars in cell & developmental biology. Elsevier; 2002.

[3] Owen SC, Shoichet MS. Design of three-dimensional biomimetic scaffolds. J Biomed Mater Res A 2010;94(4):1321–31.

[4] Veiseh M, Turley E, Bissell M. Top–down analysis of a dynamic environment: extracellular matrix structure and function. Nanotechnology and Tissue Engineering: The Scaffold 2008:6387–92.

[5] Langer R, Tirrell DA. Designing materials for biology and medicine. Nature 2004;428(6982):487–92.

[6] Moroni L, De Wijn J, Van Blitterswijk C. Integrating novel technologies to fabricate smart scaffolds. Journal of Biomaterials Science, Polymer Edition 2008;19(5):543–72.

[7] Karande T, Agrawal C. Function and Requirement of Synthetic Scaffolds in Tissue Engineering. Boca Raton, FL: CRC Press; 2008.

[8] Yoon DM, Fisher JP. Polymeric scaffolds for tissue engineering applications. Tiss Eng 2007:81–8.

[9] Jones JR, Ehrenfried LM, Hench LL. Optimising bioactive glass scaffolds for bone tissue engineering. Biomaterials 2006;27(7):964–73.

[10] Muschler GF, Nakamoto C, Griffith LG. Engineering principles of clinical cell-based tissue engineering. The Journal of Bone & Joint Surgery 2004;86(7):1541–58.

[11] Khang G, Jeon JH, Lee JW, Cho SC, Lee HB. Cell and platelet adhesions on plasma glow discharge-treated poly (lactide-co-glycolide). Biomed Mater Eng 1997;7(6):357–68.

[12] Vert M, Li S, Spenlehauer G, Guérin P. Bioresorbability and biocompatibility of aliphatic polyesters. Journal of Materials Science: Materials in Medicine 1992;3(6):432–46.

[13] Hutmacher DW. Scaffolds in tissue engineering bone and cartilage. Biomaterials 2000;21(24):2529–43.

[14] Lutolf M, Hubbell J. Synthetic biomaterials as instructive extracellular microenvironments for morphogenesis in tissue engineering. Nat Biotechnol 2005;23(1):47–55.

[15] Nuttelman CR, Mortisen DJ, Henry SM, Anseth KS. Attachment of fibronectin to poly (vinyl alcohol) hydrogels promotes NIH3T3 cell adhesion, proliferation, and migration. J Biomed Mater Res 2001;57(2):217–23.

[16] Bhati R, Mukherjee D, McCarthy K, Rogers S, Smith D, Shalaby S. The growth of chondrocytes into a fibronectin-coated biodegradable scaffold. J Biomed Mater Res 2001;56(1):74–82.

[17] Hersel U, Dahmen C, Kessler H. RGD modified polymers: biomaterials for stimulated cell adhesion and beyond. Biomaterials 2003;24(24):4385–415.

[18] Griffon DJ, Sedighi MR, Schaeffer DV, Eurell JA, Johnson AL. Chitosan scaffolds: interconnective pore size and cartilage engineering. Acta Biomater 2006;2(3):313–20.

[19] Kim HJ, Kim U-J, Vunjak-Novakovic G, Min B-H, Kaplan DL. Influence of macroporous protein scaffolds on bone tissue engineering from bone marrow stem cells. Biomaterials 2005;26(21):4442–52.

[20] Correlo V, Boesel L, Pinho E, Costa-Pinto A, Alves da Silva M, Bhattacharya M, et al. Melt-based compression-molded scaffolds from chitosan–polyester blends and composites: Morphology and mechanical properties. J Biomed Mater Res A 2009;91(2):489–504.

[21] Oh SH, Park IK, Kim JM, Lee JH. In vitro and in vivo characteristics of PCL scaffolds with pore size gradient fabricated by a centrifugation method. Biomaterials 2007;28(9):1664–71.
[22] Whang K, Healy K, Elenz D, Nam E, Tsai D, Thomas C, et al. Engineering bone regeneration with bioabsorbable scaffolds with novel microarchitecture. Tiss Eng 1999;5(1):35–51.
[23] Dehghani F, Annabi N. Engineering porous scaffolds using gas-based techniques. Curr Opin Biotechnol 2011;22(5):661–6.
[24] Wake MC, Patrick Jr C, Mikos A. Pore morphology effects on the fibrovascular tissue growth in porous polymer substrates. Cell Transplant 1993;3(4):339–43.
[25] Dhandayuthapani B, Yoshida Y, Maekawa T, Kumar DS. Polymeric scaffolds in tissue engineering application: a review. International Journal of Polymer Science 2011;2011.
[26] Fidkowski C, Kaazempur-Mofrad MR, Borenstein J, Vacanti JP, Langer R, Wang Y. Endothelialized microvasculature based on a biodegradable elastomer. Tiss Eng 2005;11(1–2):302–9.
[27] Engler AJ, Sen S, Sweeney HL, Discher DE. Matrix elasticity directs stem cell lineage specification. Cell 2006;126(4):677–89.
[28] Murphy WL, Dennis RG, Kileny JL, Mooney DJ. Salt fusion: an approach to improve pore interconnectivity within tissue engineering scaffolds. Tiss Eng 2002;8(1):43–52.
[29] Yang S, Leong K-F, Du Z, Chua C-K. The design of scaffolds for use in tissue engineering. Part I. Traditional factors. Tiss Eng 2001;7(6):679–89.
[30] Aydin H, El Haj A, Pişkin E, Yang Y. Improving pore interconnectivity in polymeric scaffolds for tissue engineering. J Tissue Eng Regen Med 2009;3(6):470–6.
[31] O'brien FJ. Biomaterials & scaffolds for tissue engineering. Materials Today 2011;14(3):88–95.
[32] Hollister SJ. Scaffold engineering: a bridge to where? Biofabrication 2009;1(1):012001.
[33] Gualandi C. Porous polymeric bioresorbable scaffolds for tissue engineering. : Springer Science & Business Media; 2011.
[34] Willians D. Definitions in Biomaterials proceeding of a Consensus Conference of the European Society for Biomaterials Chester, Progress en Biomedical Engineering. Amsterdam: Elservier; 1987.
[35] Peppas NA, Langer R. New challenges in biomaterials. Science-AAAS-Weekly Paper Edition-including Guide to Scientific Information 1994;263(5154):1715–9.
[36] Boccaccini AR, Ma PX. Tissue engineering using ceramics and polymers. Elsevier; 2014.
[37] Williams DF. March 3-5, 1986 Definitions in biomaterials: proceedings of a consensus conference of the European Society for Biomaterials. Chester, England: Elsevier Science Limited; 1987.
[38] Hench LL, Wilson J. Surface-active biomaterials. Science 1984;226(4675):630–6.
[39] Ramalingam M. Integrated Biomaterials in Tissue Engineering. : John Wiley & Sons; 2012.
[40] Chen G, Ushida T, Tateishi T. Scaffold design for tissue engineering. Macromol Biosci 2002;2(2):67–77.
[41] Nair LS, Laurencin CT. Biodegradable polymers as biomaterials. Progress in polymer science 2007;32(8):762–98.
[42] Ratner BD, Hoffman AS, Schoen FJ, Lemons JE. Biomaterials science: an introduction to materials in medicine. Academic press; 2004.
[43] Angele P, Abke J, Kujat R, Faltermeier H, Schumann D, Nerlich M, et al. Influence of different collagen species on physico-chemical properties of crosslinked collagen matrices. Biomaterials 2004;25(14):2831–41.

[44] Zeugolis D, Paul R, Attenburrow G. Factors influencing the properties of reconstituted collagen fibers prior to self-assembly: Animal species and collagen extraction method. J Biomed Mater Res A 2008;86(4):892–904.
[45] Gross RA, Kalra B. Biodegradable polymers for the environment. Science 2002;297(5582):803–7.
[46] Kanematsu A, Marui A, Yamamoto S, Ozeki M, Hirano Y, Yamamoto M, et al. Type I collagen can function as a reservoir of basic fibroblast growth factor. Journal of controlled release 2004;99(2):281–92.
[47] Pieper J, Hafmans T, Van Wachem P, Van Luyn M, Brouwer L, Veerkamp J, et al. Loading of collagen-heparan sulfate matrices with bFGF promotes angiogenesis and tissue generation in rats. J Biomed Mater Res 2002;62(2):185–94.
[48] Willoughby C, Batterbury M, Kaye S. Collagen corneal shields. Surv Ophthalmol 2002;47(2):174–82.
[49] Altman GH, Diaz F, Jakuba C, Calabro T, Horan RL, Chen J, et al. Silk-based biomaterials. Biomaterials 2003;24(3):401–16.
[50] Altman GH, Horan RL, Lu HH, Moreau J, Martin I, Richmond JC, et al. Silk matrix for tissue engineered anterior cruciate ligaments. Biomaterials 2002;23(20):4131–41.
[51] Audet J, Stanford W.L. Stem Cells in Regenerative Medicine. 2009.
[52] Dunn CJ, Goa KL. Fibrin sealant. Drugs 1999;58(5):863–86.
[53] Ye KY, Sullivan KE, Black LD. Encapsulation of cardiomyocytes in a fibrin hydrogel for cardiac tissue engineering. J Vis Exp 2011;55(e3251):1–7.
[54] Johnson PJ, Parker SR, Sakiyama-Elbert SE. Fibrin-based tissue engineering scaffolds enhance neural fiber sprouting and delay the accumulation of reactive astrocytes at the lesion in a subacute model of spinal cord injury. J Biomed Mater Res A 2010;92(1):152–63.
[55] Chen X, Aledia AS, Ghajar CM, Griffith CK, Putnam AJ, Hughes CC, et al. Prevascularization of a fibrin-based tissue construct accelerates the formation of functional anastomosis with host vasculature. Tissue Eng Part A 2008;15(6):1363–71.
[56] Le Nihouannen D, Le Guehennec L, Rouillon T, Pilet P, Bilban M, Layrolle P, et al. Micro-architecture of calcium phosphate granules and fibrin glue composites for bone tissue engineering. Biomaterials 2006;27(13):2716–22.
[57] Currie LJ, Sharpe JR, Martin R. The use of fibrin glue in skin grafts and tissue-engineered skin replacements. Plast Reconstr Surg 2001;108:1713–26.
[58] Waterhouse A, Wise SG, Ng MK, Weiss AS. Elastin as a nonthrombogenic biomaterial. Tissue Engineering Part B: Reviews 2011;17(2):93–9.
[59] Soskel NT, Wolt TB, Sandberg LB. Isolation and characterization of insoluble and soluble elastins. Methods Enzymol 1986;144:196–214.
[60] Martin SL, Vrhovski B, Weiss AS. Total synthesis and expression in Escherichia coli of a gene encoding human tropoelastin. Gene 1995;154(2):159–66.
[61] Daamen WF, Nillesen ST, Wismans RG, Reinhardt DP, Hafmans T, Veerkamp JH, et al. A biomaterial composed of collagen and solubilized elastin enhances angiogenesis and elastic fiber formation without calcification. Tissue Eng Part A 2008;14(3):349–60.
[62] Buttafoco L, Kolkman N, Engbers-Buijtenhuijs P, Poot A, Dijkstra P, Vermes I, et al. Electrospinning of collagen and elastin for tissue engineering applications. Biomaterials 2006;27(5):724–34.
[63] Hu X, Park S-H, Gil ES, Xia X-X, Weiss AS, Kaplan DL. The influence of elasticity and surface roughness on myogenic and osteogenic-differentiation of cells on silk-elastin biomaterials. Biomaterials 2011;32(34):8979–89.
[64] Wang TW, Wu HC, Huang YC, Sun JS, Lin FH. Biomimetic Bilayered Gelatin-Chondroitin 6 Sulfate-Hyaluronic Acid Biopolymer as a Scaffold for Skin Equivalent Tissue Engineering. Artif Organs 2006;30(3):141–9.

[65] Wang T-W, Spector M. Development of hyaluronic acid-based scaffolds for brain tissue engineering. Acta Biomater 2009;5(7):2371–84.
[66] Tan H, Ramirez CM, Miljkovic N, Li H, Rubin JP, Marra KG. Thermosensitive injectable hyaluronic acid hydrogel for adipose tissue engineering. Biomaterials 2009;30(36):6844–53.
[67] Perets A, Baruch Y, Weisbuch F, Shoshany G, Neufeld G, Cohen S. Enhancing the vascularization of three-dimensional porous alginate scaffolds by incorporating controlled release basic fibroblast growth factor microspheres. J Biomed Mater Res A 2003;65(4):489–97.
[68] Park SA, Park KE, Kim W. Preparation of sodium alginate/poly (ethylene oxide) blend nanofibers with lecithin. Macromolecular Research 2010;18(9):891–6.
[69] Yen CN, Lin YR, Chang MDT, Tien CW, Wu YC, Liao CJ, et al. Use of porous alginate sponges for substantial chondrocyte expansion and matrix production: effects of seeding density. Biotechnol Prog 2008;24(2):452–7.
[70] Jin R, Teixeira LM, Dijkstra PJ, Karperien M, Van Blitterswijk C, Zhong Z, et al. Injectable chitosan-based hydrogels for cartilage tissue engineering. Biomaterials 2009;30(13):2544–51.
[71] Yilgor P, Tuzlakoglu K, Reis RL, Hasirci N, Hasirci V. Incorporation of a sequential BMP-2/BMP-7 delivery system into chitosan-based scaffolds for bone tissue engineering. Biomaterials 2009;30(21):3551–9.
[72] Kucharska M, Walenko K, Butruk B, Brynk T, Heljak M, Ciach T. Fabrication and characterization of chitosan microspheres agglomerated scaffolds for bone tissue engineering. Materials Letters 2010;64(9):1059–62.
[73] Di Martino A, Sittinger M, Risbud MV. Chitosan: a versatile biopolymer for orthopaedic tissue-engineering. Biomaterials 2005;26(30):5983–90.
[74] Ishihara M., Fujita M., Kishimoto S., Hattori H., Kanatani Y. Biological, chemical, and physical compatibility of chitosan and biopharmaceuticals. Chitosan-Based Systems for Biopharmaceuticals: Delivery, Targeting and Polymer Therapeutics. 2012:93-106.
[75] Mi F-L, Shyu S-S, Wu Y-B, Lee S-T, Shyong J-Y, Huang R-N. Fabrication and characterization of a sponge-like asymmetric chitosan membrane as a wound dressing. Biomaterials 2001;22(2):165–73.
[76] Gunatillake P, Mayadunne R, Adhikari R. Recent developments in biodegradable synthetic polymers. Biotechnol Annu Rev 2006;12:301–47.
[77] Guo B, Ma PX. Synthetic biodegradable functional polymers for tissue engineering: a brief review. Science China Chemistry 2014;57(4):490–500.
[78] Cameron DJ, Shaver MP. Aliphatic polyester polymer stars: synthesis, properties and applications in biomedicine and nanotechnology. Chem Soc Rev 2011;40(3):1761–76.
[79] Hakkarainen M, Albertsson A-C. Degradation Products of Aliphatic and Aliphatic–Aromatic Polyesters Chromatography for Sustainable Polymeric Materials. Springer; 2008.85.116
[80] Jérôme C, Lecomte P. Recent advances in the synthesis of aliphatic polyesters by ring-opening polymerization. Adv Drug Deliv Rev 2008;60(9):1056–76.
[81] Athanasiou KA, Agrawal CM, Barber FA, Burkhart SS. Orthopaedic applications for PLA-PGA biodegradable polymers. Arthroscopy: The Journal of Arthroscopic & Related Surgery 1998;14(7):726–37.
[82] Seyednejad H, Ghassemi AH, van Nostrum CF, Vermonden T, Hennink WE. Functional aliphatic polyesters for biomedical and pharmaceutical applications. Journal of controlled release 2011;152(1):168–76.
[83] Gupta B, Revagade N, Hilborn J. Poly (lactic acid) fiber: an overview. Progress in polymer science 2007;32(4):455–82.

[84] Zhang R, Ma P. Degradation behavior of porous poly (alpha-hydroxy acids)/hydroxyapatite composite scaffolds. Polymer Preprints(USA) 2000;41(2):1618–9.
[85] Eling B, Gogolewski S, Pennings A. Biodegradable materials of poly (l-lactic acid): 1. Melt-spun and solution-spun fibres. Polymer (Guildf) 1982;23(11):1587–93.
[86] Pitt G, Gratzl M, Kimmel G, Surles J, Sohindler A. Aliphatic polyesters II. The degradation of poly (DL-lactide), poly (ε-caprolactone), and their copolymers in vivo. Biomaterials 1981;2(4):215–20.
[87] Woodward SC, Brewer P, Moatamed F, Schindler A, Pitt C. The intracellular degradation of poly (ε-caprolactone). J Biomed Mater Res 1985;19(4):437–44.
[88] Choi SH, Park TG. Synthesis and characterization of elastic PLGA/PCL/PLGA tri-block copolymers. Journal of Biomaterials Science, Polymer Edition 2002;13(10): 1163–73.
[89] Holland S, Jolly A, Yasin M, Tighe B. Polymers for biodegradable medical devices: II. Hydroxybutyrate-hydroxyvalerate copolymers: Hydrolytic degradation studies. Biomaterials 1987;8(4):289–95.
[90] Wolfe MS, Dean D, Chen JE, Fisher JP, Han S, Rimnac CM, et al. In vitro degradation and fracture toughness of multilayered porous poly (propylene fumarate)/β-tricalcium phosphate scaffolds. J Biomed Mater Res 2002;61(1):159–64.
[91] Torres MP, Vogel BM, Narasimhan B, Mallapragada SK. Synthesis and characterization of novel polyanhydrides with tailored erosion mechanisms. J Biomed Mater Res A 2006;76(1):102–10.
[92] Jain JP, Chitkara D, Kumar N. Polyanhydrides as localized drug delivery carrier: an update. Expert Opin Drug Deliv 2008;5(8):889–907.
[93] Jain JP, Modi S, Domb A, Kumar N. Role of polyanhydrides as localized drug carriers. Journal of Controlled Release 2005;103(3):541–63.
[94] Allcock HR. Generation of structural diversity in polyphosphazenes. Appl Organomet Chem 2013;27:620–9.
[95] Ambrosio AM, Allcock HR, Katti DS, Laurencin CT. Degradable polyphosphazene/poly (α-hydroxyester) blends: degradation studies. Biomaterials 2002;23(7):1667–72.
[96] Allcock H, Fuller T, Matsumura K. Hydrolysis pathways for aminophosphazenes. Inorg Chem 1982;21(2):515–21.
[97] Laurencin CT, El-Amin SF, Ibim SE, Willoughby DA, Attawia M, Allcock HR, et al. A highly porous 3-dimensional polyphosphazene polymer matrix for skeletal tissue regeneration. J Biomed Mater Res 1996;30(2):133–8.
[98] Conconi MT, Lora S, Baiguera S, Boscolo E, Folin M, Scienza R, et al. In vitro culture of rat neuromicrovascular endothelial cells on polymeric scaffolds. J Biomed Mater Res A 2004;71(4):669–74.
[99] Laurencin C, Ambrosio A, Sahota J, Runge C, Kurtz S, Lakshmi S, et al. Novel polyphosphazene-hydroxyapatite composites as biomaterials. IEEE engineering in medicine and biology magazine 2003;5(22):18–26.
[100] Krol P. Synthesis methods, chemical structures and phase structures of linear polyurethanes. Properties and applications of linear polyurethanes in polyurethane elastomers, copolymers and ionomers. Prog Mater Sci 2007;52(6):915–1015.
[101] Santerre J, Woodhouse K, Laroche G, Labow R. Understanding the biodegradation of polyurethanes: from classical implants to tissue engineering materials. Biomaterials 2005;26(35):7457–70.
[102] Rai R, Tallawi M, Grigore A, Boccaccini AR. Synthesis, properties and biomedical applications of poly(glycerol sebacate) (PGS): a review. Progress in polymer science 2012;37(8):1051–78.

[103] Patel A, Gaharwar AK, Iviglia G, Zhang H, Mukundan S, Mihaila SM, et al. Highly elastomeric poly (glycerol sebacate)-co-poly (ethylene glycol) amphiphilic block copolymers. Biomaterials 2013;34(16):3970–83.
[104] Masoumi N, Johnson KL, Howell MC, Engelmayr GC. Valvular interstitial cell seeded poly (glycerol sebacate) scaffolds: toward a biomimetic in vitro model for heart valve tissue engineering. Acta Biomater 2013;9(4):5974–88.
[105] Ravichandran R, Venugopal JR, Sundarrajan S, Mukherjee S, Ramakrishna S. Poly (glycerol sebacate)/gelatin core/shell fibrous structure for regeneration of myocardial infarction. Tissue Eng Part A 2011;17(9–10):1363–73.
[106] Sun Z-J, Chen C, Sun M-Z, Ai C-H, Lu X-L, Zheng Y-F, et al. The application of poly (glycerol–sebacate) as biodegradable drug carrier. Biomaterials 2009;30(28):5209–14.
[107] Khang G. Handbook of Intelligent Scaffold for Tissue Engineering and Regenerative Medicine. CRC Press; 2012.
[108] Baino F, Novajra G, Miguez-Pacheco V, Boccaccini AR, Vitale-Brovarone C. Bioactive glasses: special applications outside the skeletal system. Journal of Non-Crystalline Solids 2016;432:15–30.
[109] Miguez-Pacheco V, Hench LL, Boccaccini AR. Bioactive glasses beyond bone and teeth: Emerging applications in contact with soft tissues. Acta Biomater 2015;13:1–15.
[110] Hoppe A, Güldal NS, Boccaccini AR. A review of the biological response to ionic dissolution products from bioactive glasses and glass-ceramics. Biomaterials 2011;32(11):2757–74.
[111] Habibovic P, Barralet J. Bioinorganics and biomaterials: bone repair. Acta Biomater 2011;7(8):3013–26.
[112] Lakhkar NJ, Lee I-H, Kim H-W, Salih V, Wall IB, Knowles JC. Bone formation controlled by biologically relevant inorganic ions: role and controlled delivery from phosphate-based glasses. Adv Drug Deliv Rev 2013;65(4):405–20.
[113] Sultana N, Hassan MI, Lim MM. Composite Synthetic Scaffolds for Tissue Engineering and Regenerative Medicine. : Springer; 2015.
[114] Jarcho M. Biomaterial aspects of calcium phosphates. Properties and applications. Dent Clin North Am 1986;30(1):25.
[115] Baino F, Vitale-Brovarone C. Three-dimensional glass-derived scaffolds for bone tissue engineering: Current trends and forecasts for the future. J Biomed Mater Res A 2011;97(4):514–35.
[116] Fu Q, Saiz E, Rahaman MN, Tomsia AP. Bioactive glass scaffolds for bone tissue engineering: state of the art and future perspectives. Materials Science and Engineering: C. 2011;31(7):1245–56.
[117] Keane TJ, Badylak SF, editors. Biomaterials for tissue engineering applications. Seminars in pediatric surgery. : Elsevier; 2014.
[118] LeGeros RZ. Properties of osteoconductive biomaterials: calcium phosphates. Clin Orthop Relat Res 2002;395:81–98.
[119] LeGeros RZ. Calcium phosphate-based osteoinductive materials. Chem Rev 2008;108(11):4742–53.
[120] Yamasaki H, Sakai H. Osteogenic response to porous hydroxyapatite ceramics under the skin of dogs. Biomaterials 1992;13(5):308–12.
[121] Yuan H, Yang Z, de Bruijn JD, de Groot K, Zhang X. Material-dependent bone induction by calcium phosphate ceramics: a 2.5-year study in dog. Biomaterials 2001;22(19):2617–23.
[122] Yuan H, Fernandes H, Habibovic P, de Boer J, Barradas AM, de Ruiter A, et al. Osteoinductive ceramics as a synthetic alternative to autologous bone grafting. Proceedings of the National Academy of Sciences 2010;107(31):13614–9.

[123] Hench LL, Splinter RJ, Allen W, Greenlee T. Bonding mechanisms at the interface of ceramic prosthetic materials. J Biomed Mater Res 1971;5(6):117–41.
[124] Hench LL. Biomaterials: a forecast for the future. Biomaterials 1998;19(16):1419–23.
[125] Rahaman MN, Day DE, Bal BS, Fu Q, Jung SB, Bonewald LF, et al. Bioactive glass in tissue engineering. Acta Biomater 2011;7(6):2355–73.
[126] Rezwan K, Chen Q, Blaker J, Boccaccini AR. Biodegradable and bioactive porous polymer/inorganic composite scaffolds for bone tissue engineering. Biomaterials 2006;27(18):3413–31.
[127] Russias J, Saiz E, Deville S, Gryn K, Liu G, Nalla R, et al. Fabrication and in vitro characterization of three-dimensional organic/inorganic scaffolds by robocasting. J Biomed Mater Res A 2007;83(2):434–45.
[128] Venugopal J, Prabhakaran MP, Zhang Y, Low S, Choon AT, Ramakrishna S. Biomimetic hydroxyapatite-containing composite nanofibrous substrates for bone tissue engineering. Philosophical Transactions of the Royal Society of London A: Mathematical, Physical and Engineering Sciences 2010;368(1917):2065–81.
[129] Sahoo NG, Pan YZ, Li L, He CB. Nanocomposites for bone tissue regeneration. Nanomedicine 2013;8(4):639–53.
[130] Ambrosio A, Sahota JS, Khan Y, Laurencin CT. A novel amorphous calcium phosphate polymer ceramic for bone repair: I. Synthesis and characterization. J Biomed Mater Res 2001;58(3):295–301.
[131] Deng X, Hao J, Wang C. Preparation and mechanical properties of nanocomposites of poly (D, L-lactide) with Ca-deficient hydroxyapatite nanocrystals. Biomaterials 2001;22(21):2867–73.
[132] Xu HH, Quinn JB, Takagi S, Chow LC. Synergistic reinforcement of in situ hardening calcium phosphate composite scaffold for bone tissue engineering. Biomaterials 2004;25(6):1029–37.
[133] Tanner K. Bioactive ceramic-reinforced composites for bone augmentation. Journal of The Royal Society Interface 2010;7(Suppl 5):S541–57.
[134] Erol-Taygun M, Zheng K, Boccaccini AR. Nanoscale bioactive glasses in medical applications. International Journal of Applied Glass Science 2013;4(2):136–48.
[135] Marelli B, Ghezzi CE, Mohn D, Stark WJ, Barralet JE, Boccaccini AR, et al. Accelerated mineralization of dense collagen-nano bioactive glass hybrid gels increases scaffold stiffness and regulates osteoblastic function. Biomaterials 2011;32(34):8915–26.
[136] Valliant EM, Jones JR. Softening bioactive glass for bone regeneration: sol–gel hybrid materials. Soft Matter 2011;7(11):5083–95.
[137] Jones JR. Review of bioactive glass: from Hench to hybrids. Acta Biomater 2013;9(1):4457–86.
[138] Mikos AG, Bao Y, Cima LG, Ingber DE, Vacanti JP, Langer R. Preparation of poly (glycolic acid) bonded fiber structures for cell attachment and transplantation. J Biomed Mater Res 1993;27(2):183–9.
[139] Annabi N, Nichol JW, Zhong X, Ji C, Koshy S, Khademhosseini A, et al. Controlling the porosity and microarchitecture of hydrogels for tissue engineering. Tissue Engineering Part B: Reviews 2010;16(4):371–83.
[140] Ma Z, Kotaki M, Inai R, Ramakrishna S. Potential of nanofiber matrix as tissue-engineering scaffolds. Tiss Eng 2005;11(1–2):101–9.
[141] Li WJ, Laurencin CT, Caterson EJ, Tuan RS, Ko FK. Electrospun nanofibrous structure: a novel scaffold for tissue engineering. J Biomed Mater Res 2002;60(4):613–21.
[142] Christenson EM, Anseth KS, van den Beucken JJ, Chan CK, Ercan B, Jansen JA, et al. Nanobiomaterial applications in orthopedics. Journal of Orthopaedic Research 2007;25(1):11–22.

[143] Lu L, Mikos AG. The importance of new processing techniques in tissue engineering. Mrs Bulletin 1996;21(11):28–32.
[144] Smith L.A., Beck J.A., Ma P.X. Nanofibrous scaffolds and their biological effects. Nanotechnologies for the Life Sciences. 2006.
[145] Chen G, Ushida T, Tateishi T. Development of biodegradable porous scaffolds for tissue engineering. Materials Science and Engineering: C. 2001;17(1):63–9.
[146] Seidi A, Ramalingam M. Protocols for biomaterial scaffold fabrication. Integrated Biomaterials in Tissue Engineering 2012:1–23.
[147] Cima L, Vacanti J, Vacanti C, Ingber D, Mooney D, Langer R. Tissue engineering by cell transplantation using degradable polymer substrates. J Biomech Eng 1991;113(2):143–51.
[148] Mikos AG, Sarakinos G, Leite SM, Vacant JP, Langer R. Laminated three-dimensional biodegradable foams for use in tissue engineering. Biomaterials 1993;14(5):323–30.
[149] Mooney D, Mazzoni C, Breuer C, McNamara K, Hern D, Vacanti J, et al. Stabilized polyglycolic acid fibre-based tubes for tissue engineering. Biomaterials 1996;17(2):115–24.
[150] Freed LE, Marquis J, Nohria A, Emmanual J, Mikos A, Langer R. Neocartilage formation in vitro and in vivo using cells cultured on synthetic biodegradable polymers. J Biomed Mater Res 1993;27(1):11–23.
[151] Mikos AG, Thorsen AJ, Czerwonka LA, Bao Y, Langer R, Winslow DN, et al. Preparation and characterization of poly (L-lactic acid) foams. Polymer (Guildf) 1994;35(5):1068–77.
[152] Pego A, Siebum B, Van Luyn M, Gallego y Van Seijen X, Poot A, Grijpma D, et al. Preparation of degradable porous structures based on 1, 3-trimethylene carbonate and D, L-lactide (co) polymers for heart tissue engineering. Tiss Eng 2003;9(5):981–94.
[153] Holy CE, Dang SM, Davies JE, Shoichet MS. In vitro degradation of a novel poly (lactide-co-glycolide) 75/25 foam. Biomaterials 1999;20(13):1177–85.
[154] Suh SW, Shin JY, Kim J, Kim J, Beak CH, Kim D-I, et al. Effect of different particles on cell proliferation in polymer scaffolds using a solvent-casting and particulate leaching technique. ASAIO journal 2002;48(5):460–4.
[155] Mikos A.G., Sarakinos G., Vacanti J.P., Langer R.S., Cima L.G. Biocompatible polymer membranes and methods of preparation of three dimensional membrane structures. Google Patents; 1996.
[156] Thadavirul N, Pavasant P, Supaphol P. Development of polycaprolactone porous scaffolds by combining solvent casting, particulate leaching, and polymer leaching techniques for bone tissue engineering. J Biomed Mater Res A 2014;102(10):3379–92.
[157] Goel SK, Beckman EJ. Generation of microcellular polymeric foams using supercritical carbon dioxide. I: Effect of pressure and temperature on nucleation. Polymer Engineering & Science 1994;34(14):1137–47.
[158] Arora KA, Lesser AJ, McCarthy TJ. Preparation and characterization of microcellular polystyrene foams processed in supercritical carbon dioxide. Macromolecules 1998;31(14):4614–20.
[159] Colton J, Suh N. The nucleation of microcellular thermoplastic foam with additives: Part I: Theoretical considerations. Polymer Engineering & Science 1987;27(7):485–92.
[160] Kumar V, Suh NP. A process for making microcellular thermoplastic parts. Polymer Engineering & Science 1990;30(20):1323–9.
[161] Mooney DJ, Baldwin DF, Suh NP, Vacanti JP, Langer R. Novel approach to fabricate porous sponges of poly (D, L-lactic-co-glycolic acid) without the use of organic solvents. Biomaterials 1996;17(14):1417–22.

[162] Woods HM, Silva MM, Nouvel C, Shakesheff KM, Howdle SM. Materials processing in supercritical carbon dioxide: surfactants, polymers and biomaterials. J Mater Chem 2004;14(11):1663–78.
[163] Quirk RA, France RM, Shakesheff KM, Howdle SM. Supercritical fluid technologies and tissue engineering scaffolds. Current Opinion in Solid State and Materials Science 2004;8(3):313–21.
[164] Goel SK, Beckman EJ. Generation of microcellular polymeric foams using supercritical carbon dioxide. II: Cell growth and skin formation. Polymer Engineering & Science 1994;34(14):1148–56.
[165] Harris L.D., Kim B.-S., Mooney D.J. Open pore biodegradable matrices formed with gas foaming. 1998.
[166] Nam YS, Park TG. Porous biodegradable polymeric scaffolds prepared by thermally induced phase separation. J Biomed Mater Res 1999;47(1):8–17.
[167] Sachlos E, Czernuszka J. Making tissue engineering scaffold work. Review: on the application of solid freeform fabrication technology to the production of tissue engineering scaffolds. Eur Cell Mater 2003;5(1):29–40.
[168] Hua FJ, Kim GE, Lee JD, Son YK, Lee DS. Macroporous poly (L-lactide) scaffold 1. Preparation of a macroporous scaffold by liquid–liquid phase separation of a PLLA–dioxane–water system. J Biomed Mater Res 2002;63(2):161–7.
[169] Liu X, Ma PX. Phase separation, pore structure, and properties of nanofibrous gelatin scaffolds. Biomaterials 2009;30(25):4094–103.
[170] Wei G, Ma PX. Macroporous and nanofibrous polymer scaffolds and polymer/bone-like apatite composite scaffolds generated by sugar spheres. J Biomed Mater Res A 2006;78(2):306–15.
[171] Blaker JJ, Knowles JC, Day RM. Novel fabrication techniques to produce microspheres by thermally induced phase separation for tissue engineering and drug delivery. Acta Biomater 2008;4(2):264–72.
[172] Budyanto L, Goh Y, Ooi C. Fabrication of porous poly (L-lactide)(PLLA) scaffolds for tissue engineering using liquid–liquid phase separation and freeze extraction. Journal of Materials Science: Materials in Medicine 2009;20(1):105–11.
[173] Ma P.X., Zhang R. Synthetic nano-scale fibrous extracellular matrix. 1999.
[174] Ma PX, Zhang R, Xiao G, Franceschi R. Engineering new bone tissue in vitro on highly porous poly (α-hydroxyl acids)/hydroxyapatite composite scaffolds. J Biomed Mater Res 2001;54(2):284–93.
[175] Zhang S. Fabrication of novel biomaterials through molecular self-assembly. Nat Biotechnol 2003;21(10):1171–8.
[176] Hartgerink JD, Beniash E, Stupp SI. Self-assembly and mineralization of peptide-amphiphile nanofibers. Science 2001;294(5547):1684–8.
[177] Joshi K, Singh P, Verma S. Fabrication of platinum nanopillars on peptide-based soft structures using a focused ion beam. Biofabrication 2009;1(2):025002.
[178] Huang Y.-C, Mooney D.J. Scaffolding in Tissue Engineering. 2005.
[179] Hosseinkhani H, Hosseinkhani M, Tian F, Kobayashi H, Tabata Y. Osteogenic differentiation of mesenchymal stem cells in self-assembled peptide-amphiphile nanofibers. Biomaterials 2006;27(22):4079–86.
[180] Semino C. Self-assembling peptides: from bio-inspired materials to bone regeneration. J Dent Res 2008;87(7):606–16.
[181] Schoof H, Apel J, Heschel I, Rau G. Control of pore structure and size in freeze-dried collagen sponges. J Biomed Mater Res 2001;58(4):352–7.

[182] Mandal BB, Kundu SC. Cell proliferation and migration in silk fibroin 3D scaffolds. Biomaterials 2009;30(15):2956–65.
[183] Mandal BB, Kundu SC. Osteogenic and adipogenic differentiation of rat bone marrow cells on non-mulberry and mulberry silk gland fibroin 3D scaffolds. Biomaterials 2009;30(28):5019–30.
[184] Vert M. Encyclopedia of Biomaterials and Biomedical Engineering. Taylor & Francis; 2004.
[185] Ho M-H, Kuo P-Y, Hsieh H-J, Hsien T-Y, Hou L-T, Lai J-Y, et al. Preparation of porous scaffolds by using freeze-extraction and freeze-gelation methods. Biomaterials 2004;25(1):129–38.
[186] Liang D, Hsiao BS, Chu B. Functional electrospun nanofibrous scaffolds for biomedical applications. Adv Drug Deliv Rev 2007;59(14):1392–412.
[187] Yoo HS, Kim TG, Park TG. Surface-functionalized electrospun nanofibers for tissue engineering and drug delivery. Adv Drug Deliv Rev 2009;61(12):1033–42.
[188] Barnes CP, Sell SA, Boland ED, Simpson DG, Bowlin GL. Nanofiber technology: designing the next generation of tissue engineering scaffolds. Adv Drug Deliv Rev 2007;59(14):1413–33.
[189] Reneker DH, Chun I. Nanometre diameter fibres of polymer, produced by electrospinning. Nanotechnology 1996;7(3):216.
[190] Sill TJ, von Recum HA. Electrospinning: applications in drug delivery and tissue engineering. Biomaterials 2008;29(13):1989–2006.
[191] Yang F, Murugan R, Wang S, Ramakrishna S. Electrospinning of nano/micro scale poly (L-lactic acid) aligned fibers and their potential in neural tissue engineering. Biomaterials 2005;26(15):2603–10.
[192] Seyedjafari E, Soleimani M, Ghaemi N, Shabani I. Nanohydroxyapatite-coated electrospun poly (l-lactide) nanofibers enhance osteogenic differentiation of stem cells and induce ectopic bone formation. Biomacromolecules 2010;11(11):3118–25.
[193] Kumbar SG, Nukavarapu SP, James R, Nair LS, Laurencin CT. Electrospun poly (lactic acid-co-glycolic acid) scaffolds for skin tissue engineering. Biomaterials 2008;29(30):4100–7.
[194] Zhu X, Cui W, Li X, Jin Y. Electrospun fibrous mats with high porosity as potential scaffolds for skin tissue engineering. Biomacromolecules 2008;9(7):1795–801.
[195] Hajiali H, Shahgasempour S, Naimi-Jamal MR, Peirovi H. Electrospun PGA/gelatin nanofibrous scaffolds and their potential application in vascular tissue engineering. Int J Nanomedicine 2011;6:2133–41.
[196] Xie J, MacEwan MR, Schwartz AG, Xia Y. Electrospun nanofibers for neural tissue engineering. Nanoscale 2010;2(1):35–44.
[197] Yoon H, Kim G. A three-dimensional polycaprolactone scaffold combined with a drug delivery system consisting of electrospun nanofibers. J Pharm Sci 2011;100(2):424–30.
[198] Ji W, Sun Y, Yang F, van den Beucken JJ, Fan M, Chen Z, et al. Bioactive electrospun scaffolds delivering growth factors and genes for tissue engineering applications. Pharm Res 2011;28(6):1259–72.
[199] Bashur CA, Dahlgren LA, Goldstein AS. Effect of fiber diameter and orientation on fibroblast morphology and proliferation on electrospun poly (D, L-lactic-co-glycolic acid) meshes. Biomaterials 2006;27(33):5681–8.
[200] Murugan R, Ramakrishna S. Design strategies of tissue engineering scaffolds with controlled fiber orientation. Tiss Eng 2007;13(8):1845–66.
[201] Pham QP, Sharma U, Mikos AG. Electrospun poly (ε-caprolactone) microfiber and multilayer nanofiber/microfiber scaffolds: characterization of scaffolds and measurement of cellular infiltration. Biomacromolecules 2006;7(10):2796–805.

[202] Yeong W-Y, Chua C-K, Leong K-F, Chandrasekaran M. Rapid prototyping in tissue engineering: challenges and potential. Trends Biotechnol 2004;22(12):643–52.
[203] Leong K, Cheah C, Chua C. Solid freeform fabrication of three-dimensional scaffolds for engineering replacement tissues and organs. Biomaterials 2003;24(13):2363–78.
[204] Lee JW, Kim JY, Cho D-W. Solid free-form fabrication technology and its application to bone tissue engineering. International journal of stem cells 2010;3(2):85.
[205] Woodfield T, Guggenheim M, Von Rechenberg B, Riesle J, Van Blitterswijk C, Wedler V. Rapid prototyping of anatomically shaped, tissue-engineered implants for restoring congruent articulating surfaces in small joints. Cell Prolif 2009;42(4):485–97.
[206] Cooke MN, Fisher JP, Dean D, Rimnac C, Mikos AG. Use of stereolithography to manufacture critical-sized 3D biodegradable scaffolds for bone ingrowth. J Biomed Mater Res Part B Appl Biomater 2003;64(2):65–9.
[207] Lan PX, Lee JW, Seol Y-J, Cho D-W. Development of 3D PPF/DEF scaffolds using micro-stereolithography and surface modification. Journal of Materials Science: Materials in Medicine 2009;20(1):271–9.
[208] Zein I, Hutmacher DW, Tan KC, Teoh SH. Fused deposition modeling of novel scaffold architectures for tissue engineering applications. Biomaterials 2002;23(4):1169–85.
[209] Chim H, Hutmacher D, Chou A, Oliveira A, Reis R, Lim TC, et al. A comparative analysis of scaffold material modifications for load-bearing applications in bone tissue engineering. Int J Oral Maxillofac Surg 2006;35(10):928–34.
[210] De Mulder EL, Buma P, Hannink G. Anisotropic porous biodegradable scaffolds for musculoskeletal tissue engineering. Materials 2009;2(4):1674–96.
[211] Rai B, Teoh S-H, Hutmacher D, Cao T, Ho K. Novel PCL-based honeycomb scaffolds as drug delivery systems for rhBMP-2. Biomaterials 2005;26(17):3739–48.
[212] Hutmacher DW, Schantz T, Zein I, Ng KW, Teoh SH, Tan KC. Mechanical properties and cell cultural response of polycaprolactone scaffolds designed and fabricated via fused deposition modeling. J Biomed Mater Res 2001;55(2):203–16.
[213] Rimell JT, Marquis PM. Selective laser sintering of ultra high molecular weight polyethylene for clinical applications. J Biomed Mater Res 2000;53(4):414–20.
[214] Tan K, Chua C, Leong K, Cheah C, Gui W, Tan W, et al. Selective laser sintering of biocompatible polymers for applications in tissue engineering. Biomed Mater Eng 2005;15(1, 2):113–24.
[215] Williams JM, Adewunmi A, Schek RM, Flanagan CL, Krebsbach PH, Feinberg SE, et al. Bone tissue engineering using polycaprolactone scaffolds fabricated via selective laser sintering. Biomaterials 2005;26(23):4817–27.
[216] Tan K, Chua C, Leong K, Cheah C, Cheang P, Bakar MA, et al. Scaffold development using selective laser sintering of polyetheretherketone–hydroxyapatite biocomposite blends. Biomaterials 2003;24(18):3115–23.
[217] Cheah C, Chua C, Leong K, Chua S. Development of a tissue engineering scaffold structure library for rapid prototyping. Part 1: investigation and classification. The International Journal of Advanced Manufacturing Technology 2003;21(4):291–301.
[218] Mironov V, Boland T, Trusk T, Forgacs G, Markwald RR. Organ printing: computer-aided jet-based 3D tissue engineering. Trends Biotechnol 2003;21(4):157–61.
[219] Xu T, Jin J, Gregory C, Hickman JJ, Boland T. Inkjet printing of viable mammalian cells. Biomaterials 2005;26(1):93–9.

Naturally based and biologically derived nanobiomaterials

4

Mehdi Razavi[1,*], *Kai Zhu*[2,3,4,*] *and Yu S. Zhang*[2]
[1]Stanford University, Palo Alto, CA, United States
[2]Harvard Medical School, Cambridge, MA, United States
[3]Fudan University, Shanghai, China
[4]Shanghai Institute of Cardiovascular Disease, Shanghai, China

4.1 Introduction

Over the past decades, nanotechnologies have emerged and matured with a potential to revolutionize the field of medicine, in improving the quality of healthcare owing to the myriad of applications stemming from their unique properties at the nanoscale [1–5]. With typical sizes ranging from 1 to 100 nm nanomaterials have undergone rapid development for diverse biomedical applications, for instance, biomaterials, tissue engineering, drug delivery, and regenerative medicine [3,6–8]. Recently, there are increasing attention on the development of natural-based and biologically derived nanobiomaterials such as polysaccharide-, protein-, and carbon-based nanomaterials [9–11].

Polysaccharides include chitin, chitosan, and cellulose, which are plentiful in nature, renewable, resorbable, biocompatible, and quite low-cost, which can be utilized in drug delivery, cell-encapsulating biomaterials, and tissue engineering [12,13]. The chitin nanoparticles were also found to possess antibacterial property and its ferromagnetic performance allow for its possible application in drug-tracking systems [14,15]. Chitosan is also a most important derivative of chitin and a natural biopolymer [16], which is more suitable for the biological applications compared to chitin owing to its superior solubility in organic solvents and water [17,18]. It is simply processed into nanofibers [19], nanoparticles [20], and has greater chemical and physical properties such as high surface area, porosity, tensile strength, conductivity, photoluminescent, and better mechanical properties compared to pure chitosan [16]. Chitosan nanofibers have several usages for the development of wound dressing and for bioscaffolds [19,21]. With new encouragements proposed by new properties of chitosan-based nanomaterials and vast advanced prospects brought by nanotechnology, it is realistic to foresee the substantial developments that will revolutionize nanotechnology in the near future [16]. Cellulose is also the most abundant form of living terrestrial biomass and finds many applications in modern industry. Nanocellulose has a high surface area and negative charge of crystalline suggesting that high amounts of drugs can be bound to its surface with the potential for high payloads and

[*] These authors contributed equally to this work.

Nanobiomaterials Science, Development and Evaluation. DOI: http://dx.doi.org/10.1016/B978-0-08-100963-5.00004-5

optimal control of dosing [22]. Development of nanoscale cellulose fibers and their application in composite materials is attractive matter because of their high strength and stiffness as well as low weight, biodegradability, and renewability. Application of cellulose nanofibers in polymer reinforcement is a quite new research area [23]. Presently, nanocellulose has been known as the eye of biomaterial applicable for biomedical industry [22].

In particular, recent years have seen increasing attention in devising protein-based nanobiomaterials, which are considered as the natural counterparts to those of synthetic origins, with tunable biodegradability, low antigenicity, high nutritional value, and abundant sources [24]. As naturally occurring components that can be metabolized, protein nanobiomaterials are likely to be well tolerated in vivo with minimal deleterious side effects, whereas synthetic polymers on the other hand, may generate degradation products that induce adverse side effects of the host tissues [25]. Moreover, due to the rich functional groups on the primary sequences of polypeptides, protein-based nanobiomaterials can be exploited to generate effective interactions with cells [26]. The multiple binding sites of proteins can efficiently interact with active molecules, enabling high loading capacity of various drug cargos [27]. In addition, protein nanomaterials can be easily prepared and scaled up during the manufacture procedure, facilitating their translation into the clinics [26,28]. As with conventional synthetic polymer-based nanoparticles, the fabrication of protein-based nanobiomaterials can be divided into three general strategies, including coacervation/phase-separation, emulsion/solvent extraction, and complexation (Fig. 4.1), which may be further altered according to the specific types of proteins and needs involved.

Carbon nanomaterials such as carbon nanotubes and graphene are widely explored as new nanobiomaterials for drug delivery and developing the bioscaffolds to regenerate particular tissue [29]. It was indicated that carbon nanomaterials may be successfully delivered into nucleus and other organelles [30] where the hollow structure and intracellular transportation make them ideal to load and deliver drugs to cancerous cells. However, the important thing that needs to be addressed prior to commercializing the carbon-based nanobiomaterials is occupational health safety and health issues in production [31].

Herein, we provide an overview of polysaccharide-, protein-, and carbon-based nanobiomaterials and specifically discuss those derived from chitin, chitosan, and cellulose, collagen, gelatin, silk, fibrin, plant proteins, carbon nanotubes, and graphene, which have been extensively investigated in the past decade. We further illustrate the applications of these nanobiomaterials in tissue engineering and drug delivery. We finally summarize with perspectives and future directions on the widespread use and translation of these nanobiomaterials.

4.2 Polysaccharide-based nanomaterials

Polysaccharides are biodegradable and biocompatible materials that have a high content of functional groups, which include hydroxyl, amino, and carboxylic acid groups. The mentioned functional groups can be utilized for extra surface treatment

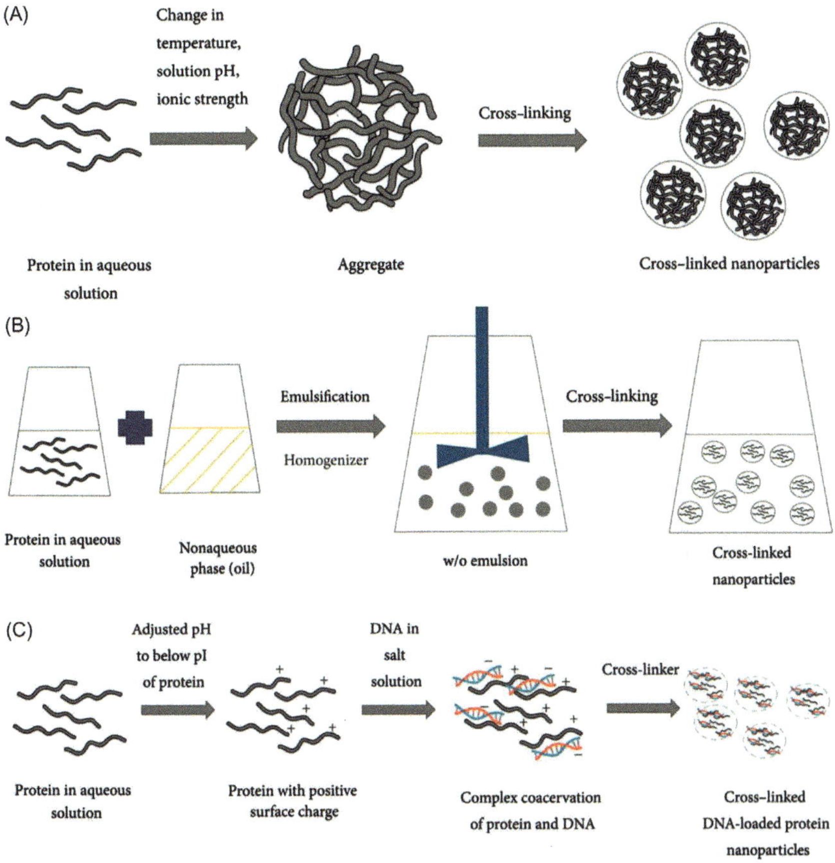

Figure 4.1 Three different strategies to prepare protein-based nanoparticles.
(A) Coacervation or phase-separation method. (B) Emulsion/solvent extraction method.
(C) Complexation method.
Source: Adapted with permission from Lohcharoenkal, W., et al., Protein nanoparticles as drug delivery carriers for cancer therapy. BioMed research international, 2014. 2014, copyright Hindawi Publishing Corporation 2014.

of the polysaccharides. Such structures have attracted a high attention to make polysaccharide-based biomaterials for numerous applications such as drug delivery, cell-encapsulating biomaterials, bioscaffolds for tissue engineering, and regenerative medicine [12].

However, polysaccharides also have some weaknesses that are their broad distribution of molecular weight and suffering from batch-to-batch variability. Additionally, most polysaccharides normally indicate restricted solubility in common organic solvents [32].

Because of the aforementioned favorable uses and to overcome the limitations, different routes through polymerization and well-defined organic synthesis have been extensively explored, and the modified polysaccharides were employed as effective building blocks to manufacture the cross-linked microgels/nanogels, self-assembled micelles, fibrous meshes, and three-dimensional (3D) hydrogels [12]. Typical examples of polysaccharides include chitin, chitosan, and cellulose are discussed in this chapter as follows.

4.2.1 Chitin

Chitin (poly (β-(1–4)-N-acetyl-D-glucosamine)) is a natural polysaccharide, which is synthesized by several living organisms and finds in nature to form structural constituents in the exoskeleton of arthropods or in the cell walls of yeast and fungi. Since a high amount of chitin is synthesized per annum in the world, it is the most plentiful polymer after cellulose. It is also made by many living organisms in the animal kingdoms and lower plant, serving in various aims where reinforcement and strength are necessary. By partial deacetylation of chitin in the solid state, chitosan is obtained as the most-known derivative chitin [14].

In a research, water-soluble carboxymethyl chitin (CMC) was used for drug delivery [19]. Through the cross-linking approach by $CaCl_2$ and $FeCl_3$, CMC nanoparticles were synthesized [15] and they were found to be compatible to fibroblast L929 cells. Furthermore, the 5-fluorouracil (5-FU) drug as a hydrophobic anticancer was loaded into CMC nanoparticles by emulsion cross-linking method and drug release studies confirmed that the CMC nanoparticles offered a sustained and controlled drug release at pH-6.8. The prepared nanoparticles were also found to have antibacterial property and its ferromagnetic performance allows its possible use in drug-tracking systems for cancer therapy.

In a research, Shalumon et al. [33] developed nanofibers from chitin and found that the nanofibers are bioactive and biocompatible. They also reported an electrospun water-soluble CMC/PVA (polyvinyl alcohol) blend for tissue engineering to attain nanofibers followed by cross-linking with glutaraldehyde vapors and thermal treatment processes.

Chitin can also be utilized as bone substitute for bone regeneration only if its mechanical behavior can be enhanced with incorporation of biomaterials such as hydroxyapatite (HA), bioactive glass ceramic (BGC), and so on. Adding a material such as silica can also improve the bioactivity and biocompatibility of chitin [14]. Madhumathi et al. [34] produced chitin composite bioscaffolds containing nanosilica using chitin hydrogel and their bioactivity, swelling ability, and cytotoxicity were analyzed in vitro. These bioscaffolds were found to be biocompatible and bioactive when tested with MG63 cell line. Biocompatibility was seen to enhance with increasing amount of powdered chitin/nanosilica bioscaffolds added to the media. These findings propose that chitin/nanosilica composite bioscaffolds can be beneficial for bone tissue engineering.

Also, Madhumathi et al. [35] synthesized novel α-chitin/nanosilver composite bioscaffolds for wound healing and these α-chitin/nanosilver composite bioscaffolds were found to possess outstanding antibacterial activity against *Staphylococcus aureus* and *Escherichia coli*, combined with good blood-clotting ability. These in vitro results recommended that α-chitin/nanosilver composite bioscaffolds could be utilized for wound healing. Similarly, Sudheesh Kumar et al. [36] developed and characterized β-chitin/nanosilver composite bioscaffolds for wound healing by β-chitin hydrogel containing silver nanoparticles. The antibacterial, whole blood clotting, swelling as well as cytotoxicity of the developed composite bioscaffolds were investigated. These β-chitin/nanosilver composite bioscaffolds were found to be antibactericidal against *E. coli* and *S. aureus* and demonstrated suitable blood-clotting ability as well. Furthermore, β-chitin/nanosilver composite bioscaffolds were assessed for their cell adhesion behavior using epithelial cells (Vero cells). The attachment of the Vero cells to the surface of the β-chitin/nanosilver composite bioscaffolds confirmed that nanosilver incorporated bioscaffolds are encouraging matrices offering good cell attachment apart from their antibacterial activity, which is ideal for wound healing [14].

4.2.2 Chitosan

Over the last era, research in functional biomaterials such as chitosan has resulted in the advances of new drug delivery system and superior regenerative medicine, now one of the most fast growing fields in the area of health science [16]. Chitosan is a unique biopolymer since it can be modified with different functional groups to control hydrophobic, cationic, and anionic behaviors. The most interesting properties of chitosan come from the presence of primary amines along with its backbone. Such structures impart to these polysaccharides are not only greatly valuable physicochemical behavior but also specific interactions with cells and biomolecules [16]. Chitosan-based nanobiomaterials possess superior chemical and physical properties including high surface area, porosity, mechanical strength, conductivity, and photoluminescence compared to pure chitosan. However, owing to the insolubility in a neutral and basic media, its uses are restricted [16]. Chitosan nanofibers have many different applications for the development of wound dressing [19], which can be prepared from trifluoroacetic acid and dichloromethane mixtures [37,38].

Besides, nano-HA together with chitosan (CS), Jiang et al. [39] have reported sodium carboxymethyl cellulose hybrid membrane that was curled in a concentric manner to realize an anisotropic spiral–cylindrical bioscaffold. The cylinder-shaped bioscaffold had similarity to natural bone accelerated complete infiltration of bone tissues in vivo and ultimately recognized osteointegration and functional reconstruction of damage bone, as indicated in Fig. 4.2A. The silk fibroin-hydroxybutyl chitosan-blended nanofibers successfully provided bioscaffold for the growth of porcine iliac endothelial cells. The nanofibers provided typical Extra Cellular Matrix (ECM) to cells, where these cells formed endothelial monolayer with higher confluency [40]. In Fig. 4.2B, Tang et al. [41] developed apatite-collagen-polycaprolactone (Ap-Col-PCL) composites that exhibited outstanding bioactivity to stimulate fast bone regeneration in rabbit model with fractional long bone defect. They mixed rapid prototyping fabrication technology and 3D functionalization strategy for biomimetic deposition and collagen incorporation. These composite materials presented excellent mechanical properties similar to cancellous bone, suitable biodegradability, and hierarchical architecture of three nano–micro–macro levels [41,42].

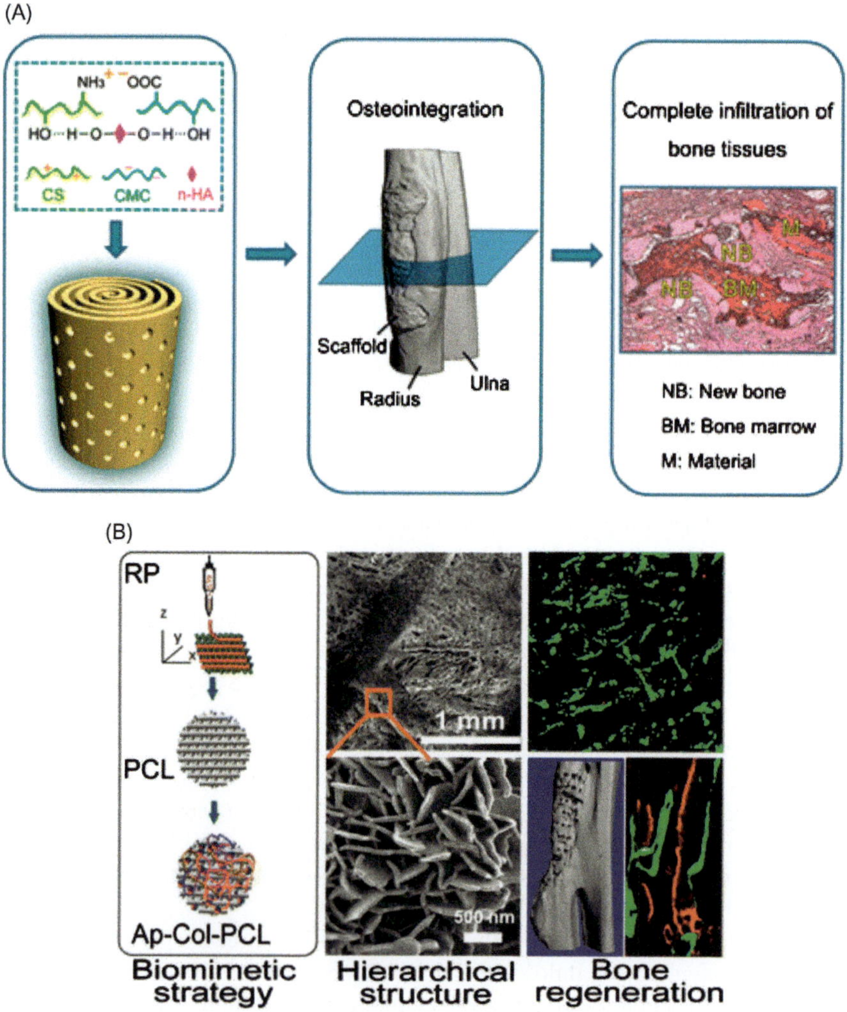

Figure 4.2 (A) Chitosan/cellulose/nano-hydroxyapatite biomimetic spiral–cylindrical bioscaffold hybrid membrane. (B) Biomimetically ornamented rapid prototyping fabrication of an apatite–collagen–polycaprolactone construct with nano–micro–macro hierarchical structure.
Reprinted with permission from ref. [39] ACS Publishing Group and ref. [41] ACS Publishing Group.

Chitosan nanoparticles (CNPs) are prepared by the ionotropic gelation technique where the reaction between the amino group of chitosan and negatively charged tripolyphosphates forms nanoparticles. CNPs can also be formulated by a micro-emulsion route, an emulsion solvent diffusion method followed by high-pressure homogenization [43].

A brushite chitosan system with vascular endothelial growth factor (VEGF) and platelet-derived growth factor (PDGF) controlled release displayed improved bone healing; however, PDGF was more rapidly delivered in rabbit femurs, than VEGF. Both growth factors were detected around the implantation site (5 cm) with negligible systemic exposure, leading to a peak concentration of VEGF of 5.5 ng/g at 1 week [44]. Teng et al. [45] developed carboxymethyl chitosan (CMCS) and soy protein isolate (SPI) nanoparticles by a simple ionic gelation technique. The effect of Ca21 concentration, pH, and CMCS/SPI mass ratio on the formation of nanoparticles was systematically studied. Vitamin D3 was incorporated into the polymeric complex (162 and 243 nm). The combination of nanoparticles reached 96.8% encapsulation efficiency, probably because of their compact structure and high capability of hydrogen bonding. These nanoparticles can also be loaded onto the bioscaffold for delivery of vitamin D3. In another study, chitosan fibrin nanocomposites (CFNs) were found to be appropriate candidates for drug delivery and for usage as a wound-healing agent. CFNs (24 28 nm) loaded with methotrexate [46] showed antibacterial activity against *E. coli* and *S. aureus* and nanocomposite presented dose-dependent toxicity in both HeLa and MCF-7 cells. Alternatively, topical application of CFNs for 10 days could totally heal the wounds in 14 days. Histological and biochemical analyses witnessed enhanced synthesis of collagen with active migration of fibroblasts and epithelial cells in CFN-treated wounds. Another drug delivery technique was investigated by chitosan and functionalized CNPs [47], as a bioscaffold material with superior efficiency together with PLGA (poly[lactic-co-glycolic acid]) nanoparticles [43,48].

Dev, Binulal, et al. [49] synthesized poly(lactic acid) (PLA)/CS nanoparticles by emulsion technique for anti-HIV drug delivery systems. The hydrophilic antiretroviral drug lamivudine was loaded into PLA/CS nanoparticles. The encapsulation efficiency and in vitro drug release behavior of drug-loaded PLA/CS nanoparticles were studied using absorption spectrophotometry. Furthermore, the cytotoxicity of PLA/CS nanoparticles using 3-(4,5-dimethylthiazol-2-yl)-2,5-diphenyltetrazolium bromide (MTT) assay was also explored. The in vitro drug release studies indicated that the drug release rate from PLA/CS nanoparticles reduced when the pH of the medium changed from alkaline to acidic to neutral. The drug release rate was lower in the acidic pH when compared to alkaline pH, which is because of the repulsion between H^+ ions and cationic groups present in the nanoparticles. These results confirmed that the PLA/CS nanoparticles are an encouraging carrier system for controlled delivery of anti-HIV and cancer drugs [14,49].

4.2.3 Cellulose

Cellulose is the most abundant form of living terrestrial biomass and finds numerous usages in modern industry. It is a long-chain polymer with repeating units of Dglucose, a simple sugar that appears in almost pure form in cotton fiber while, in wood, plant leaves, and stalks, it is found in combination with other materials such as hemicelluloses and lignin. Some bacteria are also found to synthesize cellulose.

Nanocellulose has a large surface area and negative charge of crystalline suggesting that high amounts of drugs can be bound to its surface with the potential for high payloads and optimal control of dosing. The abundant hydroxyl groups on the surface of crystalline nanocellulose provide surface modification sites with a range of chemical groups through applying the different techniques. Surface modification may be used to modulate the release and loading of drugs that would not typically bind to nanocellulose, including nonionized and hydrophobic drugs [22].

Cellulose macro- and nanofibers have attracted much attention because of the high strength and stiffness, biodegradability, and renewability, and their production and use in composite developments. Fabrication of cellulose nanofibers is a relatively new research area. Cellulose nanofibers may be used as filler in composite materials owing to the enhanced mechanical and biodegradation behavior of composites. The fibers are naturally hydrophilic, so it is necessary to increase their roughness to make the composites with better properties. Production of nanoscale cellulose fibers and their application in composites is interesting due to their high strength and stiffness coupled with low weight as well as its biodegradability. Application of cellulose nanofibers as polymer filler is also a novel research area [23]. The main reason to use cellulose nanofibers in composite materials is because one can possibly attain the high stiffness of the cellulose crystal, which can be done by breaking down the hierarchical structure of the plant into individualized nanofibers of high crystallinity, with a decrease in amorphous parts [50]. Many researches have been conducted on isolation and analysis of cellulose nanofibers from various sources. Cellulose nanofibers can be extracted from the cell walls by simple mechanical or a combination of both mechanical and chemical methods [22].

Currently, nanocellulose has been identified as the eyes of biomaterial particularly suitable for biomedical industry, which includes skin substitutes for wounds and burns; drug delivery system; blood vessel growth; nerves, gum, and duramater reconstruction; tissue engineered bioscaffolds; stent covering and bone repair [37,38,51,52].

Nanocellulose mats are very efficient in promoting autolytic debridement, declining the pain, and accelerating the granulation, all of which are crucial for a good wound healing. These nanobiocellulose membranes can be synthesized in any shape and size, which is beneficial for treatment and coverage of large areas of the body. Odontology is challenged to find a perfect material as the bones substitute in several procedures, as bones malformation, maxillary, and facial deformities; for example, loss of alveolar bone has been the main challenge. Nanocellulose having fitting porosity, which gives the mat an infection barrier, loss of fluids, painkiller effect, allows medicines to be easily applied and it also absorbs the purulent fluids during all inflammatory stages, expelling it later on in a controlled and painless manner [53]. Furthermore, nanocellulose has been improved by immersion in solutions of gelatin and polyacrylamide-yielding hydrogels with increased toughness [54]. Similarly, immersion of nanocellulose into poly (vinyl alcohol) has made hydrogels with a wide range of mechanical behavior for cardiovascular diseases [55]. Nasal reconstruction is also another application of nanocellulose. Nose, centrally located in the face, is more exposed to traumas, deformities, and so social disorders. Even since having a major breathing function, it has an esthetic function. Amorim et al. [56] evaluated the tissue response to the presence of nanocellulose in the nose bone. It had been used in 22 rabbits, being that, in 20 a cellulose blanket was implanted in the nasal dorsum, and 2 were kept as control. Nanocellulosic blanket showed an acceptable biocompatibility, therefore a proper biomaterial to raise the nose bone. Moreover, nanocellulose was observed in dental tissue regeneration. Microbial cellulose, produced by the *Glucanacetobacter xylinus* strain, may be used to regenerate the human dental tissues. In dentistry, nanocellulose product Gengiflex and Gore-Tex has intended applications where it has been produced with the aim of periodontal tissue repair [57]. An explanation was given of a complete repair of an osseus defect around an Intramobile Cylinder (IMZ) implant related to a Gengiflex therapy. The advantages included the reestablishment of aesthetics and function of the mouth and that fewer surgical steps were required [57].

4.3 Collagen-based nanobiomaterials

Collagens account for 20%–30% of all the proteins in the human body and have been widely used in biomedical applications due to their strong biocompatibility, weak antigenicity, and fast biodegradability [58]. However, some disadvantages of using collagen-based systems do exist toward their biomedical applications. For instance, they can potentially cause alterations of cell growth or motility, have poor mechanical strength, and may undergo contraction [59]. The predominant form of collagens used in biomedicine is type I collagen, which possesses self-assembled triple helix structure following a multiscale process and can be found almost ubiquitously in the body, including most commonly, skin and bone [60].

Collagens can form hydrogel networks without the mediation of chemical cross-linking but only by physical denaturation [61]. However, the preparation of stable collagen nanoparticles usually requires additional chemical treatments owing to the innate low mechanical strength of collagens [62]. Electrostatic interactions are often applied to prepare collagen nanoparticles using sodium sulfate as a desolvating agent [63]. Another strategy is based on lipid vesicle–assisted methods, by which lipid vesicles are used as molds to produce spherical particles with controlled sizes [64].

Owing to their large specific surface areas, high adsorption capacity, and dispersion ability in water, collagen nanoparticles have been commonly used for drug loading and delivery [65]. The collagen-based nanoparticles can be easily taken up by the reticuloendothelial system (RES) in vivo, enabling enhanced uptake of loaded drugs into a number of cells, making collagen-based nanoparticles as a class of good candidates for systemic drug delivery [66]. Besides, collagen-based nanoparticles have also been used as sustained release vectors for antimicrobial agents or steroids [67]. Recently, collagens were further used as bioconjugates with metal nanoparticles to develop biologically based hybrid biomaterials toward a range of therapeutic and diagnostic applications. For example, Yan and colleagues synthesized stable colloidal gold-collagen core-shell nanoconjugates in an aqueous solution at room temperature, without use of any reducing agents and stabilizing agents (Fig. 4.3) [68]. The mechanism for the formation of the core-shell nanoconjugates could be explained by an electrostatic interaction between the negatively charged gold surfaces with the positively charged collagen chains and subsequent reduction by hydroxyproline residues of collagen (Fig. 4.3E). After layer-by-layer assembly with polylysine (PLL) film on a substrate, cell adhesion, growth, and differentiation were significantly improved (Fig. 4.3F).

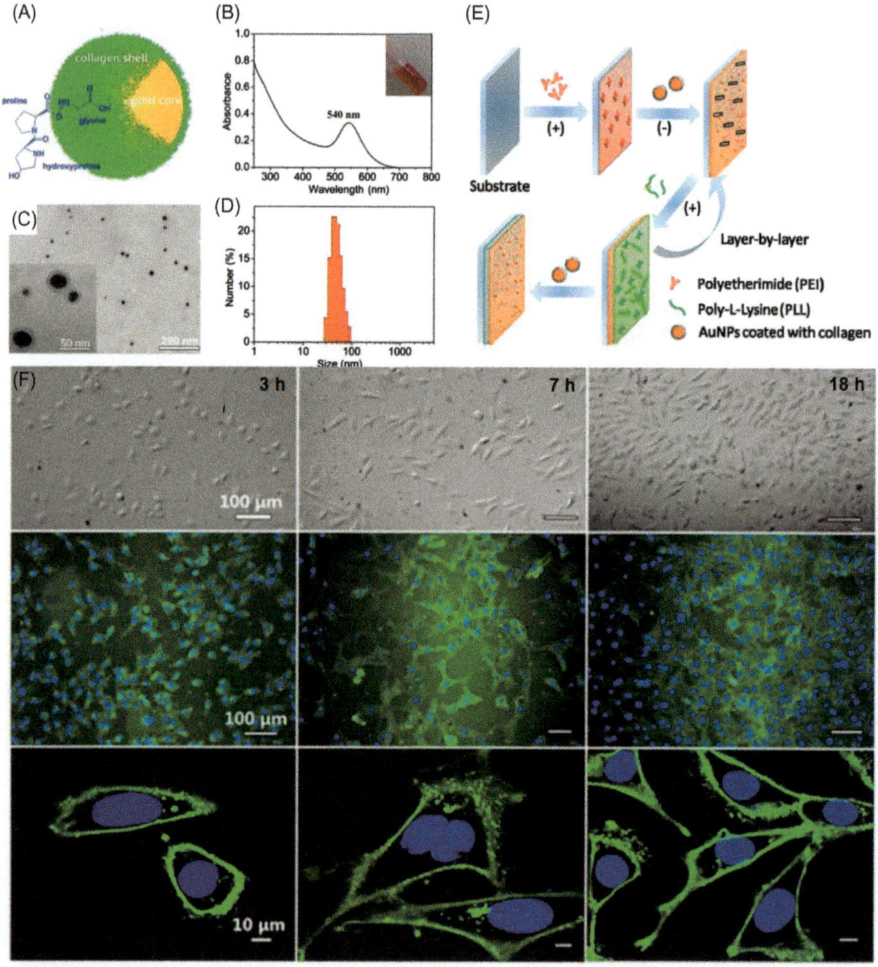

Figure 4.3 (A) Schematic of the colloidal gold-collagen nanoconjugates. (B) UV–vis absorption spectrum of colloidal gold-collagen nanoconjugates and photograph of an aqueous solution containing the nanoconjugates (inset). (C) Transmission electron microscopy (TEM) image of the colloidal gold-collagen core-shell nanoconjugates at lower and higher (inset) magnifications. (D) Size distribution diagram of the nanoconjugates. (E) Schematic of layer-by-layer assembled film. (F) The gold-collagen core-shell nanoconjugates were demonstrated to improve cell attachment and growth.
Source: Adapted with permission from Xing, R., et al., Colloidal Gold–Collagen Protein Core–Shell Nanoconjugate: One-Step Biomimetic Synthesis, Layer-by-Layer Assembled Film, and Controlled Cell Growth. ACS applied materials & interfaces, 2015; 7(44): 24733–40, copyright American Chemical Society 2015.

4.3.1 Gelatin

As a denatured protein, gelatin is obtained from collagen by acid/alkaline hydrolysis. It is a safe biomaterial approved by United States Food and Drug Administration (FDA) and has been widely used in pharmaceuticals, cosmetics, as well as food products [69]. Owing to its denatured property, it has a relatively low antigenicity when used in vivo. Gelatin nanoparticles have been reported for use in successful delivery of various drugs, protein synthesis inhibitors, tissue-type plasminogen activator, as well as therapeutic genes [70,71]. After chemical modification on its functional groups, gelatin can be further developed into targeted drug delivery vehicles [72].

Gelatin nanoparticles can be prepared using desolvating agents, such as alcohol or acetone [73]. However, these desolvating agents could result in the formation of large nanoparticles with a wide size range. Therefore, Kreuter and colleagues reported a two-step desolvation process to fabricate smaller nanoparticles with a narrow size distribution [74]. Glutaraldehyde can be used as a cross-linker to improve the mechanical properties and stability of gelatin nanoparticles. However, the cytotoxicity of residual glutaraldehyde limits the biomedical applications of these nanoparticles. The use of nontoxic cross-linkers has thus been pursued as alternatives [75]. Genipin is a compound found in gardenia fruit extract and has been adopted as cross-linker without obvious cytotoxicity [76]. In one study, recombinant human gelatin nanoparticles were prepared using genipin as a cross-linker and showed a sustained release for protein drug delivery [77]. Another less-toxic cross-linker relies on the carbodiimide reaction. It was demonstrated that the efficiency of drug entrapment and loading was significantly higher in the carbodiimide-cross-linked nanoparticles than that of nanoparticles cross-linked with glutaraldehyde [75]. Although the release kinetics of glutaraldehyde-cross-linked nanoparticle was a little bit faster than carbodiimide-cross-linked one, they showed similar release trends at pH 7.4, which may be attributed to the similar intensities of interactions between the drug and two types of nanoparticles. Moreover, Coester and colleagues used the recombinant enzyme microbial transglutaminase as a cross-linker to produce gelatin nanoparticles with sizes below 250 nm and a narrow size distribution [78].

Gelatin nanoparticles can also be prepared by coacervation-phase separation [30], emulsification-solvent evaporation [79], reverse-phase evaporation [80], and nanoprecipitation [81]. A coacervation-phase separation method was reported to prepare paclitaxel-loaded gelatin nanoparticles, where an aqueous solution of sodium sulfate was added slowly to a gelatin solution containing Tween-20 followed by the addition of isopropanol-containing paclitaxel. The resultant nanoparticles showed longer retention and higher accumulation in tissues than the conventional paclitaxel formulation using cremophor/ethanol as solubilizers [82]. For the emulsification-solvent evaporation method, gelatin nanoparticles can be prepared by mixing an aqueous phase of both gelatin and drug with an oil phase such as polymethylmethacrylate and then cross-linked with glutaraldehyde-saturated solvent (e.g., toluene) [79]. Reverse-phase evaporation method was used to prepare gelatin nanoparticles inside the inner aqueous core of reverse micellar droplets formed by dissolving the surfactant (e.g., sodium bis(2-ethylhexyl) sulfosuccinate) in the solvent (e.g., *n*-hexane) [80].

In another study, Lim and colleagues prepared drug-loaded gelatin nanoparticles by nanoprecipitation method using water as a solvent, ethanol as a nonsolvent, and poloxamer as a stabilizer [81]. Recently, a novel water-in-water emulsion technique was further successfully applied to prepare D,L-glyceraldehyde-cross-linked gelatin-poloxamer 188 nanoparticles as pulmonary insulin-administration system. The nanoparticles promoted effective pulmonary absorption of insulin and showed good relative pharmacological availability [83].

Recently, it has also been shown that gelatin can be mixed with polysaccharides or synthetic polymers as hybrid nanocomplexes for drug delivery applications. The nanocomplexes can be formed by ionic gelation and self-assembly. For instance, Sánchez and colleagues developed new hybrid nanoparticles via ionic gelation between cationized gelatin and the anionic polysaccharides, dextran sulfate, and chondroitin sulfate, for delivery of plasmid DNA to the ocular surface [84]. Furthermore, composite nanoparticles based on glycidyl methacrylated dextran and gelatin were fabricated by a facile synthesis method assisted by self-assembly without using any organic solvents, where the release of bone morphogenetic protein was maintained for more than 12 days under degradative conditions by dextranase [85]. Another strategy is using modified gelatin to fabricate functional nanoparticles. For example, Amiji et al. conjugated 2-iminothiolane to primary amine groups on type B gelatin to fabricate a redox-responsive thiolated gelatin-based nanoparticle that could efficiently deliver its payload in the presence of glutathione-mediated reducing intracellular environment [86].

4.3.2 Silk protein

Silk is a protein spun by some lepidoptera larvae, such as silkworms, spiders, scorpions, mites, and flies. Silk proteins are promising biomaterials for drug delivery and tissue engineering applications due to their biocompatibility, slow biodegradability, self-assembly, excellent mechanical properties, and controllable structure and morphology [87].

Fibroin is a fibrous protein constituting the core of silk [88]. Zhang and colleagues developed a type of insulin-loaded silk fibroin nanoparticles, where the crystalline silk nanoparticles could be covalently conjugated with insulin via the cross-linking reagent glutaraldehyde through the primary amine groups present on the surface of the nanoparticles [89]. The bioconjugation of insulin with silk fibroin nanoparticles improved their in vitro stability in both human serum and trypsin solutions. In another study, silk fibroin nanoparticles of controllable sizes were obtained in an all-aqueous process by salting out with potassium phosphate and could be loaded with small-molecule drugs through simple electrostatic interactions between the negatively charged nanoparticles and the positively charged small molecules (Fig. 4.4) [90]. Another common fabrication strategy of silk nanoparticles is the desolvation technique using dimethyl sulfoxide as a desolvating agent. The active amino groups and tyrosine residues of the resultant silk fibroin favored its bioconjugation with VEGF leading to a sustained release profile of over 3 weeks [91]. A phase-separation method using PVA as a continuous phase was also utilized to separate silk solution into micro- and nanoparticles [92]. The porous interior space and amphiphilic nature of

	N-terminus	Repetitive part	C-terminus	Light chain
Charge ratio (-/+)	(20/12)	(34/5)	(1/9)	(22/15)
PI	4.6	3.80	10.5	5.1
Size (aa)	151	5062	50	262
Hydropathicity	-0.35	0.24	-0.48	0.05

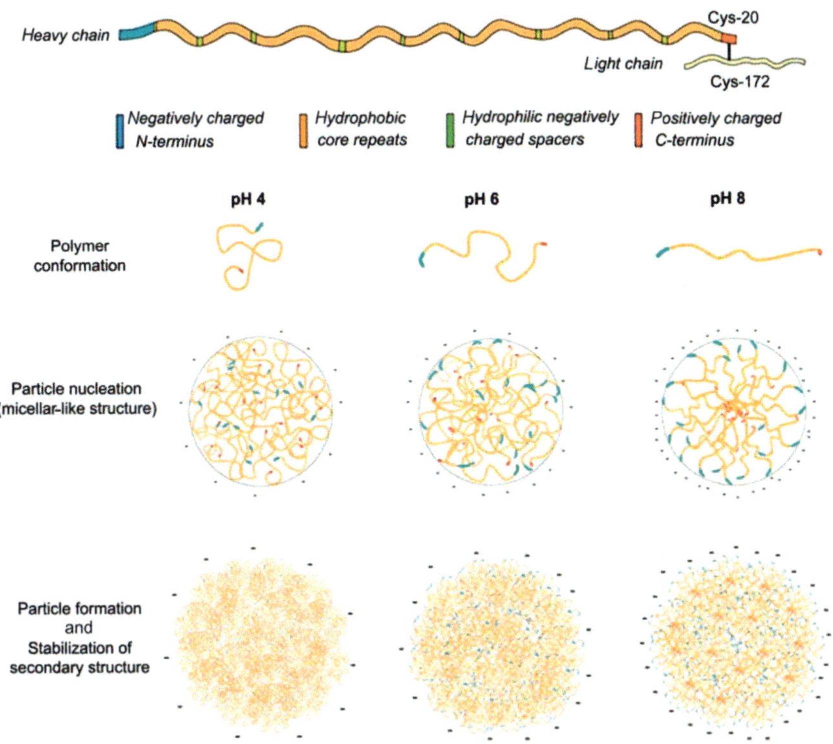

Figure 4.4 Schematic showing formation of silk fibroin nanoparticles using an all-aqueous process. (A) Characteristics of silk fibroin considering the charge distribution along the amino acid chain. pI, isoelectric point. (B) Top: Silk fibroin molecule conformation at different pH values. Middle: Particle nucleation into micellar-like structures. Bottom: Particle formation and stabilization of secondary structures through clustering of micellar-like structures in the presence of potassium phosphate.
Source: Adapted with permission from Lammel, A.S., et al., Controlling silk fibroin particle features for drug delivery. Biomaterials, 2010; 31(16): 4583–91, copyright Elsevier 2010.

silk spheres facilitated the entrapment of drugs with different molecular weights and hydrophobicity.

Silk fibroin was also blended with other nanobiomaterials for improved efficacy. For example, silk was blended with Pluronic F-127 and F-87 in the presence of solvents to achieve self-assembled micellar nanostructures, which enabled co-loading of both hydrophilic (insulin) and hydrophobic (anticancer paclitaxel) drugs to the targeted sites [93].

4.3.3 Fibrin

Fibrin is a fibrous and nonglobular protein involved in the blood coagulation cascade; together with platelets, the polymerized fibrin can form a hemostatic clot over the wound site [94]. Owing to its biocompatible and biodegradable properties, fibrin serves as an attractive matrix for cell growth and differentiation [95]. Besides, fibrin has also been exploited to process into various nanomaterials for sustained release of drugs and proteins [96].

An approach of synthesizing fibrin nanoparticles was previously reported, using a process wherein fibrinogen was first mixed with thrombin and then introduced to an oil emulsion to obtain fibrin microbeads with size from 60 to 180 μm, which were subsequently homogenized to derive fibrin nanoparticles [97]. Alternatively, a surfactant-free, water-in-oil emulsification-diffusion technique was used to synthesize fibrin nanoparticles with high yield [98]. Recently, Jayakumar and colleagues developed chitosan-hyaluronic acid composite sponge incorporated with fibrin nanoparticles loaded with VEGF as a dressing for diabetic wounds (Fig. 4.5) [99]. More than 60% of the loaded VEGF was released in 3 days and induced effective angiogenesis at the wound site.

4.3.4 Plant proteins

Animal protein-based nanoparticles are usually difficult to achieve sustained drug release due to their hydrophilic nature and rapid solubilization in aqueous environments. These nanoparticles could absorb water and swell, thus making drugs rapidly diffuse out. Chemical cross-linkers typically used to harden protein nanoparticles suffer from the presence of unreacted residuals within the nanoparticles leading to the risk of formation of toxic products by reaction with the tissues during in vivo biodegradation. This problem could be potentially overcome by using hydrophobic plant proteins with no need for cross-linking. Plant proteins represent a new class of natural biomaterials, such as those derived from zein, gliadin, soy proteins, and lectins [100]. Compared to hydrophilic animal proteins, hydrophobic plant proteins such as zein and gliadin have the capability of yielding sustained drug release [101,102]. They are less expensive than their animal equivalents but also possess functional groups that can be easily used either to adsorb or to covalently couple molecules capable of modifying the targeting properties of nanoparticles. In addition, plant protein–based nanobiomaterials may reduce the risk of spreading animal protein-related diseases such as bovine spongiform encephalitis [103].

Several methods have been reported for the preparation of nanoparticles from plant protein raw materials. Coacervation or controlled desolvation methods have been developed using solvent or electrolyte as the coacervation agent or by adjusting the pH or the ionic strength. Plant protein-based nanobiomaterials are promising

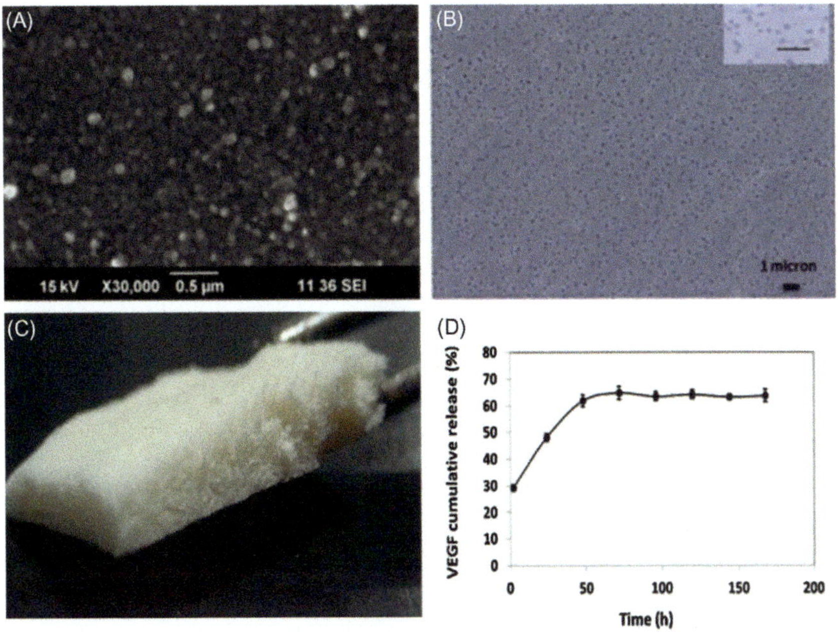

Figure 4.5 Schematic of chitosan-hyaluronic acid (HA) sponge encapsulating VEGF-loaded fibrin nanoparticles (VnF) for enhancing angiogenesis in wounds. (A) Scanning electron microscopy (SEM) image and (B) phosphotungstic acid hematoxylin staining of VEGF-loaded fibrin nanoparticles (VnF). (C) Photograph of the composite sponge. (D) Release profile of VEGF from the composite sponges.
Source: Adapted with permission from Mohandas, A., et al., Chitosan–hyaluronic acid/VEGF loaded fibrin nanoparticles composite sponges for enhancing angiogenesis in wounds. Colloids and Surfaces B: Biointerfaces, 2015; 127: 105–13, copyright Elsevier 2015.

candidates for drug delivery due to some of their unique properties. For instance, Guo and colleagues demonstrated the targeting potential of zein nanoparticles to the liver. Following intravenous injection of 5-FU-loaded zein nanoparticles, they were found to mostly accumulate in the liver and adequately remained in the blood circulation for at least 24 h due to their relatively high molecular weight and small particle sizes achievable [102].

4.4 Carbon-based nanobiomaterials

Carbon nanomaterials are defined as sp^2-carbon-bonded structures including zero-dimensional, one-dimensional (1D), and two-dimensional (2D) forms, such as fullerenes, carbon nanotubes, and graphene [104]. Carbon nanomaterials such as carbon nanotubes and graphene are widely explored as novel nanobiomaterials for drug delivery and developing the bioscaffolds to restore tissue. Carbon-based nanobiomaterials, mainly in the form of nanotubes and graphene, have attracted much attention recently because of their distinctive physical and chemical behavior such as their hollow structure, their high surface area/volume ratio, thermal conductivity, electrical conductance, mechanical stiffness, and the potentials of functionalizing them to alter their inherent behavior [105].

Carbon nanomaterials such as single-wall and multiwall carbon nanotubes, carbon nanofibers, fullerenes (C60), activated carbons, and graphene, are usually created by various routes including plasma-enhanced chemical vapor deposition (CVD), electric arc discharge, laser ablation, thermal or epitaxial growth, and mechanical exfoliation [29].

Another exciting property of carbon-based nanomaterials is their electrical conductivity, which has been indicated to promote nerve restoration [106]. Two special applications of carbon nanobiomaterials to neurobiologists are repairing the damaged nervous tissues by the scaffolding technology and biocompatible electrodes for recording from or stimulating nervous tissues [29]. Currently, carbon nanobiomaterials have been studied as a different material for neural electrode since they have exceptional mechanical and electrical properties in comparison with the conventional electrode materials. Moreover, deposited carbon nanotubes on neural electrodes increase the recording abilities of the electrodes [107].

As one of the carbon-based nanobiomaterials, graphene, the elementary structure of graphite, is an atomically thick sheet composed of sp^2-carbon atoms arranged in a flat honeycomb structure [108], which can be wrapped into spherical structures (zero-dimensional fullerenes), rolled into 1D structures (carbon nanotubes, CNTs) or stacked into 3D layered structures (graphite) [109]. Each carbon atom has three σ-bonds and an out-of-plane π-bond that can bind with neighboring atoms [110] and the strong carbon/carbon bonding in the plane, aromatic structure, presence of free π electrons and reactive sites for surface reactions have made graphene a unique material with exceptional mechanical, physicochemical, thermal, electronic, and optical properties. Hence, it is not surprising that graphene has generated great interest in nanomedicine and biomedical applications (Fig. 4.6) [111].

Besides, by physical and chemical modifications, graphene sheets can be transformed into single and multilayered graphene, graphene oxide (GO), and reduced GO (rGO), each of which has unique tunable properties [110]. Many researchers have utilized different techniques include coating, hydrogel blending, wet/dry-spinning processes, and 3D printing to make 2D or 3D graphene-based constructs. Graphene and its derivatives can also be tethered with other biomaterials [110]. Some examples of the reported advantages of graphene-based materials are: (a) enhancement of biomaterials mechanical/electrical properties, (b) improvement in cellular attachment and growth at biomaterials surface, and (c) production of more efficient biosensors [108].

Several biomedical applications have been studied, such as biosensing/bioimaging, drug delivery, cancer photothermal therapy, and antibacterial materials [108]. These applications used the properties of graphene in different ways. For example, while the excellent optical properties are appropriate for bioimaging, graphene's large surface area and availability of free π electrons are beneficial in gene and

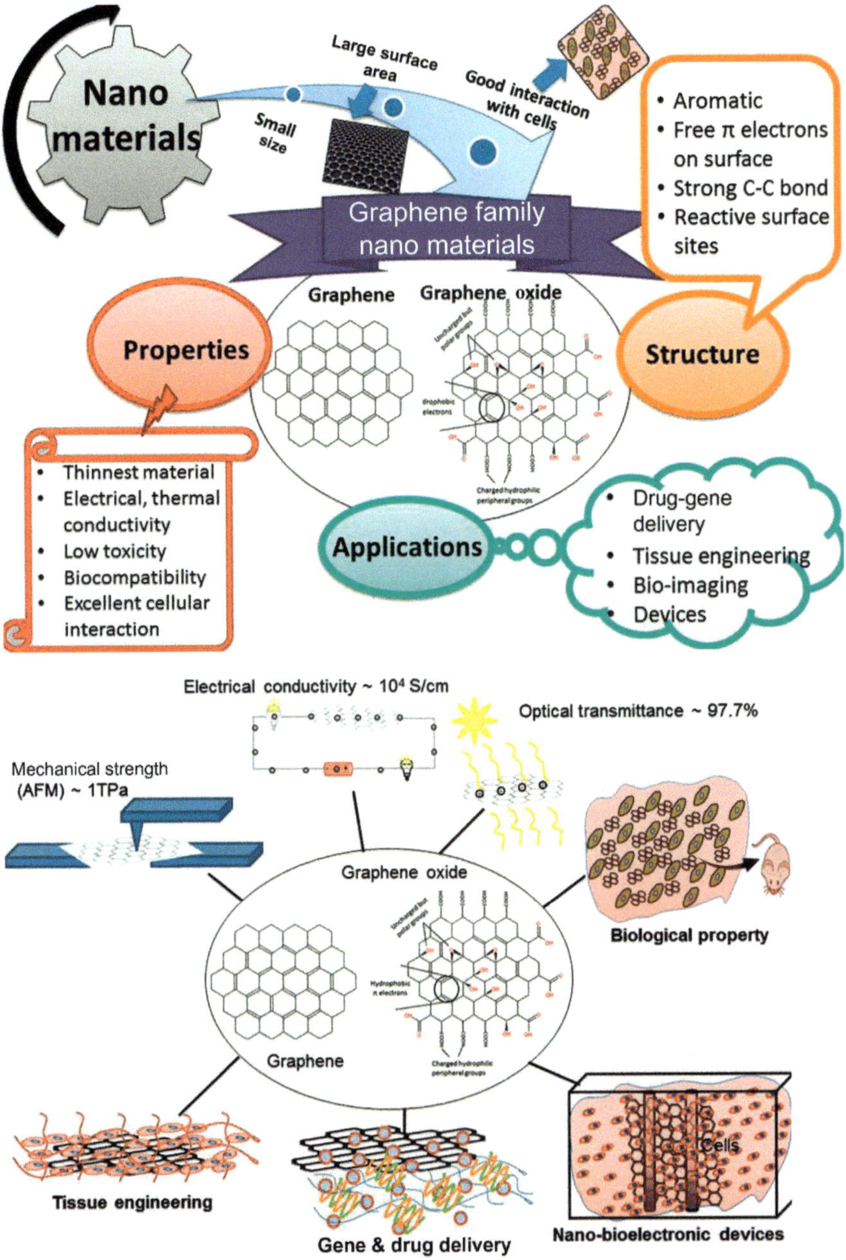

Figure 4.6 Schematic overview of various applications of graphene showing its structure, properties, and applications. Graphene-based nanomaterials have been used for different nonmedical and biomedical applications because of their excellent mechanical, electrical, and optical properties.
Source: Adapted with permission from Goenka, S., V. Sant, and S. Sant, Graphene-based nanomaterials for drug delivery and tissue engineering. Journal of Controlled Release, 2014; 173: 75–88, copyright Elsevier 2016.

drug delivery platforms. Furthermore, excellent mechanical strength, stiffness, and electrical conductivity make graphene-based nanobiomaterials a good candidate for engineering the bone and neural tissue [110]. GO has also been utilized as a photothermal agent for cancer treatment with encouraging therapeutic results owing to its high, intrinsic near-infrared (NIR) absorbance [112]. Also, advances for applications in bioengineering, regenerative medicine, and biotechnology are under study [108].

For example Li et al. [113] produced 3D graphene bioscaffold by CVD method using Ni foam template. Scanning electron microscopy (SEM) observation (Figs. 4.7A and 4.7B) indicates that graphene bioscaffolds indicated a monolith of continuous and porous structure, which copied and inherited the interconnected 3D structure of the Ni foam template. The porosity of 3D-GFs was around 99.5% and had a pore size of 100–300 μm. Although the graphene layers were very thin, the network had excellent mechanical properties and flexibility, and can stand alone. Moreover, compared with the structure of graphene bioscaffolds prepared by freeze-drying or template assembly techniques, the monolith of graphene network by CVD ensured a high conductivity owing to the lack of defects and intersheet junction contact resistance [113].

Also neural stem cells (NSCs) adhesion on 3D-GFs was first studies. For no more than 10 h after cell seeding, almost no free-floating cell could be found in the culture medium, showing a quick cell attachment on the graphene. After another 5 days of culture, NSCs cultured on 3D-GFs formed a well neural network and presented excellent cell adhesion (Figs. 4.7C and 4.7D). High-resolution SEM image demonstrates that the cells spread widely and formed strong filopodia/GF interaction (inset of Fig. 4.7B). Furthermore, in the cross-section fluorescence image of graphene bioscaffold with NSCs (DAPI (4′,6-diamidino-2-phenylindole) staining), a number of cells were seen inside the scaffold as well as on the surface, clearly indicating that the cells grew in a 3D fashion. Additionally, the SEM observation presents that the 3D-GFs remained intact during cell culture process over 2 weeks. Fig. 4.7C indicates that almost 90% of the cells cultured on 3D-GFs for 5 days were viable. The cells were also stained with antibody against nestin, a protein marker of NSCs. Fig. 4.7D indicates that almost all of cells on graphene bioscaffold were immunopositive for nestin (*green*), with no obvious difference from that on 2D graphene films, showing that NSCs proliferated well on 3D-GFs while maintaining their stemness [113].

Drug delivery by using graphene is also another booming area. Graphene nanoparticle sheets decorated with strontium metallic nanoparticles have showed to be advantageous in bone tissue engineering [114]. Reduced graphene oxide nanoparticles coated with strontium (rGO-Sr) are produced from the reduction of GO and strontium nitrate. The rGO-Sr (200–300 nm) coated with 22% strontium has been incorporated into macroporous tissue bioscaffolds of PCL. The PCL/rGO-Sr bioscaffolds presented high and distinct osteoblast proliferation due to the release of strontium from hybrid nanoparticles. The bioscaffolds, furthermore, indicated good mechanical behavior and so they can be utilized for designing biomaterials in tissue regeneration.

Sol–gel-driven HA nanoparticles and graphene nanoflakes incorporated with PCL were electrospun at different spinning conditions such as electrical potential, pump speed, distance, and viscosity [115]. The HA nanoparticles were initially amorphous and hence were annealed at 750°C for 2 h to crystallize them. The HA nanoparticles

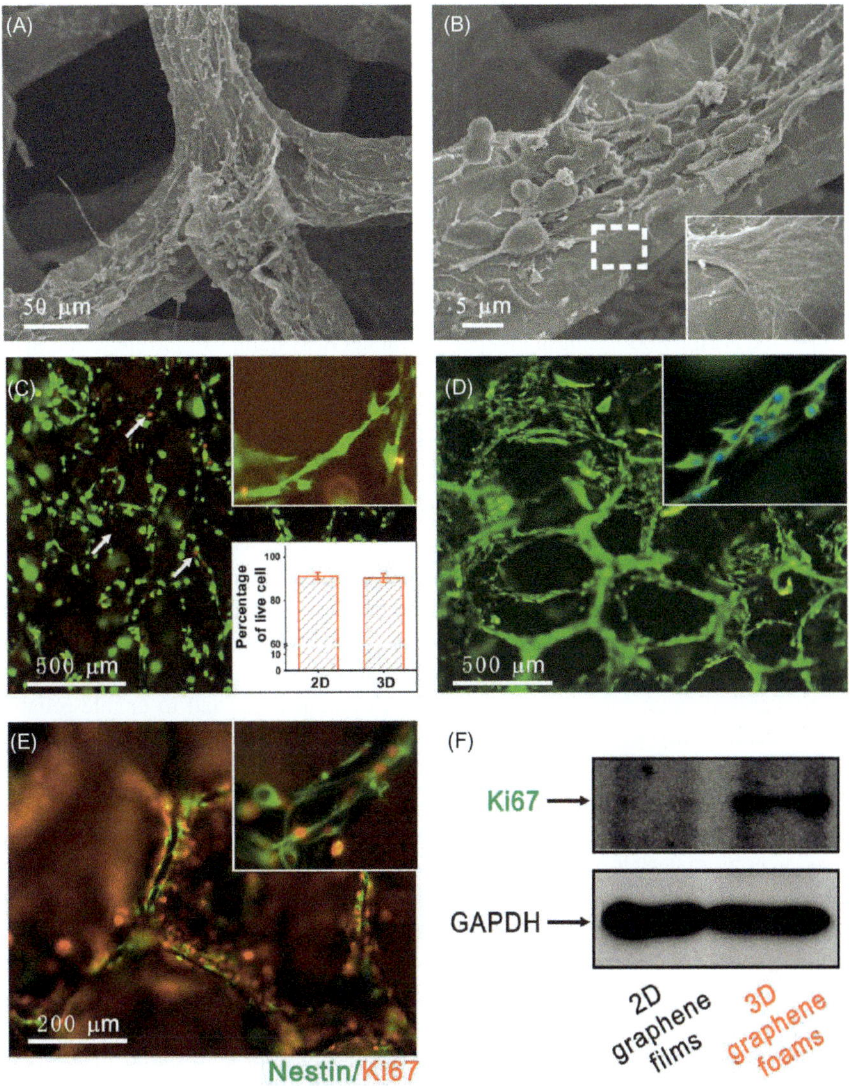

Figure 4.7 NSC adhesion and proliferation on graphene bioscaffold. (A) Low- and (B) high-magnified SEM images of NSCs cultured on graphene bioscaffold. The inset illustrates the interaction between the cell filopodia and the surface of material. (C) Cell viability assay of NSCs after 5 days of culture as determined by live/dead assay, live cells are stained *green* and dead cells are *red*, *white* arrow points to dead cell. The lower right inset indicates the percentage of live cell on graphene films (2D) and graphene bioscaffolds (3D). (D) Fluorescence images of NSCs proliferated on 3D-GFs for 5 days, immunostaining markers were nestin (*green*) for NSCs and DAPI (blue) for nuclei. (E) NSCs were double-immunostained with anti-Ki67 (*red*) and antinestin (*green*) antibodies, Ki67 is a marker for cell proliferation. (F) Western blot analysis of Ki67 expression on 2D graphene films and 3D graphene bioscaffold.
Source: Adapted with permission from Li, N., et al., Three-dimensional graphene foam as a biocompatible and conductive scaffold for neural stem cells. Scientific reports, 2013, copyright Nature Publishing Group 2013.

and graphene distributed in the PCL fibers and accelerated bone regeneration. Many other researches have also proved that graphene and GO are both potential compounds in bone tissue engineering [43,116].

However, the thing that needs to be addressed before commercializing the carbon nanomaterials in the biomedical and pharmaceutical markets is health and safety issues [31]. Carbon-based nanomaterials can be exposed in the body by the different pathways such as lung, skin, nose, eyes, and digestive tract. Upon inhalation, they can be translocated readily to extrapulmonary sites and reach other target organs, for example the lymph node, central and peripheral nerve system, liver, kidney, and heart. Hence, further research targeting relevant exposures to carbon-based nanobiomaterials are required prior to their mass production [29].

4.5 Conclusions and future perspectives

Naturally based and biologically derived nanobiomaterials are still in its infancy but upward strides are being made to advance and enhance protocols for clinical applications and continued research in both biomedical engineering and biochemical engineering will be needed to understand the potential of this type of nanobiomaterials for medicine and surgery. Moreover, process development is needed to enable reliable, cost-effective, scaled-up fabrication of bioderived polymers with desired physical, mechanical, chemical, and biological properties.

The success stories of polysaccharide-based nanobiomaterials for tissue engineering illustrate the versatility and capability of naturally based and biologically derived nanobiomaterials as biological implants. Even more types of naturally derived materials are on the horizon for clinical medicine. Synthesizing new polymers using monomers obtained from agricultural resources is one avenue for future innovation. Agricultural resources such as cellulose may also provide useful starting materials for implantable medical devices. Moreover, additional polymers derived from microbial production are under exploration.

We have also provided an overview of the emerging protein-based nanobiomaterials derived from collagen, gelatin, silk, fibrin, and plant proteins, with a focus on their applications in drug delivery. While these protein nanobiomaterials possess superior advantages such as biocompatibility and ease of functionalization, limitations still exist. For example, as natural polymers protein-based nanobiomaterials are heterogeneous of molecular weights, thus oftentimes yielding wider nanoparticle size distribution and exhibiting more batch-to-batch variations than their synthetic counterparts [117]. Therefore, there is limited standard scaling-up process for protein-based nanobiomaterials. An attractive strategy is to use the recombinant protein technology. The monodispersed molecular weight, precisely defined physicochemical properties, as well as the predictable placement of functional groups, binding moieties, or their programmable degradation profiles potentially make the recombinant proteins useful for drug delivery and tissue engineering applications [118]. In addition, further studies are needed to investigate new and safe cross-linkers for stabilizing protein nanoparticles as alternatives to the toxic ones currently widely used. In the future, a better fundamental understanding of the mechanisms of protein–drug interactions at the molecular level will provide a basis for their further optimization to ensure the design of ideal protein nanocarriers and open more exciting opportunities for their use in the area of drug and gene delivery.

Whether and how the carbon-based nanobiomaterials influence the long-term immune-response to downstream events of foreign body reaction have not yet been systemically addressed. Additional in vivo examinations and preclinical experiments are certainly required before these materials can be translated into the market.

4.6 Conflict of interest

The authors declare that there is no conflict of interests regarding the publication of this book chapter.

4.7 Acknowledgment

Y.S.Z. acknowledges funding from the National Cancer Institute of the National Institutes of Health Pathway to Independence Award (K99CA201603). K.Z. acknowledges the National Science Foundation of China (Grant No. 81301312), and the "Chen Guang" Project supported by Shanghai Municipal Education Commission and Shanghai Education Development Foundation (Grant No. 14CG06).

References

[1] Sun T, et al. Engineered nanoparticles for drug delivery in cancer therapy. Angew Chem Int Ed 2014;53(46):12320–64.
[2] Zhu K, et al. Nanoparticles-Assisted Stem Cell Therapy for Ischemic Heart Disease. Stem Cells Int 2016;2016(2016):1384658.
[3] Razavi M, et al. Nanobiomaterials in periodontal tissue engineering Nanobiomaterials in hard tissue engineering: applications of nanobiomaterials. Kidlington, Oxford: William Andrew; 2016. p. 323.
[4] Kheirkhah M, et al. Surface modification of stainless steel implants using nanostructured forsterite (Mg_2 SiO_4) coating for biomaterial applications. Surf Coat Technol 2015;276:580–6.
[5] Razavi M, et al. In vivo biocompatibility of Mg implants surface modified by nanostructured merwinite/PEO. J Mater Sci: Mater Med 2015;26(5):1–7.
[6] Jang HL, Zhang YS, Khademhosseini A. Boosting clinical translation of nanomedicine. Nanomedicine 2016 (0).
[7] Razavi M, et al. In vivo study of nanostructured akermanite/PEO coating on biodegradable magnesium alloy for biomedical applications. J Biomed Mater Res A 2015;103(5):1798–808.

[8] Razavi M, et al. Regenerative influence of nanostructured bredigite (Ca 7 MgSi 4 O 16)/ anodic spark coating on biodegradable AZ91 magnesium alloy implants for bone healing. Mater Lett 2015;155:97–101.
[9] Jazayeri HE, et al. Dental Applications of Natural-Origin Polymers in Hard and Soft Tissue Engineering. J Prosthodontics 2016.
[10] Yazdimamaghani M, et al. Significant degradability enhancement in multilayer coating of polycaprolactone-bioactive glass/gelatin-bioactive glass on magnesium scaffold for tissue engineering applications. Appl Surf Sci 2015;338:137–45.
[11] Fahmy MD, et al. Three-dimensional bioprinting materials with potential application in preprosthetic surgery. J Prosthodontics 2016.
[12] Wen Y, Oh JK. Recent strategies to develop polysaccharide-based nanomaterials for biomedical applications. Macromol Rapid Commun 2014;35(21):1819–32.
[13] Heidari F, et al. Preparation of natural chitosan from shrimp shell with different deacetylation degree. Mater Res Innovations 2016:1–5.
[14] Jayakumar R, et al. Biomedical applications of chitin and chitosan based nanomaterials—A short review. Carbohydr Polym 2010;82(2):227–32.
[15] Dev A, et al. Novel carboxymethyl chitin nanoparticles for cancer drug delivery applications. Carbohydr Polym 2010;79(4):1073–9.
[16] Shukla SK, et al. Chitosan-based nanomaterials: a state-of-the-art review. Int J Biol Macromol 2013;59:46–58.
[17] Mima S, et al. Highly deacetylated chitosan and its properties. J Appl Polym Sci 1983;28(6):1909–17.
[18] Heidari F, et al. Mechanical properties of natural chitosan/hydroxyapatite/magnetite nanocomposites for tissue engineering applications. Mater Sci Eng C 2016;65:338–44.
[19] Jayakumar R, et al. Novel chitin and chitosan nanofibers in biomedical applications. Biotechnol Adv 2010;28(1):142–50.
[20] Anitha A, et al. Synthesis, characterization, cytotoxicity and antibacterial studies of chitosan, O-carboxymethyl and N, O-carboxymethyl chitosan nanoparticles. Carbohydr Polym 2009;78(4):672–7.
[21] Croisier F, Jérôme C. Chitosan-based biomaterials for tissue engineering. Eur Polym J 2013;49(4):780–92.
[22] Kalia S, et al. Cellulose-based bio-and nanocomposites: a review. Int J Polym Sci 2011;2011.
[23] Siró I, Plackett D. Microfibrillated cellulose and new nanocomposite materials: a review. Cellulose 2010;17(3):459–94.
[24] Elzoghby AO, Samy WM, Elgindy NA. Protein-based nanocarriers as promising drug and gene delivery systems. J Controlled Release 2012;161(1):38–49.
[25] Chen L, Remondetto GE, Subirade M. Food protein-based materials as nutraceutical delivery systems. Trends Food Sci Technol 2006;17(5):272–83.
[26] Sengupta D, Heilshorn SC. Protein-engineered biomaterials: highly tunable tissue engineering scaffolds. Tissue Eng B Rev 2010;16(3):285–93.
[27] MaHam A, et al. Protein-based nanomedicine platforms for drug delivery. Small 2009;5(15):1706–21.
[28] Lohcharoenkal W, et al. Protein nanoparticles as drug delivery carriers for cancer therapy. BioMed Res Int 2014;2014.
[29] Yun Y. Carbon nanomaterials: from therapeutics to regenerative medicine. J Nanomed Biother Discov 2012;2012.
[30] Minchin R. Nanomedicine: sizing up targets with nanoparticles. Nat Nanotechnol 2008;3(1):12–13.

[31] Lam C-W, et al. A review of carbon nanotube toxicity and assessment of potential occupational and environmental health risks. Crit Rev Toxicol 2006;36(3):189–217.
[32] Payen A. Mémoire sur la composition du tissu propre des plantes et du ligneux. Comptes Rendus 1838;7:1052–6.
[33] Shalumon K, et al. Electrospinning of carboxymethyl chitin/poly (vinyl alcohol) nanofibrous scaffolds for tissue engineering applications. Carbohydr Polym 2009;77(4):863–9.
[34] Madhumathi K, et al. Novel chitin/nanosilica composite scaffolds for bone tissue engineering applications. Int J Biol Macromol 2009;45(3):289–92.
[35] Madhumathi K, et al. Development of novel chitin/nanosilver composite scaffolds for wound dressing applications. J Mater Sci Mater Med 2010;21(2):807–13.
[36] Kumar PS, et al. Preparation and characterization of novel β-chitin/nanosilver composite scaffolds for wound dressing applications. Carbohydr Polym 2010;80(3):761–7.
[37] Czaja WK, et al. The future prospects of microbial cellulose in biomedical applications. Biomacromolecules 2007;8(1):1–12.
[38] Klemm D, et al. Bacterial synthesized cellulose—artificial blood vessels for microsurgery. Prog Polym Sci 2001;26(9):1561–603.
[39] Jiang H, et al. Biomimetic spiral-cylindrical scaffold based on hybrid chitosan/cellulose/nano-hydroxyapatite membrane for bone regeneration. ACS Appl Mater Interfaces 2013;5(22):12036–44.
[40] Zhang K, et al. Electrospun silk fibroin–hydroxybutyl chitosan nanofibrous scaffolds to biomimic extracellular matrix. J Biomater Sci Polym Ed 2011;22(8):1069–82.
[41] Tang W, et al. Bioinspired trimodal macro/micro/nano-porous scaffolds loading rhBMP-2 for complete regeneration of critical size bone defect. Acta Biomaterialia 2016;32:309–23.
[42] Yi H, et al. Recent advances in nano scaffolds for bone repair. Bone Res 2016;4:16050.
[43] Sawant S, Shegokar R. Bone scaffolds: what's new in nanoparticle drug delivery research? Nanobiomater Hard Tissue Eng Appl Nanobiomater 2016:155.
[44] De la Riva B, et al. Local controlled release of VEGF and PDGF from a combined brushite–chitosan system enhances bone regeneration. J Controlled Release 2010;143(1):45–52.
[45] Teng Z, Luo Y, Wang Q. Carboxymethyl chitosan–soy protein complex nanoparticles for the encapsulation and controlled release of vitamin D 3. Food Chem 2013;141(1):524–32.
[46] Vedakumari WS, Prabu P, Sastry TP. Chitosan-fibrin nanocomposites as drug delivering and wound healing materials. J Biomed Nanotechnol 2015;11(4):657–67.
[47] Kumari S, Singh RP. Glycolic acid functionalized chitosan–Au–Fe 3 O 4 hybrid nanoparticle based nanohybrid scaffold for drug delivery. Int J Biol Macromol 2013;54:244–9.
[48] Kutlu C, Çakmak AS, Gümüşderelioğlu M. Double-effective chitosan scaffold-PLGA nanoparticle system for brain tumour therapy: in vitro study. J Microencapsulation 2014;31(7):700–7.
[49] Dev A, et al. Preparation of poly (lactic acid)/chitosan nanoparticles for anti-HIV drug delivery applications. Carbohydr Polym 2010;80(3):833–8.
[50] Eichhorn SJ, et al. Review: current international research into cellulose nanofibres and nanocomposites. J Mater Sci 2010;45(1):1–33.
[51] Fontana J, et al. Acetobacter cellulose pellicle as a temporary skin substitute. Appl Biochem Biotechnol 1990;24(1):253–64.
[52] Mello LR, et al. Use of lyophilized cellulose in peripheral nerve lesions with loss of substance. Arquivos de neuro-psiquiatria 2001;59(2B):372–9.
[53] Czaja W, et al. Microbial cellulose—the natural power to heal wounds. Biomaterials 2006;27(2):145–51.

[54] Yasuda K, et al. Biomechanical properties of high-toughness double network hydrogels. Biomaterials 2005;26(21):4468–75.
[55] Millon L, Wan W. The polyvinyl alcohol–bacterial cellulose system as a new nanocomposite for biomedical applications. J Biomed Mater Res B Appl Biomater 2006;79(2):245–53.
[56] Amorim WL, et al. Experimental study of the tissue reaction caused by the presence of cellulose produced. Braz J Otorhinolaryngol 2009;75(2):200–7.
[57] Novaes Jr AB, Novaes AB. Soft tissue management for primary closure in guided bone regeneration: surgical technique and case report. Int J Oral Maxillofac Implants 1997;12:1.
[58] Lee CH, Singla A, Lee Y. Biomedical applications of collagen. Int J Pharm 2001;221(1):1–22.
[59] Friess W. Collagen–biomaterial for drug delivery. Eur J Pharm Biopharm 1998; 45(2):113–36.
[60] Bosman FT, Stamenkovic I. Functional structure and composition of the extracellular matrix. J Pathol 2003;200(4):423–8.
[61] Gentleman E, et al. Mechanical characterization of collagen fibers and scaffolds for tissue engineering. Biomaterials 2003;24(21):3805–13.
[62] Lv Q, et al. Fibroin/collagen hybrid hydrogels with crosslinking method: preparation, properties, and cytocompatibility. J Biomed Mater Res A 2008;84(1):198–207.
[63] Marty J, Oppenheim R, Speiser P. Nanoparticles – a new colloidal drug delivery system. Pharmaceutica Acta Helvetiae 1978;53(1):17.
[64] Papi M, et al. Controlled self assembly of collagen nanoparticle. J Nanopart Res 2011;13(11):6141–7.
[65] Nicklas M, et al. Preparation and characterization of marine sponge collagen nanoparticles and employment for the transdermal delivery of 17β-estradiol-hemihydrate. Drug Dev Ind Pharm 2009;35(9):1035–42.
[66] Bender AR, et al. Efficiency of nanoparticles as a carrier system for antiviral agents in human immunodeficiency virus-infected human monocytes/macrophages in vitro. Antimicrob Agents Chemother 1996;40(6):1467–71.
[67] El-Samaligy M, Rohdewald P. Reconstituted collagen nanoparticles, a novel drug carrier delivery system. J Pharm Pharmacol 1983;35(8):537–9.
[68] Xing R, et al. Colloidal gold–collagen protein core–shell nanoconjugate: one-step biomimetic synthesis, layer-by-layer assembled film, and controlled cell growth. ACS Appl Mat Interf 2015;7(44):24733–40.
[69] Veis A. The macromolecular chemistry of gelatin. New York: Academic Press; 1964.
[70] Shutava TG, et al. Layer-by-layer-coated gelatin nanoparticles as a vehicle for delivery of natural polyphenols. ACS nano 2009;3(7):1877–85.
[71] Elzoghby AO. Gelatin-based nanoparticles as drug and gene delivery systems: reviewing three decades of research. J Controlled Release 2013;172(3):1075–91.
[72] Zwiorek K, et al. Gelatin nanoparticles as a new and simple gene delivery system. J Pharm Pharm Sci 2004;7(4):22–8.
[73] Azarmi S, et al. Optimization of a two-step desolvation method for preparing gelatin nanoparticles and cell uptake studies in 143B osteosarcoma cancer cells. J Pharm Pharm Sci 2006;9(1):124–32.
[74] Coester C, et al. Gelatin nanoparticles by two step desolvation a new preparation method, surface modifications and cell uptake. J Microencaps 2000;17(2):187–93.
[75] Qazvini NT, Zinatloo S. Synthesis and characterization of gelatin nanoparticles using CDI/NHS as a non-toxic cross-linking system. J Mater Sci Mater Med 2011;22(1): 63–9.

[76] Liang HC, et al. Genipin-crosslinked gelatin microspheres as a drug carrier for intramuscular administration: In vitro and in vivo studies. J Biomed Mater Res A 2003;65(2):271–82.
[77] Won Y-W, Kim Y-H. Recombinant human gelatin nanoparticles as a protein drug carrier. J Controlled Release 2008;127(2):154–61.
[78] Fuchs S, et al. Transglutaminase: new insights into gelatin nanoparticle cross-linking. J Microencaps 2010;27(8):747–54.
[79] Bajpai A, Choubey J. Design of gelatin nanoparticles as swelling controlled delivery system for chloroquine phosphate. J Mater Sci Mater Med 2006;17(4):345–58.
[80] Gupta AK, et al. Effect of cellular uptake of gelatin nanoparticles on adhesion, morphology and cytoskeleton organisation of human fibroblasts. J Controlled Release 2004;95(2):197–207.
[81] Lee EJ, et al. Studies on the characteristics of drug-loaded gelatin nanoparticles prepared by nanoprecipitation. Bioprocess Biosys Eng 2012;35(1-2):297–307.
[82] Yeh TK, et al. Formulating paclitaxel in nanoparticles alters its disposition. Pharm Res 2005;22(6):867–74.
[83] Zhao Y-Z, et al. Experiment on the feasibility of using modified gelatin nanoparticles as insulin pulmonary administration system for diabetes therapy. Acta diabetologica 2012;49(4):315–25.
[84] Zorzi GK, et al. Hybrid nanoparticle design based on cationized gelatin and the polyanions dextran sulfate and chondroitin sulfate for ocular gene therapy. Macromol Biosci 2011;11(7):905–13.
[85] Chen F-m, et al. Composite glycidyl methacrylated dextran (Dex-GMA)/gelatin nanoparticles for localized protein delivery. Acta Pharmacologica Sinica 2009;30(4):485–93.
[86] Xu J, Singh A, Amiji MM. Redox-responsive targeted gelatin nanoparticles for delivery of combination wt-p53 expressing plasmid DNA and gemcitabine in the treatment of pancreatic cancer. BMC Cancer 2014;14(1):1.
[87] Numata K, Kaplan DL. Silk-based delivery systems of bioactive molecules. Adv Drug Delivery Rev 2010;62(15):1497–508.
[88] Altman GH, et al. Silk-based biomaterials. Biomaterials 2003;24(3):401–16.
[89] Yan H-B, et al. Biosynthesis of insulin-silk fibroin nanoparticles conjugates and in vitro evaluation of a drug delivery system. J Nanopart Res 2009;11(8):1937–46.
[90] Lammel AS, et al. Controlling silk fibroin particle features for drug delivery. Biomaterials 2010;31(16):4583–91.
[91] Kundu J, et al. Silk fibroin nanoparticles for cellular uptake and control release. Int J Pharm 2010;388(1):242–50.
[92] Wang X, et al. Silk nanospheres and microspheres from silk/pva blend films for drug delivery. Biomaterials 2010;31(6):1025–35.
[93] Mandal BB, Kundu S. Self-assembled silk sericin/poloxamer nanoparticles as nanocarriers of hydrophobic and hydrophilic drugs for targeted delivery. Nanotechnology 2009;20(35):355101.
[94] Schenone M, Furie BC, Furie B. The blood coagulation cascade. Curr Opin Hematol 2004;11(4):272–7.
[95] Ahmed TA, Dare EV, Hincke M. Fibrin: a versatile scaffold for tissue engineering applications. Tissue Eng B Rev 2008;14(2):199–215.
[96] Whelan D, Caplice N, Clover A. Fibrin as a delivery system in wound healing tissue engineering applications. J Controlled Release 2014;196:1–8.
[97] Zangi, L., et al. Isolation with fibrin microbeads of bone marrow-derived pluripotent cell lines. In: Cell transplantation. Cognizant Communication Corp 3 Hartsdale Road, Elmsford, NY 10523-3701 USA; 2003.

[98] Praveen G, et al. Fibrin nanoconstructs: a novel processing method and their use as controlled delivery agents. Nanotechnology 2012;23(9):095102.
[99] Mohandas A, et al. Chitosan–hyaluronic acid/VEGF loaded fibrin nanoparticles composite sponges for enhancing angiogenesis in wounds. Colloids Surf B 2015;127:105–13.
[100] Scheller J, Conrad U. Plant-based material, protein and biodegradable plastic. Curr Opin Plant Biol 2005;8(2):188–96.
[101] Ezpeleta I, et al. Gliadin nanoparticles for the controlled release of all-trans-retinoic acid. Int J Pharm 1996;131(2):191–200.
[102] Lai L, Guo H. Preparation of new 5-fluorouracil-loaded zein nanoparticles for liver targeting. Int J Pharm 2011;404(1):317–23.
[103] Moire L, Rezzonico E, Poirier Y. Synthesis of novel biomaterials in plants. J Plant Physiol 2003;160(7):831–9.
[104] Geim AK, Novoselov KS. The rise of graphene. Nat Mater 2007;6(3):183–91.
[105] Schulz MJ, Shanov VN, Yun Y. Nanomedicine design of particles, sensors, motors, implants, robots, and devices. artech house; 2009.
[106] Ghasemi-Mobarakeh L, et al. Application of conductive polymers, scaffolds and electrical stimulation for nerve tissue engineering. J Tissue Eng Regener Med 2011;5(4):e17–35.
[107] Keefer EW, et al. Carbon nanotube coating improves neuronal recordings. Nat Nanotechnol 2008;3(7):434–9.
[108] Pinto AM, Gonçalves IC, Magalhães FD. Graphene-based materials biocompatibility: a review. Colloids Surf B 2013;111:188–202.
[109] Liu J, Cui L, Losic D. Graphene and graphene oxide as new nanocarriers for drug delivery applications. Acta Biomaterialia 2013;9(12):9243–57.
[110] Shin SR, et al. Graphene-based materials for tissue engineering. Adv Drug Delivery Rev 2016;105:255–74.
[111] Goenka S, Sant V, Sant S. Graphene-based nanomaterials for drug delivery and tissue engineering. J Controlled Release 2014;173:75–88.
[112] Yang Y, et al. Graphene based materials for biomedical applications. Mater Today 2013;16(10):365–73.
[113] Li N, et al. Three-dimensional graphene foam as a biocompatible and conductive scaffold for neural stem cells. Sci Rep 2013:3.
[114] Kumar S, Chatterjee K. Strontium eluting graphene hybrid nanoparticles augment osteogenesis in a 3D tissue scaffold. Nanoscale 2015;7(5):2023–33.
[115] Jabbarnia A, et al. Electrospun Fibers Incorporated With Hydroxyapatite Nanoparticles and Graphene Nanoflakes for Bone Scaffolding ASME 2012 International Mechanical Engineering Congress and Exposition. American Society of Mechanical Engineers; 2012.
[116] Dinescu S, et al. In vitro cytocompatibility evaluation of chitosan/graphene oxide 3D scaffold composites designed for bone tissue engineering. Biomed Mater Eng 2014;24(6):2249–56.
[117] Malafaya PB, Silva GA, Reis RL. Natural–origin polymers as carriers and scaffolds for biomolecules and cell delivery in tissue engineering applications. Adv Drug Delivery Rev 2007;59(4):207–33.
[118] Langer K, et al. Human serum albumin (HSA) nanoparticles: reproducibility of preparation process and kinetics of enzymatic degradation. Int J Pharm 2008;347(1):109–17.

Nanogels for biomedical applications: Drug delivery, imaging, tissue engineering, and biosensors

5

Magdalini Tsintou[1,2,*], *Cang Wang*[3,*], *Kyriakos Dalamagkas*[1,2,4], *Ding Weng*[5], *Yi-Nan Zhang*[6,**] *and Wanting Niu*[1,7,**]
[1]Harvard Medical School, Boston, MA, United States
[2]University College of London, London, United Kingdom
[3]Zhejiang University, Hangzhou, China
[4]Weiss Memorial Hospital, Chicago, IL, United States
[5]Tsinghua University, Beijing, China
[6]University of Toronto, Toronto, ON, Canada
[7]VA Boston Healthcare System, Boston, MA, United States

Abbreviations

AuNPs	gold nanoparticles
BA	boronic acid
BBB	blood brain barrier
BSA	bovine serum albumin
CAs	contrast agents
CNS	central nervous system
CuAAC	copper catalyzed azide/alkyne cycloaddition
ECM	extracellular matrix
EPR	enhanced permeation retention
GI	gastrointestinal
GSH	Glutathione
HA	hyaluronic acid
HAases	hyaluronidases
HPC–PAA	hydroxypropylcellulose–poly(acrylic acid)
IM	intramuscular
IONPs	iron oxide nanoparticles
IPNs	interpenetrated polymeric networks
IUPAC	International Union of Pure and Applied Chemistry
IV	intravenous
LCST	lower critical solution temperature

* Co-first authors and they contribute equally in this work.
** Corresponding authors.

Nanobiomaterials Science, Development and Evaluation. DOI: http://dx.doi.org/10.1016/B978-0-08-100963-5.00005-7

MMPs	matrix metalloproteinases
MRI	magnetic resonance imaging
MWNT	multiwalled nanotube
NDs	nanodiamonds
NIR	near-infrared irradiation
NPs	nanoparticles
PAA	poly(acrylic acid)
PBA	phenylboronic acid
PCL	poly(εε-caprolactone)
PDT	photodynamic therapy
PE	polyelectrolyte
PEG	poly(ethylene glycol)
PET	poly(ethylene terephthalate)
pHex	extracellular pH
PL	photoluminescence
PMAA	poly(methacrylic acid)
PNIPAM	poly(*N*-isopropylacrylamide)
P(NIPAM-co-RhBUA)	poly(*N*-isopropylacrylamide) nanogel covalently labeled rhodamine B urea derivatives
P(VPBA-DMAEA)	poly(4-vinylphenylboronic acid-co-2-(dimethylamino) ethylcrylate)
PTT	photothermal therapy
PTs	photothermal transductors
QDs	quantum dots
RH	relative humidity
SAW	surface acoustic wave
semi-IPNs	semi-interpenetrated polymeric networks
SM	single molecule
SPIONs	superparamagnetic iron oxide nanoparticles
UCST	upper critical solution temperature

5.1 Introduction

Nanogels, also known as nano-sized hydrogels or hydrogel nanoparticles (NPs), are defined as polymer gels with a sub-micrometer size (typically in the range of 20–200 nm) formed by physical or chemical cross-linking methods. In the recent decade, sudden outbreaks in nanotechnology have introduced nanogels into medical sciences, for the applications of drug delivery, gene delivery, imaging, biosensors, and so on. With the combined properties of both hydrogel and NP systems, nanogels have gained noticeable research and application interests in recent years. Nanogels have high colloidal stability, both in vitro and in vivo; they also offer the opportunity to load large amounts of drugs without chemical reactions and they have unique, easily tunable release behavior [1]. Their nano-scale size and tailored special surface properties offer nanogels many advantages as vehicles for delivery of small molecules, proteins, genes, and composite drugs since they have the abilities of reaching the capillary vessels, passing blood brain barrier (BBB). Even though some nanogels may escape from the recognition of immune system to perform their duties, the majority of the administrated dose is still sequestrated by the mononuclear phagocyte system [2–4].

Nanogels could be classified as stimuli-responsive or nonresponsive gels. The nonresponsive gels simply swell after absorbing water, but the volume or structure of stimuli-responsive gels changes with response to the fluctuation of environmental factors, such as temperature, pH, pressure, electric and magnetic field, molecular species, ionic strength, and the combination of more than one factors [1,2]. Most of the functional nanogels are developed based on those sensibilities of the stimuli-responsive polymers.

This chapter introduces the material types and properties of broadly used nanogel systems, then explore their biomedical applications in the fields of drug delivery, imaging, tissue engineering, regenerative medicine, and biosensors.

5.2 Materials and methods for selected nanogel systems

Hydrogels are usually built up with three dimensional (3D) cross-linked hydrophilic polymers, which could be classified as natural and synthetic materials, or as positively and negatively charged polymers. This polymer backbone forms the hydrated network which mimics the porous native tissue microenvironment and is friendly in terms of encapsulating molecules or cells [4]. Gelation time, gel stiffness, and degradability are key factors that must be considered in the design processes. Gelation method could be selected based on the functional groups attached to the polymeric backbones.

Two distinct designs of nanogel systems are polymer hydrogel NPs and functional inorganic NPs entrapped in a hydrogel shell. The polymer framework could also be designed as regular continuous networks, interpenetrated networks (IPNs), or semi-interpenetrated polymer networks (semi-IPNs).

The International Union of Pure and Applied Chemistry (IUPAC) defines IPNs as "two or more networks that are at least partially interlaced on a molecular scale, but not covalently bonded to each other and cannot be separated unless chemical bonds are broken" [5]. The final products of IPNs require enhanced mechanical properties and phase stabilities. The network will not be ruined if one component is degraded. Noncovalent semi-IPN is termed as only one component of the polymeric network cross-linked with the other one in a linear form. Covalent semi-IPN has two independent polymeric systems cross-linked together as a single network [6]. Core-cell polymeric nanogels are heterogeneous, but stable complexes that are made of completely distinct, covalently bound compartments.

The typical methods of nanogel preparation could be summarized as physical methods (i.e., emulsification and diffusion method, double homogenization method, self-assembling method) and chemical cross-linking methods (i.e., photo-cross-linking, enzyme catalyzed cross-linking, electromagnetic radiation polymerization).

5.2.1 Chitosan-based nanogels

Chitosan is one of the most common hydrophilic cationic polysaccharide, which is usually prepared through *N*-deacetylating chitin. Because of D-glucosamine and

N-acetyl-D-glucosamine units, chitosan presents a pKa value around 6.5 that can easily aggregate under physiological conditions. Therefore, nanogels based on chitosan can be divided into three main catalogs: self-assembled, ionic cross-linked, and chemically cross-linked. In self-assembled chitosan nanogels, chitosan is usually given amphiphilic property through the modification of hydrophobic groups, which is the simplest way to prepare chitosan nanogels without surfactant or cross-linker that may cause side effects [7]. However, its strong cationic charge still cause aggregation under physiological conditions. Therefore, Makhlof et al. employed ethylene glycol group to increase chitosan's water solubility and prepared self-assembled chitosan nanogels with deoxycholic acid as hydrophobic moity [8]. On the other hand, this strong cationic charge makes chitosan cross-linkable with anionic (PEs), for example, alginate, DNA, hyaluronic acid (HA), tripolyphosphate, etc. to form ionic cross-linked nanogels [9–14]. Size, surface charge, and stability of formed nanogel can be adjusted by the solution concentration, molecular weight of chitosan, the nonstoichiometric ratio of anionic/cationic polymers, and the ionic strength [15–18].

Chitosan nanogels can also be prepared by chemically cross-linking amino groups on its backbone with various cross-linkers, which offer better stability, structure, and drug release properties [7]. PEG-based cross-linker are commonly used to react with amino groups on chitosan molecules. For instance, Jin et al. reported that dialdehyde-caped poly(ethylene glycol) (PEG) were applied with ultrasonic spray to form urokinase-loaded chitosan nanogels without using surfactant [19]. In another study, Yong and Gan used PEG dicarboxylic acid to fix reversed mini-emulsion of chitosan, which resulted in mono-dispersed nanogels and tunable sizes [20].

5.2.2 Gelatin based nanogels

Gelatin, as a valuable protein-based natural biopolymer, is widely used in tissue engineering, drug delivery, food industries, costume and drug industries, etc. Gelatin is mainly obtained from hydrolyzed triple-helix collagen, which grants it great biocompatibility and biodegradability.

Gelatin is a polyampholyte protein and can be easily modified and cross-linked since it contained large amounts of amino groups and acid groups. Gelatin nanogel can be prepared using simple desolvation method. Saraogi et al. added acetone as nonsolvent into gelatin water solution and fixed with glutaraldehyde, which resulted in gelatin nanogels with a size around 260 nm [21]. Reversed mini-emulsion is another approach to prepare gelatin nanogels. Briefly, gelatin was first cross-linked with *N,N′*-methylenebis(acrylamide), then radically polymerized to form semi-IPN structure. The products were further cross-linked by glutaraldehyde to complete IPN nanogels with a mono-dispersed size around 255 nm [22].

5.2.3 Hyaluronic acid based nanogels

Hyaluronic acid, as the only nonsulfated glycosaminoglycan, is a special polysaccharide in synovial fluid and extracellular matrix (ECM) [23]. Similar to the situation of chitosan, HA nanogel can be prepared by self-assembly by increasing its hydrophobicity via conjugating with tetradecylamine [24]. The size of nanogels decreases when the degree of substitution of hydrophobic moieties increases due to their smaller and tighter hydrophobic core in physiological conditions. Moreover, anionic HA in physiological also allows ionic bond forming with cationic polymers like chitosan, PEI, and polyarginine [13,14,25,26].

5.2.4 Poly(ethylene glycol) based nanogels

PEG, also known as poly(oxyethylene) or poly(ethylene oxide) (PEO), depending on the molecular weights (Mw <100,000 are called PEGs, while higher Mw polymers are classified as PEOs). It is a synthetic amphiphilic polymer which is soluble in water and many organic solvents (e.g., methylene chloride, ethanol, toluene, acetone, and chloroform). PEGs with Mw < 1000 are viscous liquids which are nontoxic and could be quickly cleaned from the body. It has been approved for biomedical application by Food and Drug Administration (FDA). The terminal $–CH_2OH$ groups and the interior $–CH_2OCH_2–$groups of PEG are expected to have chemical interactions with various functional groups of proteins [27], thus PEG is considered to be a perfect candidate of protein drug delivery vehicles, tissue engineering scaffolds, and biosensing membranes.

To accomplish targeted delivery of anticancer drugs to the tumor adjacent area (where pH is lower than normal tissue), with long blood circulation time and reduced nonspecific interactions with serum proteins, a novel design of PEG-based nanogels (PEGylated gels) with core–shell structure was prepared by using emulsion polymerization method. The derived poly(2-*N*,*N*-(diethylamino)ethyl methacrylate) (PEAMA) cores had hydrodynamic diameters in the range of 93–103 nm, with zeta potential of 3.4–6.4 mV under physiological pH 7.4; while with larger size of 115–141 nm and zeta potential of 0.03–0.3 mV under lower pH at 5.5 when the PEG-based gel NPs are in the swollen status. Thereafter, the PEAMA cores were covered via the Menschutkin reaction using bromobenzyl-terminated short PEG, and the nanogel half-life in the bloodstream can be prolonged [28].

5.2.5 Poly(N-isopropylacrylamide) based nanogels

Poly(*N*-isopropylacrylamide) (PNIPAM) is a “smart” polymer which has been most extensively investigated for environmentally sensitive applications, for example, drug delivery and biosensing membrane, because of its temperature and pH-responsive properties. PNIPAM can be easily modified with N-hydroxysuccinimide (NHS) ester, carboxylic acid, amine, and maleimide groups. It can also be copolymerized with other molecules, such as methacrylic acid. Based on this concept, a series of functional polymers have been developed based on PNIPAM [29]. PNIPAM’s volume phase transition (VPT) temperature is at 32°C in water. Heating above this lower critical solution temperature (LCST) leads to a rapid phase transition from hydrophilic to hydrophobic, and a collapsed state [30].

In order to reduce the cytotoxicity of nano-sized airborne pollutes, melatonin loaded PNIPAM nanogels were developed by mixing monomers of *N*-isopropylacrylamide

(NIPAM) and acrylic acid (AAc) with cross-linker poly(ethylene glycol) diacrylate, then gelated by adding ammonium persulfate (APS) under mechanical agitation. The final products of PNIPAM nanogels have hydrodynamic diameters in a range of 765–955 nm, with surface zeta potential about −10 mV at 25°C, while the size decreased to 178–450 nm when temperature increased to 37°C [31]. In another study [30], doxorubicin (DOX), a potential anticancer drug, was delivered using thermoresponsive N,O-carboxymethyl chitosan-conjugated PNIPAM-based nanogels, called poly(*N*-isopropylacrylamide-co-1-propene-2-3-dicarboxylate-co-2-acrylamido-2-methyl-1-propanesulfonate [poly(NIPAAm-IA-AMPS)]. These nanogels were chemically cross-linked with co-monomers NIPAM and itaconic acid (IA), with cross-linkers of 2-acrylamido-2-methylpropanesulfonic acid (AMPS) and ethylene glycol dimethacrylate at 75°C, then initiated gelation by adding APS slowly under vigorous stirring. After dialysis purification, the derived poly(NIPAAm-IA-AMPS) nanogels showed hydrodynamic diameters of 221 ± 3 nm and 198 ± 3 nm, with surface zeta potential about −30 mV and −32 mV (with high colloidal stability) at temperatures of 25°C and 37°C, respectively. The derived nanogels could be further grafted by N,O-carboxymethyl chitosan (NOCC) via classical 1-ethyl-3-(3-(dimethylamino) propyl)-carbodiimide-mediated coupling chemistry.

5.2.6 Hydrogel-nanoparticle composites

Nowadays, many kinds of NPs have found applications in biomedical fields and they have been commercialized, while most of them are still facing the concerns regarding the stability and cytotoxic issues. These challenges are expected to be overcome by incorporating nanogel technologies into the hydrogel-NP composites that have demonstrated enhanced properties, in order to further advance the resulting products.

Encapsulating metal NPs, especially optical or magnetic responding metals, with colloidal polymer shells, to construct core–shell nanogels is of great interest for biomedical imaging. There are in general two methods to construct functional metal NP–hydrogel composites: by using polymers containing strong metal binding ligands or by depositing polymers from the metal surface via covalent attachment or electrostatic interactions [32].

Nanogel contrast agents (CAs) have been developed for magnetic resonance imaging (MRI) [6] and positron emission tomography (PET) [33] in recent years, with most of them being based on metal chelating cross-linked nanogel technique. T_1 MRI CA, gadolinium (Gd)-chelating self-assembled pullulan NPs were prepared by cross-linking the surface acryloyl groups of cholesteryl-modified pullulan with 1,4,7,10-tetraazacyclododecane-1,4,7,10-teraacetic acid, then formulating Gd with UV irradiation. The hydrodynamic size of this product was 65 ± 7 nm, which is efficiently retained in tumors over 7 days, and provide sixfold higher T_1 relaxivity than Magnevist and Dotarem in a 1.4 T imaging system. The pullulan nanogels could be cleared from the body ~20 days post-injection, without organ dysfunction [34]. By using similar metal chelating skills, the same group successfully trapped ^{64}Cu into the backbones of polyacrylamide, and prepared nanogel particles with hydrodynamic size in the range of 56–65 nm with different cross-linkers. This nanogels could be accumulated in tumors and be used as PET/MRI CAs [33].

5.3 Nanogels as carriers for bioactive molecules delivery

5.3.1 The clinical problem and the ideal platform for bioactive molecules delivery

A drug delivery system is defined as "a formulation or a device that enables the introduction of a therapeutic substance in the body and improves its efficacy and safety by controlling the rate, time, and place of release of drugs in the body" [35]. Conventional drug delivery methods involve the formulation of a drug into a form which is suitable based on the route of delivery. For example, a compressed tablet would be developed if the drug is needed for per os (oral) administration, whereas a solution would be developed for parenteral use, for example, intravenous (IV) or intramuscular (IM) use. There are several routes for systemic drug delivery, such as gastrointestinal (GI)/enteral, parenteral, transmucosal, transnasal, pulmonary, transdermal, and intra-osseous. Each route of delivery is inherently linked to certain advantages and disadvantages [36].

Especially when a drug is being administered per os, the concentration of the administered drug needs to be much higher in order to accomplish therapeutic effects to the end organ due to several obstacles that the drug has to overcome until the destination is reached, like the significant first pass metabolism of the drug after an oral dose (for many drugs this occurs in the liver) [37]. Parenteral drug administration might be advantageous in terms of the rapid onset of action and the predictable and almost complete bioavailability of the drug due to the bypass of GI tract metabolism. The pain related to the injection of the drug (sometimes in multiple areas to avoid tissue damage due to repeated local tissue exposure to the drug) is a major problem though that lead to poor patients' compliance compared to per os administration. In addition, sustained release of the drugs and targeted delivery through parenteral route of administration is still a challenge. An extensive overview of the conventional drug delivery platforms is beyond the scope of this section.

In General, the conventional drug delivery methods demonstrate lower effectiveness and are linked to toxicity and adverse effects due to the generalized effect that can extend to the healthy tissue, especially in high doses. Therefore, there has been a significant clinical need for the development of other more advanced drug delivery systems in order to overcome the current limitations linked to the conventional methods. The newly developed systems are mostly aiming in effective, controlled drug delivery, and targeted effect to a specific tissue or even to specific cells.

Key aspects that would define an ideal drug or protein delivery platform would relate to: (1) the encapsulation stability of the delivery system, so that the drug does not leak prematurely to the circulation causing unwanted effects to other tissues; (2) the effective response to certain stimuli that would allow the release of the drug only within the desired tissue or under certain circumstances; (3) the size-controlled passive targeting of certain impaired tissues (e.g., cancerous tissues) due to the enhanced permeation retention (EPR) effect that allows the local permeation of macromolecules in the range of 20–200nm; (4) the active targeting of certain disease phenotypes, using specific ligands that are incorporated within the structure of the carrier, in order to interact with the microenvironment and reduce adverse effects; (5) the biodegradability that would leave no "leftovers" that could induce inflammation/toxicity in the body and the lack of toxicity of the directly used delivery system, but also of its indirectly produced byproducts after metabolic processing in the body; and, finally, (6) the ease of synthesis that would be crucial for scaling up production and for the ultimate approval by regulatory bodies such as the FDA [38].

With the recent advances in the field of nanotechnology, nanogels and/or nanocomposite gels for biomolecules delivery applications seem to be ticking most of the boxes of the "ideal" delivery platform. Therefore, in the future, we can only expect that nanomedicine will be more and more implemented in clinical practice to improve the patients' medical care.

5.3.2 Hydrogels versus nanogels for bioactive molecules delivery

Originally, hydrogels were developed in order to be used as stand-alone biomaterials due to their inherent low protein absorption that allowed them to minimize host response (which is part of the umbrella term of biocompatibility) or as devices for controlled release applications [5,6,39,40]. Nevertheless, hydrogels were also used for cell encapsulation approaches opening new pathways in the field, and starting a trend to aim much more for bioactive than for bioinert materials. Based on the needed application, the classification category of a hydrogel (its porosity, physical structure, source, ionic charge, crosslinks, etc.) gives a lot of information on whether a hydrogel is appropriate for a specific tissue repair attempt or the delivery of a bioactive substance (e.g., drug, growth factors, cells, etc.) to the cells or tissues may promote a certain effect.

Hydrogels that are biocompatible, biodegradable, porous (to allow sustained local delivery of cells or biomolecules), and functionalized with certain molecules gradually become available with encouraging outcomes. No matter how promising this may be, after extensive studies for controlled drug release, most hydrogels seem to demonstrate a slower hydration response to changes in stimuli compared to the needed reaction time that would allow therapeutic clinical applications [39,41–44]. This has motivated researchers to gradually shift their attention to develop hydrogels in the micro- or nano-scale [45]. For the time being, nanogels are considered the best vehicles for drug delivery due to their nano-scale-related properties (e.g., longer circulation times).

Nanogels are nano-sized hydrogel, this does not imply that nanogels escape the natural barriers of the human body and the natural metabolic processing due to their nano-scale related properties. The routes of administrations are still the same for nanogels as described above, thereafter there are certain limitations that researchers have been trying to overcome. Fig. 5.1 demonstrates the physical barriers obstructing the effective administration of the drug to the end organ, even via the use of nanogels delivery systems [46]. Nevertheless, the superiority of nanogels lies in their multifunctionality, stability, and flexibility. Each nanogel's characteristics (e.g., size, charge, porosity, amphiphilicity, softness, and biodegradability) can be easily tuned

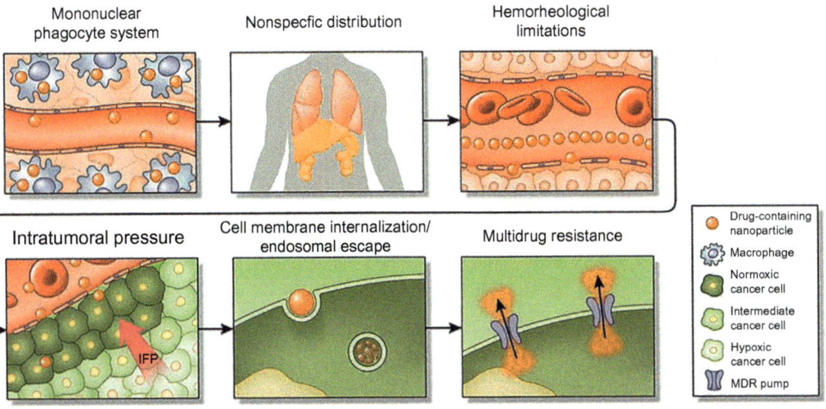

Figure 5.1 This is an illustrative demonstration of the barriers that the nanogels encounter after parenteral administration. Under normal circumstances NPs would undergo the process of opsonization that is mediated by residual macrophages. This would lead to a nonspecific distribution of the nanogel in healthy tissues such as the liver and the spleen. In addition, due to vascular dynamics, spherical particles in the nano-scale would limit their interactions with the endothelial cells of the blood vessels, reducing their distribution in the tissues (either via active or passive targeting mechanisms). Another significant barrier that impedes the nanogels accumulation in the desired tissues (e.g., cancerous tissues) regards the high intratumoral pressure that can stem from impaired vasculature, aggressive cellular proliferation, fibrosis, dense ECM formation, and impaired lymphatics. In addition, endocytosis can follow different routes (e.g., via clathrin-coated pits or caveolae) depending on the size and surface decoration of the nanogels, thereby directly affecting the fate of the carrier. After the process of endocytosis, endolysosomal degradation in a low pH environment is detrimental to the cargo, especially for genetic material. Last but not least, if the nanocarrier survives up to that point, it may be expelled by certain drug efflux pumps that have been correlated with multidrug resistance (i.e., MDR pumps), inhibiting the effective release of the therapeutic. Reproduced with permission from Schmitt F, Lagopoulos L, Kauper P, Rossi N, Busso N, Barge J, et al. Chitosan-based nanogels for selective delivery of photosensitizers to macrophages and improved retention in and therapy of articular joints. J Control Release 2010:144;242–50. Copyright © 2015 Macmillan Publishers Limited, part of Springer Nature.

through changes in the chemical composition of the gel, directly affecting its loading capacity, metabolic processing, and spatial distribution in the human body [47–49]. Thus, certain design implementations, as presented in Fig. 5.2, have addressed initial limitations discussed in Fig. 5.1.

Functionalization of the nanogel's membrane with biomimetic molecules (e.g., grafting PEG or CD47 "self" peptides to the surface, coating with biomimetic extracted membranes from autologous leukocytes or red blood cells) is an example of one of the most classically used strategies in more new nanogel delivery systems that has allowed escape of the nanogels from phagocytic opsonization and sequestration processes. Likewise, endolysosomal degradation of the nanogel and/or the embedded therapeutic molecule has been avoided with the use of membrane-destabilizing

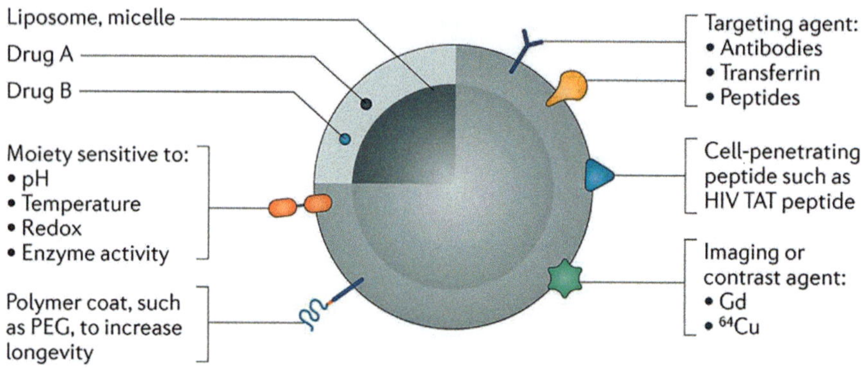

Figure 5.2 If drug A and drug B are two different drugs that are loaded within the nanocarrier, this is a representation of the potential agents that can be added to the initial structure in order to maximize the therapeutic or diagnostic potentials. Depending on the purpose of the nanocomposite, certain targeting agents can be added to increase specificity of the carrier for a particular tissue or to improve blood circulation times and cell penetration. Other added agents may enable imaging applications providing the opportunity for a theranostics platform or may induce specific stimuli-based reactions (e.g., stimuli-based controlled drug release).
Reproduced with permission from Gwak SJ, Jung JK, An SS, Kim HJ, Oh JS, Pennant WA, et al. Chitosan/TPP-hyaluronic acid nanoparticles: a new vehicle for gene delivery to the spinal cord. J Biomater Sci Polym Ed. 2012:23;1437 – 50. Copyright © 2014 Macmillan Publishers Limited, part of Springer Nature.

peptides, which induces an escape mechanism, or with the use of biomimetic ligands or membranes, which allows cellular internalization and safe transportation of the nanocarrier. To the same direction, the utilization of nontraditional geometries has led to improved vascular dynamics. Blanco et al. have published an extensive analysis of the different strategies that have been used to address the initially discovered limitations linked to NP-based drug delivery [46].

Last but not least, an important and unique advantage of the use of nanogels regards the ability of the nanogels to incorporate a wide range of entities that vary in physical properties (from biomacromolecules such as proteins or drugs, up to inorganic materials, allowing the use not only in theranostics but also in imaging/screening applications and combinatorial approaches). This property stems from the versatility of the nanogels' architecture and this is what makes nanogels such a promising tool in the field of nanomedicine, with potential clinical applications that are not limited to therapeutic interventions, but also to the field of diagnostology and imaging (with the use of the newly developed class of agents named "nanohybrids," incorporating inorganic materials for imaging applications) [50,51].

5.3.3 Nanogels as therapeutic drug carriers

As previously discussed, nanogels simultaneously possess features and characteristics of hydrogels and nano-scale systems. Smart nanogels have attracted much attention for their translational medical therapeutic potentials, due to their capacity to respond to multiple diverse environmental stimuli such as pH, temperature, ionic force, redox environment, etc. by changing their volume, refractive index, and hydrophilicity/hydrophobicity [52].

When compared to macroscopic hydrogels, nanogels demonstrate faster responsiveness. They also allow the penetration of the BBB, demonstrating safe and efficient delivery of macromolecules across the barrier. This can be highly impactful in terms of clinical applications such as for the treatment of malignant brain tumors. Nanogels are also considered to be excellent carriers for drugs when sustained, prolonged drug release is desired. For example, when inhaled, it has been postulated that the swellable nanogels are poorly cleared in the lungs, increasing the circulation times, thereafter maximizing the time of the biomolecule sustained release [53,54]. In terms of their loading potentials, they are considered to have a great loading capacity with the ability to carry a wide variety of drugs (e.g., drugs of both low and high molecular weight, both hydrophobic and hydrophilic drugs) for several clinical applications [55].

As mentioned above, many NPs are designed as core–shell structures for drug delivery applications. The core–shell polymeric nanogels are inhomogenous, but stable complexes that are made of completely distinct, but covalently bound compartments. Therefore, such nanocomposite hydrogel matrices are thought to be innovative means for optimized modulation of the parameters linked to the drug/protein release rate from the matrix [56]. Given the design-specific compartmentalization of the nanocomposite systems, a multistimuli-response has become feasible using nanocomposite hydrogel matrices, allowing the targeted release of bioactive substances under certain conditions in different parts of the body, significantly enhancing previously used hydrogel models. These targeted drug delivery systems have captivated increasing attention, mainly in cancer therapy. The higher temperature and lower pH linked to cancer tissues compared to normal tissues makes the use of thermo- and pH-responsive nanocomposite systems useful for cancer theranostics [57–59]. They also allow the effective incorporation of hydrophobic drugs [60,61], which was previously known to be challenging with other carriers. The major advantage of those advanced matrices is the tunability, given the higher allowed level of control, which is required for effective tissue engineering applications. Nagahama et al. recently reported a novel controlled drug release system [62], highlighting the high levels of control that can be obtained with such advanced systems. The injectable gel he developed via the method of self-assembly of copolymer micelles clay nanodisks and doxorubicin gave a dual property to the drug; in particular the drug was not only acting as a cross-linker for the formation of gel networks, but it also enabled control over its own release.

An interesting approach that is meant to enable optimal, controlled external stimulation of the drug release from the nanogel or nanocomposite gel to enable a controlled external stimulation for initiating the drug release from such hydrogels (e.g., via light or electrical and magnetic fields exposure) have been increasingly studied [63–65].

Photothermal therapy (PTT) and photodynamic therapy (PDT) are currently the most promising techniques for the treatment of cancer [66]. They are mostly based on the utilization of plasmonic hybrid nanogels (e.g., nanogels hybridized mostly with gold or silver NPs) that efficiently absorb and scatter light. The nanogels' increasing use towards that direction could potentially revolutionize the oncology clinical practice.

Another major breakthrough in the field of nanotechnology has been the recent development of self-healing injectable nanogels or nanocomposite hydrogels. In general, self-healing materials are commonly found in living organism, but some years ago, it was unimaginable that such a self-healing system would be possible to be created artificially. Contrary to traditional injectable hydrogels, transient and reversible interactions governing the conformation of self-healing nanocomposites allow them to flow and deform into liquids under excessive strain and recover back into hydrogels when higher strain is removed [67–71], demonstrating new potentials for tissue engineering applications.

5.3.4 Nanogels in diagnostics and imaging

Theranostics is a combinatorial therapeutic and diagnostic approach using multifunctional platforms (e.g., nanogels) [72]. In the clinical setting, theranostics is an important field that can significantly benefit oncology-related pathologies. MRI is one of the most effective tools for the timely diagnosis of cancer in early stages. Nevertheless, MRI is relatively insensitive, frequently requiring the use of tailored CAs in order to enhance image contrast, thereby effectively highlighting anatomical and pathological features of the imaged tissues [73]. Just like small therapeutic biomolecules, CAs suffer from short blood circulating times, nonspecific biodistribution, and noncontrolled release, while they can also exhibit cytotoxic effects [74]. For example, gadolinium (Gd^{3+}) ion is toxic, but in order to be safe for clinical administration for imaging purposes, it is given in the form of chelates. Even chelates though have been found to be more sensitive to transmetallation reactions that can displace the chelated metal ion by another competing ion, leading to toxic effects. Contrary to that, certain nanogels have been reported to be more inert to transmetallation reactions, reducing that possibility further [75].

As mentioned before, it is the unique characteristics of nanogels that make them ideal carriers for a variety of imaging probes and CAs, opening a new pathway in theranostics and imaging applications. Nanogels that have recently been used for theranostic and/or imaging applications belong to another category of hybrid inorganic–organic materials (the so-called "nanohybrids"). These nanogels are hybridized with inorganic NPs (e.g., plasmonic, magnetic, and carbonaceous materials-based NPs). The inorganic NPs can either interact with the nanogel through strong chemical bonds like covalent or Lewis acid–base bonds or solely through weak forces like hydrogen bonding, van der Waals and electrostatic forces [76,77]. Fig. 5.3 is an illustrative presentation of such a hybrid nanogel, aiming at theranostic applications for cancer. In this particular example, imaging-guided drug delivery is targeted towards the cancerous cells upon exposure to ultrasound signals [78].

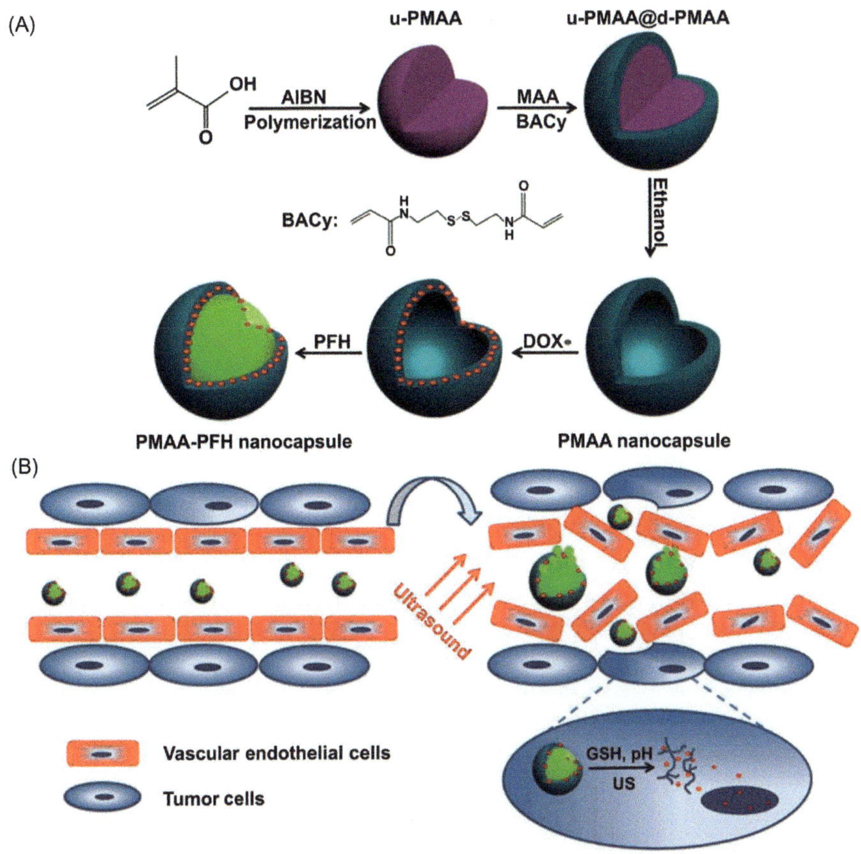

Figure 5.3 (A) Schematic representation of the preparation of doxorubicin (DOX)-loaded poly (methacrylic acid)-perfluorohexane (PMAA-PFH) nanocapsules as described by Vashist et al. [54]. (B) Schematic illustration of an imaging-guided drug delivery system based on the previously seen biodegradable PMAA-PFH nanocapsules. Drug delivery is triggered by ultrasound signals exposure.
Reproduced with permission from Ghasemi A, Mohtashami M, Sheijani SS, Aliakbari K. Chitosan-genipin nanohydrogel as a vehicle for sustained delivery of alpha-1 antitrypsin. Res Pharm Sci 2015;10(6):523–34. Copyright © 2016 Elsevier.

Given the promising applications of nanohybrids in the field of theranostics and nanomedicine, there has been an increasing number of studies exploring the development of more advanced hybrids for combinatorial applications [79]. The ability of plasmonic NPs to absorb and scatter light has increased the popularity of the nanogels that are hybridized with gold nanoparticles (AuNPs), acting as phototherapeutic agents that target malignant cells [80–83]. Apart from the encouraging results in the field of PTT and PDT, plasmonic NPs also have imaging properties, along with their controlled drug release profile, when combined with nanogels [84].

Another interesting nanohybrid that has great potential in theranostic applications is a result of the hybridization with magnetic NPs. Such hybridization allows manipulation of the carrier via magnetic fields. This allows nanohybrids to be guided by magnetic fields directly to the tumor site, thereby improving the efficacy and reducing any cytotoxic effects of the incorporated substances [85–87]. A common approach to create these nanohybrids is to combine the nanogels with superparamagnetic iron oxide nanoparticles (SPIONs) [88]. The magnetic field can, simultaneously, induce multiple potential reactions, such as chemotherapy delivery, hyperthermia therapy, and diagnostic imaging contrast in MRI [89]. On the other hand, quantum dots (QDs), which exhibit unique optical and electronic properties (e.g., wideband excitation, phenomenal photostability, and high quantum yield) have attracted intensive interest in the biomedical field, while having their own role in diagnostic imaging applications. Entrapment of semiconductor QDs that emit fluorescent light into the polymeric nanogel can also confer imaging properties to the nanohybrids [90,91].

Carbonaceous NPs were not traditionally implemented in theranostics applications. Nevertheless, a particular allotropic form of carbon (i.e., nanodiamonds, NDs) has been considered for bio-imaging, biosensing, and therepautic applications lately. Apart from the unique properties that NDs gain due to their distinctive surface architecture [92,93], they are also proven to be biocompatible in several in vitro and in vivo studies, providing an alternative for theranostics approaches [94,95].

Undoubtedly, utilization of the aforementioned techniques would lead to the development of smart nanogels that could, in turn, address a variety of currently incurable diseases from different angles. Thus, there has been an increasing number of studies that have summarized the preparation of different multifunctional hybrid NPs and their applications in theranostics.

5.4 Tissue engineering applications—potential applications of nanogels in selected fields

Nanogels have been increasingly used in several fields such as sensing, diagnostics, and biomedical engineering, but their most impactful applications are in the area of drug/biomolecules delivery.

Traditionally, tissue engineering scaffolds were based on degradable macroporous materials that could induce a "passive" reparative process through the release of therapeutics. Contrary to that, the current trend in the field is the use of bioactive materials with nano-topographical features that closely resemble the native tissue (e.g., natural ECM), aiming at directly affecting and guiding the restorative process. This comes as no surprise, given the fact that tissue engineering scaffolds are meant to act as temporary, supportive, artificial ECM to accommodate cells, and guide 3D tissue formation [39].

The sectors of tissue engineering and drug delivery are two closely related areas. Tissue engineering is mostly used as a means of combinatorial therapeutic approaches. It does not only provide the scaffolds/hydrogels for structural support to, physically, help bridging the damaged area, but it also allows the scaffolds/hydrogels to act as sustained release biomolecules vehicles in order to guide cellular responses and/or directly engage in the reparative process. The induced cellular response in the microenvironment can, subsequently, enhance the efficacy of the supportive scaffold/hydrogel [39]. Therefore, many times tissue engineering can be viewed as a special case of advanced drug delivery. We can actually realize that when talking about nanogels or nanocomposite gels, the terms drug delivery and tissue engineering applications can be used interchangeably. This is because nanogels are already nano-engineered carriers that provide not only a highly efficient platform for therapeutics encapsulation, but also a versatile, protected and controlled delivery system that can be autoregulated based on certain stimuli.

Although tissue engineering constructs can be developed in the micro- or macro-scale based on the required application, incorporation of NPs within a scaffold or hydrogel (e.g., nanocomposite hydrogels) and/or the ability to manipulate nano-scale parameters of the scaffold (i.e., via 3D nanoprinting technique) are crucial for the effective reparative outcome. Not only the implementation of nano-scale factors (e.g., NPs) can greatly improve the field of tissue engineering, but also tissue engineering methodologies can directly affect and improve nano-scale parameters. In particular, the tremendous problem of the poor reproducibility of reported research results, which has been expressed several times in the medical research literature, also affects the field of nanotechnology [96]. It is very hard to precisely control nano-scale elements of a nanogel/nanocomposite hydrogel obtaining a highly standardized and reproducible model.

To that direction, there has been an increasing interest for the development of 3D nanoprinting technology, which is thought to lead the field to a future revolution. The attempts to accomplish a good reproducibility in a nano-scale level though 3D printing have already become more intense, leading to the recent emergence of a new pending patent on 3D nanoprinting via scanning probe lithography-delivered layer-by-layer deposition. This protocol enables the conduction of 3D printing with nanometer precision and inter-layer registry in all three dimensions, using PE inks and atomic force microscopy [97].

Therefore, the accomplishments in the field of nanomedicine with the use of nanogels are already significant and promising, but, they can be enhanced through the utilization of tissue engineering advancements. This way the field can advance further, moving towards clinical translation, in order to improve the quality of care in many different medical areas in the future.

This section aims at introducing some nanogel-based tissue engineering applications in different medical areas analyzing the rationale behind nanogels' use. Nanogels can obviously be used in a wide range of medical areas such as oncology, radiology, neurology, dermatology, infectious diseases, pulmonology, gene therapy, and many more, while this list will keep expanding more and more due to the introduction of novel nanogel-based systems based on clinical needs. Therefore, we mainly focus our attention, thereby dedicating a significant portion of this section to oncology-related applications, due to the significant contribution of nanogels to this field of nanomedicine. Other applications in systems like musculoskeletal, central nervous system (CNS), and cardiovascular are also noted but the extensive analysis within seperate sub-sections goes beyond the scope of this chapter. Key aspects on the rationale behind the nanogels' use in the analyzed fields of tissue engineering and nanomedicine are of high importance for the deeper understanding of the field, but also for the future advancement of developed nano-engineered materials, therefore they are highlighted in each sub-section.

5.5 Nanogels in oncology

5.5.1 The clinical need and current limitations in oncology theranostics

Although cancer therapeutics have greatly advanced to the point that many oncology patients are able to live a normal and long life, surviving cancer, cancer remains one of the major examples of ineffective therapeutic strategies in current clinical practice. To be more specific, chemotherapy is a commonly used therapeutic approach, applicable for many types of cancer. Nevertheless, the delivery of conventional chemotherapeutics is still challenging and it is also directly linked to significant adverse effects [98] that have urged many patients with advanced cancers to decline therapy in order to "respectfully" live their lives with their families. Different chemotherapeutic agents may cause different side effects like fatigue, pain, mouth and throat sores, change in bowel habits, nausea and vomiting, blood disorders, nervous system effects, cognitive alterations, sexual and reproductive issues, appetite loss, hair loss, or other long term effects damaging certain tissues (e.g., heart, liver, kidneys, etc.). The toxicity of those drugs and adverse effects are related to issues with the drugs solubility, poor pharmacokinetics, and in vivo stability.

To avoid the unwanted side effects and promote targeted delivery of therapeutics to the cancerous tissues, immunomodulatory methods have emerged. These methods use antigenic proteins, peptides, or nucleic acids for direct targeting of the cancerous cells-related abnormalities (e.g., defects in antiapoptotic proteins, inducing uncontrollable cell proliferation) in order to promote a more effective reaction, specifically aiming for the anomalous cells [99]. However, there are certain downsides linked to traditional immunomodulatory biologics, such as the low transfection efficacy, serious adverse effects (e.g., serious infections, malignancy, cytokine release syndrome, anaphylaxis, and immunogenicity), as well as uncontrollable and untraceable gene transfer [100]. Thus, the clinical need for the development of efficient tools for cancer-related theranostics remains. This has shifted scientific attention to the field of nanotechnology, with a focus on nanogels due to their versatile, promising properties that may help to minimize adverse effects, maximize targeted therapeutics uptake, and overcome physical normal or disease-related barriers.

5.5.2 Rationale for use of nanogels: Advantages over conventional methods

Nanogels and nanocomposite gels seem to be uniquely qualified for the development of novel oncology-related theranostics, overcoming most of the limitations that are linked to the use of conventional therapeutics. The tunability and multifunctionality of the nanogels as discussed in the section of drug delivery is of high importance for nanomedicine and tissue engineering applications. In particular, using versatile surface modifications and altering the size and shape of the nanogels, passive or active drug targeting can be accomplished, despite the presence of multiple physical barriers that would normally halt delivery [38]. Surface biofunctionalization techniques also allow controlled and targeted release of the embedded biomolecule, while the increased surface/volume ratio of NPs facilitate the transfer of large cargos to the desired area. A significant advantage linked to the effective nanogels-based drug release regards the capability of the nanogels to load large amounts of payload without the need of chemical reactions that might be detrimental for the drug's bioactivity. Finally, the use of nanocarriers in oncology provide an advanced vehicle for drug delivery, enabling improved solubility, stability, and penetration of the embedded drug, regardless of the obstacles that are associated with the particular route of drug administration used. Challenging issues that are used to raise problems in the delivery of therapeutics (e.g., hydrophilicity/hydrophobicity of the embedded molecule) have now been resolved thanks to nanocarriers design.

Therefore, systemic efforts have been made in order to develop novel theranostics based on the advantageous use of nanogels. Nanogels are mainly used as more efficient, targeted, and safe delivery systems for theranostics substances [101,102] or even for cancer vaccines for immunomodulatory purposes [103,104] in oncology. The flexibility of their design can offer nano-scale systems that respond to single or multiple stimuli, enabling premium control over the release pattern of the embedded substances. Delivery of two or more molecules that have different characteristics (i.e., one hydrophilic and one hydrophobic molecule) has become feasible and efficient regulation of each substance's release can be internally or externally induced [102]. Thus, it is evident that the challenges that the field of oncology has been facing for so many years can partially be overcome with the advances in nanotechnology.

To develop efficient therapeutics though, a deeper understanding of the clinical need and the pathophysiological background of the targeted disorder is required first. The nanogels-based delivery systems that have been developed are directly associated with the pathophysiological characteristics of cancerous tissues. In specific, it is known that the disrupted local vasculature, coupled with diffusion anomalies due to tumor-related vascular dynamics and reduced total oxygen (O_2) blood capacity secondary to the disease- or treatment-induced anemia lead to an imbalance of O_2 supply and consumption in the cancerous tissues. Secondary to the low oxygen levels, the tissues produce energy via anaerobic pathways and lactic acid production is increased [105,106]. This subsequently causes a mild decrease in the extracellular pH (pHex) of a tumor (i.e., $pH_{ex} \sim 6.5$ compared to the normal of ~ 7.4) [107]. Even though the hypoxia and the hypoxia-induced acidic microenvironment of cancerous tissues pose major challenges in the treatment of cancer and can negatively affect therapeutic outcomes [105], they can be also used to our advantage for the development of targeted tissue-specific therapies. This is the basis for the development of pH-responsive nanogels.

A recent example of a pH-responsive nanogel was reported by Steinhilber et. al. [108], utilizing benzacetal bonds for generating biodegradable protein-resistant polyglycerol nanogels. In this study, it was reported that the encapsulation efficiencies of the developed nanogels were more than 99% for labile macromolecules (e.g., proteins and enzymes) when the nanogel was intact. The nanogel was capable of remaining stable in physiological pH values for a long time but it could rapidly degrade into low molecular fragments within acidic microenvironments, like the ones found in malignancies. There have been a series of studies [109–111] that gradually improve similar nanogels, aiming at prolonging the drugs' availability in the local tissues and targeting cancerous cells.

Effectively targeting the cancerous cells may be essential in order to minimize the side effects caused by cytotoxic drugs and maximize bioavailability of the drugs in the desired areas only. Nevertheless, after successfully reaching the tumor site, it is important that the carrier is able to penetrate the cancerous mass. Solid tumors are normally hard to penetrate due to the abnormal vasculature and the dense ECM that surround the tumor [112]. To tackle this obstacle, novel pH-dependent reversible swelling–shrinking nanogels have been developed [112,113]. These nanogels are slightly negatively charged under physiological conditions (i.e., pH ~ 7.4), but during the opsonization process, after they get exposed to the highly acidic endolysosomal environment (i.e., pH of 5.0–6.0) of the cells, they become swollen in the core area due to the protonation of core-embedded amino groups that turn the core's charge positive. The subsequent massive volume expansion leads not only to the release of the drug, but also to endolysosomal bursting, allowing escape of the carrier in the cytosol. The normal pH within the cytosol induces another transformation of the nanogel, which eventually shrink and return to their original state. While the released drug keeps killing cancerous cells, the nanogel returns to the original size, escapes from the dead cell, and penetrates deeper into the tumor tissue due to the repeated "infection" of the cells.

Other pH-dependent nanogels that aim at deeper penetration into malignant tissues have also been developed, like the recent example for dual pH-triggered multistage drug delivery system of Zan et al. [114]. In that case, an initial reduction of the pH close to the usual malignant tissue levels (i.e., pH ~ 6.5) induced the reorganization of the nanogels into much smaller NPs that could easily penetrate deeper into the cancerous tissue, while in parallel a further reduction of the pH value (i.e., pH ~ 5.0) triggered the drug release within the endolysosomal environment of the targeted cells.

Apart from pH values, temperature also seems to possess an important place in the pathophysiology and treatment of cancer. It has been suggested that mild increase in the local tissues temperature can be caused in malignant tissues [115]. Therefore, similarly to the pH-sensitive nanogels, thermoresponsive nanogels have been developed that respond only to temperature alterations (e.g., drug release upon exposure to higher temperature in malignant tissues). For the development of such nanogels, the choice of materials is based on their good thermosensitivity and LCST. PNIPAM is the most commonly used thermosensitive material used for the development of thermosensitive drug delivery systems, demonstrating a LCST of around 32°C in distilled water [116].

Although initial attempts focused on the LCST effect on the nanogel efficacy, it is now known that the upper critical solution temperature (UCST) also plays an important role in the temperature-induced response of the nanogel. UCST-like behavior that is characterized by swelling rather than de-swelling of the nanogel at increased temperatures was found to be beneficial for the efficient release of the drug. Thermoresponsive nanogels that were formed from a combination of acrylic acid and acrylamide have been studied as an example of a UCST-like system due to the weak nature of the hydrogel bonds between acrylic acid and acrylamide, causing the bonds to break in higher temperature. These nanogels were found to be remarkably more efficient at slightly higher temperatures [117], providing an alternative for cancer-related applications.

Despite promising preliminary findings, pH-thermal dually responsive nanogels are still considered a better approach to effectively target cancerous cells [118]. In order to accomplish dually responsive hybrid nanogels with little interference between stimuli, IPNs are mostly utilized due to their native design characteristics (see Section 5.3.2.3 for more details on IPNs) [119–122]. The potentials and tunability of such hybrid dual-responsive nanogel systems can be seen in a recent study of Chen et al. [122]. In this study a novel pH-thermal dual-responsive nanogel of hydroxypropylcellulose–poly(acrylic acid) (HPC–PAA) particles in the form of IPN structure was developed and after being loaded with anticancer drugs, it demonstrated encouraging results. The novelty of this system lied in the fact that, depending on the chemical composition and the degree of cross-linking, the thermoresponsive behavior could be shifted from the UCST to the LCST.

Other nanogels have focused on targeting other aspects of the pathophysiological changes observed in cancer. Redox-responsive nanogels are single-response delivery systems that are meant to be sensitive in the so-called redox reactions. Redox reactions are oxidation–reduction reactions that are highly significant for the cell's survival. It comes as no surprise that there is a local alteration in redox reactions when there is a malignancy. Glutathione (GSH) is a crucial tripeptide that is needed to alleviate oxidative stress through redox reactions. GSH is capable of reducing disulfide bonds by acting as an electron donor [123]. The cytoplasmic concentration of GSH has been found to be about 1000-fold the GSH concentration of the extracellular environment [114] and in tumor tissues it has been estimated that these concentrations become about 4-fold higher compared to normal tissues [124]. Thus, this leads to the development of a reducing intracellular environment in malignant tissues. Other pathophysiological mechanisms (e.g., high content of endolysosomal reducing enzymes, such as γ-interferon-inducible lysosomal thiol reductase, that can act at low pH values) have also been thought to contribute to the reducing intracellular cancerous environment [125]. This have given the opportunity for redox-responsive nanogels, which commonly employ disulfide bonds (easy to be broken down in the reducing environment), to effectively target the tumor site.

Several studies have proceeded with the development of redox-responsive nanogels to enhance accumulation at the target sites and reduce the chance of premature leakage of the embedded drug in the delivery pathway [126–128]. The employment of redox-sensitive disulfide bonds is a common practice for the development of smart delivery vaccines, providing a potential vehicle for more effective immunomodulatory treatments. Bioreducible (disulfide cross-linked) cationic nanogels have successfully mediated antigen or gene delivery to the desired tissues [103,129,130].

On the other hand, other studies have dedicated their efforts in developing nanogels that respond to the presence of certain enzymes in the targeted tissues. For instance, an abundance of HA receptors have been observed on the surface of numerous tumor cells. This is consistent with the overexpression of enzymes belonging to the family of hyaluronidases (HAases). The enzymes are known to degrade HA intracellularly and extracellularly [131]. Therefore, HA is kind of natural biodegradable biomaterial with an inherent active tumor targeting property and this is the reason why it is commonly used as a means to reach the tumor site. Indeed, HA nanogels containing enzyme-sensitive groups were proven to prolong anticancer drugs circulation times and promote their accumulation in the tumor site. Yim et al. [132] took advantage of the action of HAases in order to gain deeper penetration of the drug to malignant tissues. In that case, HA degradation enabled the action of their degradable cationic nanogel, which could subsequently induce cancerous cell death. The induced necrosis would in turn reduce cell density within the cancerous mass, facilitating paracellular transport of the nanogels, allowing deeper penetration to heterogenous tumors.

Similarly, tumors are known to excrete a significant amount of proteolytic enzymes (e.g., matrix metalloproteinases, MMPs). These enzymes are thought to indirectly promote the tumor's growth by degrading the basement membrane and natural ECM, providing free space for the cancerous cells uncontrollable proliferation. On this basis, MMPs-sensitive core–shell nanogels prepared by the method of self-assembly were designed [133]. Thanks to the core–shell like structure of such nanogels, effective and stable encapsulation of hydrophobic drugs has become feasible. This way the drugs are only released when they reach areas overexpressing MMPs (i.e., malignant tissues).

However, perhaps the currently most promising techniques for cancer therapies, namely the PTT and PDT [66], have been based on light responsive nanogels or nanohybrids. As illustrated in Fig. 5.4, in that case, photothermal transductors (PTs) with absorption in the biological optical window are incorporated within the nanogels. Therefore, near-infrared irradiation (NIR), also known as "biological optical window" due to the combination of high tissue penetration with low damage, can be utilized to externally regulate the impact of the nanogels in the targeted tissues. In specific, PDT is based on PTs that can use NIR light in order to produce reactive oxygen species, subsequently causing tissue destruction. On the other hand, PTT utilizes specific PTs that can transform NIR light into local heat [135]. Local hyperthermia (rise in tumor temperature) has a long history in the annals of cancer treatment. This is because hyperthermia (40–45°C) is thought to initiate a cascade of subcellular events, thereby rendering the malignant cells susceptible to radiation and chemotherapy [136,137]. The targeted delivery of nanogels-induced heat to the cancerous mass is certainly advantageous compared to traditionally used methods such as hot-water bath or heated blood perfusion [135]. Nanogels incorporating PTs within their structure are ideal nano-engineered devices for PTT because of their tunable size and architecture, biocompatibility, biodegradability, loading capacity, post-synthetic modification, and capability of targeted accumulation within the tumor site [138].

Recent advancements in the field of nanotechnology have also improved the nanohybrids that incorporate the PTs, after utilization of thermoresponsive polymeric materials that are meant to induce a simultaneous chemotherapeutic effect. To be

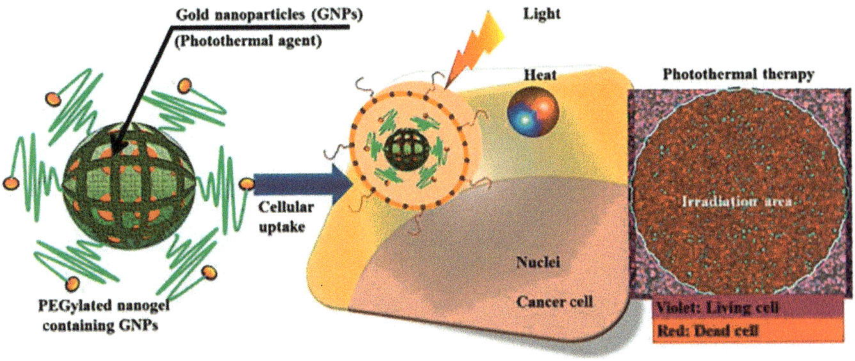

Figure 5.4 Schematic representation of the principles of photothermal therapy. PEGylated gold NPs with incorporated photothermal agents internalized by the targeted cells. Upon irradiation NPs react both to heat and light causing malignant cells that include the NPs to get killed.

Reproduced with permission from Lakshmanan S, Gupta GK, Avci P, Chandran R, Sadasivam M, Jorge AES, et al. Physical energy for drug delivery; poration, concentration and activation. Adv Drug Deliv Rev 2014;71:98–114. Copyright © 2013 Elsevier.

more specific, employment of thermoresponsive polymeric materials within the nanogel's structure can induce a swelling/de-swelling effect, depending on the fluctuations of local temperature, thereby enabling targeted and regulated release of an embedded chemotherapeutic agent [139]. Thus, this provides a "two-hit" therapeutic possibility for the treatment of cancer: (1) initially the incorporated PTs increase the local temperature upon external stimulation with NIR light, targeting only malignant tissues, thereby making the cells susceptible to damage (first hit) and (2) the increase in local temperature induces a structural change to the thermoresponsive nanogel. This subsequently, enables the regulated release of anticancer drugs, targeting only the already susceptible to chemotherapy-induced damage cancerous mass (second hit).

Last but not least, the use of multiresponsive nanogels (e.g., pH-thermal or pH-redox dually responsive nanogels) became more and more common in the field of nanomedicine [58,140–143], providing more versatile system allowing premium level of control. This can gradually help in developing more and more effective nanogels, being directly guided by the clinical needs and relying on observed disease-specific pathophysiological alterations.

5.6 Biosensor

Biosensor is an analytical device used for the detection of an analyte with chemical or biochemical detector [144]. Nanogels have gained great attention for application in biosensors because of their stability, biocompatibility, stimuli-response, swelling translation, and large surface area. In recent years, a great variety of nanogels have been used in biosensors. According to the roles nanogels have played, the applications on biosensor mainly focus in three sections: nanogels as encapsulation vehicles for biosensor detectors; nanogels as multifunctional stimuli-responsive materials for biosensor detectors; and nanogels as sensory membrane of biosensors.

5.6.1 Nanogels as encapsulation vehicles for biosensor detectors

Nanogels are now playing an important role in biosensors because of their unique properties. Like gels and microgels, the hydrophilicity of nanogels offers great biocompatibility and physical–chemical stability. The small size of nanogels ($<0.2\,\mu m$) [145] confers on high responsiveness to various stimuli as well as quick response time. These characteristics make nanogels good candidates as encapsulation vehicles for biosensor detectors. Nanogels as encapsulation vehicles could be used as scaffolds to support both inorganic and organic functional NPs.

Inorganic functional NPs, such as QDs, magnetic, and metallic nanoparticles are always used for biosensors due to their own special properties: they act as optical identification code, increase sensor sensitivity, and expand sensor detection range [149]. However, there are still many disadvantages to be addressed. For example, QDs placed into live cells exhibit aggregation which may interfere with cell function, thus, causing cell toxicity [146]; magnetic NPs easily tend to aggregate without special surfactant; metallic NPs have the great disadvantage of being reactive to oxidizing agents and having potential risk of chronical nanotoxicity. Since inorganic functional nanoparticals rarely meet the requirement of biosensor, research on nanogels as the scaffold/encapsulation for inorganic functional NPs continuously grow. Riedinger et al. [147] used pH-responsive poly(2-vinylpyridine-co-divinylbenzene) nanogels as scaffold for allyl-PEG capped inorganic NPs, including magnetic iron oxide nanoparticles (IONPs), fluorescent CdSe/ZnS QDs, and metallic gold, as illustrated in

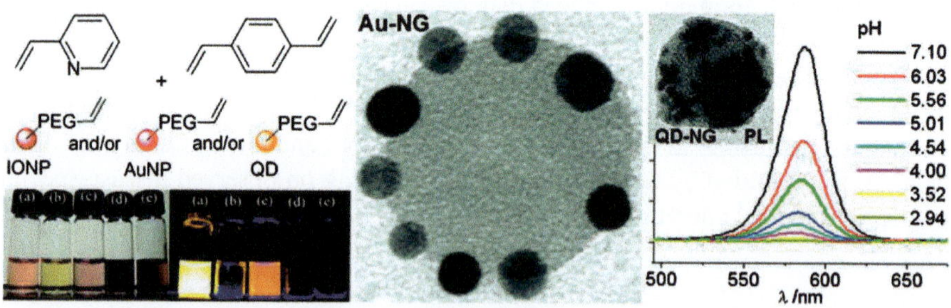

Figure 5.5 Allyl-PEG capped inorganic NPs, including magnetic IONPs, fluorescent CdSe/ZnS QDs, and metallic gold (AuNPs of 5 and 10 nm) individually and in combination were covalently attached to pH-responsive poly(2-vinylpyridine-co-divinylbenzene) nanogels. Adapted from Weng J, Ren J. Luminescent quantum dots: a very attractive and promising tool in biomedicine. Curr Med Chem 2006;13(8):897–909. Reprinted with permission from American Chemical Society, Copyright (2011).

Fig. 5.5. Another attempt that goes beyond the fabrication of discrete inorganic NPs is the one of Goswami et al. [148] who designed a novel luminescent sensor by encapsulating luminescent Au nanoclusters with chitosan nanogels. This sensor showed nearly threefold photoluminescence (PL) intensity compared to the one of nonchitosan nanogel. Similarly, Chen et al. [80] developed near infrared (NIR) luminescent gold cluster–poly(acrylic acid) (PAA) hybrid nanogels by in situ reduction of gold salt in the core-hollow and shell-porous PAA nanogels. Taking PAA nanogels as scaffold, the quantum yield of Au–PAA nanogels is determined to be 0.9%, twofold higher in magnitude than the one of other synthesized Au clusters, while the excitation wavelength is in the NIR range. With these characteristics, it is evident that Au-PAA nanogels exhibit tumor imaging ability without any target group.

Organic functional NPs/molecules, such as enzymes, fluorescent probes, and DNA, are widely used for the biosensor because of high catalytic ability, mild reaction conditions, and specificity of the reactions. However, there are still many disadvantages of taking organic functional NPs as detectors in a biosensor. Organic NPs, especially enzymes, require strict monitoring of several parameters (e.g., solvent pH, local environmental temperature, purity of solvent) to maintain fully operational physical environments. Even tiny shift in the working environment could cause great fluctuation in the activity of organic NPs. Furthermore, biosensors formed by organic NPs rely heavily on immobilization technology. Leakage of organic NPs seriously impacts biosensor sensitivity because of the high catalytic efficiency and finite lifetime of organic NPs. In order to tackle these disadvantages, nanogels have been explored as an alternative due to their unique characteristics, attracting increasing attention based on promising preliminary findings. The nanosize of the gels provide great surface area and plenty cross-linkable sites for organic-NPs-loading or covalent cross-linking [150]. These characteristics result in highly catalytic activity and immobilization

Table 5.1 Recent studies on immobilization of organic NPs on nanogels

Nanogel	Organic nanoparticles	Immobilization technique	Ref.
Poly(acrylic acid)-based nanogels	Glucose oxidase	Covalent	[151]
Polyacrylamide nanogel	Bovine carbonic anhydrase	Covalent	[152]
Polyacrylamide nanogel	Lipase	Encapsulation	[153]
Fe_3O_4/chitosan nanogel	Glucoamylase	Adsorption	[154]
Polyethyleneglycol	Lipase	Imprinted	[155]
Pluronic F127	Fluorescent probe (DMDP-M)	Adsorption	[156]
Polyurethane nanogel	Coumarin 6/Nile Red	Adsorption	[157]
Polyurethane nanogel	8-Hydroxypyrene-1-carbaldehyde	Adsorption	[158]
Poly(ethylene glycol) nanogel	2-Methacryloyloxyethyl phosphorylcholine copolymer bearing oligonucleotides	Physical interaction	[159]

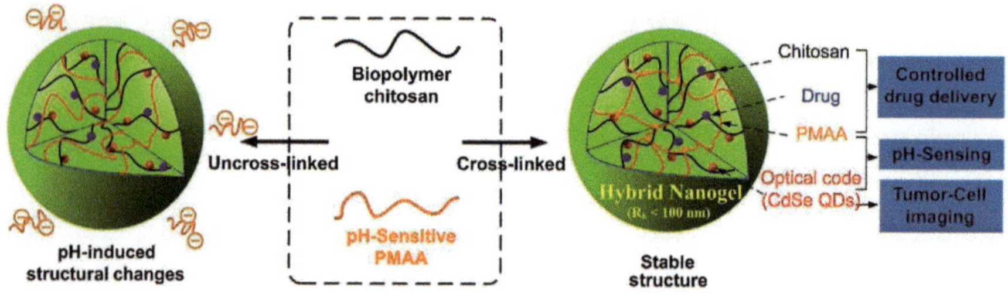

Figure 5.6 Schematic representation of the concept for designing multifunctional chitosan–PMAA–CdSe hybrid nanogel and its potential extending applications in biomedical field. Adapted from Wu W, Shen J, Banerjee P, Zhou S. Chitosan-based responsive hybrid nanogels for integration of optical pH-sensing, tumor cell imaging and controlled drug delivery. Biomaterials 2010:31(32);8371–81. Reprinted with permission from Elsevier Publishing Group, Copyright (2010).

stability of organic NPs. In addition, the biocompatibility and great water-retention capability of nanogels provide a favorable microenvironment for organic NPs. An overview of the growing research about immobilizing organic NPs on nanogels can be seen in Table 5.1, which summarizes recent representative reports.

As shown in Table 5.1, varieties of organic NPs are reported being immobilized on nanogels acting as detectors for the biosensor. According to the literature reports, frequently immobilized organic NPs can be divided into three classes: enzymes, fluorescent probes, and DNA. Using a variety of immobilization methods, these kinds of organic NPs were encapsulated in nanogels, exhibiting enhanced activity and stability.

5.6.2 Nanogels as multifunctional stimuli-responsive materials for biosensor detectors

As mentioned in the introduction, nanogels simultaneously possess advantageous properties of a hydrogel system and NPs. Multifunctional stimuli-responsive hydrogels, which are able to dramatically change their volume and other properties in response to environmental stimuli such as temperature [160,161], redox [162], pH [163], light [160], glucose concentration [164,165], and magnetic field [166] are increasingly attracting attention in the biosensor area. Mingle structured and core–shell structured are the two main composite structure-based categories of multifunctional stimuli-responsive nanogels.

Mingle structured multifunctional nanogels, which are commonly used for multifunction biosensors, contain two parts: stimuli-responsive nanogel and functional particles. Take the multifunctional chitosan–poly(methacrylic acid) (PMAA)–CdSe hybrid nanogel as an example: as illustrated in Fig. 5.6, chitosan–PMAA–CdSe nanogel is made up of a pH responsive nanogel and CdSe QDs. The cross-linked PMAA together with semi-interpenetrating chitosan were prepared as a pH-responsive nanogel, which can sufficiently undergo a pH-induced volume phase transition. CdSe QDs, which are mixed homogeneously in the nanogel system, can translate the

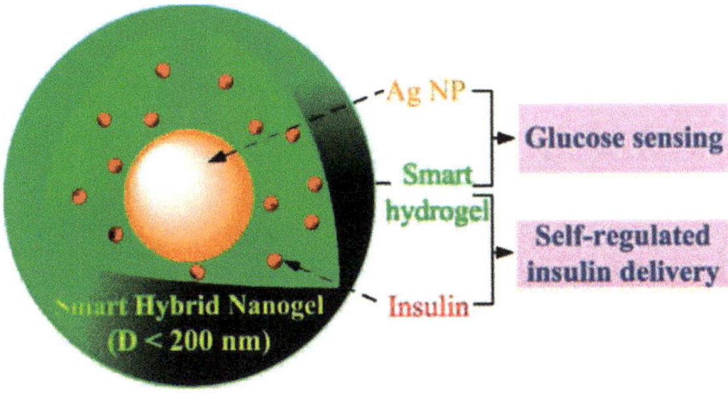

Figure 5.7 Schematic illustration of smart hybrid nanogels that can integrate optical glucose detection and self-regulated insulin delivery at physiological pH and temperature into a single nano-object.
Adapted from Wu W, Mitra N, Yan EC, Zhou S. Multifunctional hybrid nanogel for integration of optical glucose sensing and self-regulated insulin release at physiological pH. ACS Nano 2010:4(8);4831–9. Reprinted with permission from American Chemical Society, Copyright (2010).

volume phase transition into optical codes. These two parts make chitosan–PMAA–CdSe hybrid nanogel a good detector candidate for pH-biosensor. Additionally, the functional-NPs/mingle-structured-gels composite nanogels facilitate favorable interactions between each subcomponent. Zhu et al. [168] reported a temperature-responsive hybrid nanogel system, in which immobilized Bi_2O_3 QDs can work cooperatively with nanogel networks of poly(vinyl alcohol). Li and Lu [169] successfully developed nanogel-based temperature and Hg^{2+} ions dual fluorescent sensors, in which the thermo-induced collapse of PNIPAM nanogel was successfully utilized to further enhance the Hg^{2+} detection sensitivity. Coincidentally, Li and Lu [169] developed a thermoresponsive nanogel-based sensitive and selective fluorescent sensor for Cr^{3+} detection with PNIPAM nanogel, which was covalently labeled using rhodamine B urea derivatives (P(NIPAM-co-RhBUA)). Upon heating above the phase transition temperature, enhanced fluorescence intensity of P(NIPAM-co-RhBUA) was observed ($\approx$61-fold increase at 45°C), accompanied by an improved detection sensitivity.

Core–shell is one special structure of multifunctional nanogels, which has gained significant attention from an increasing number of researchers because of the improved biocompatibility, biostability, and convenient manufacturing process. Compared with mingle multifunctional nanogels, core–shell structured nanogels' sensitive properties mainly depend on the nature of the encapsulated cores. As shown in Fig. 5.7, small AgNPs (10 ± 3 nm) core is covered by poly(4-vinylphenylboronic acid-co-2-(dimethylamino) ethyl acrylate)[p(VPBA-DMAEA)]gel shell. AgNPs, being noble-metal-based NPs, can provide strong fluorescence without bleaching. While boronic acid (BA)-based ligands coupled with polymers (such as phenylboronic acid copolymer) can be used for glucose sensing, p(VPBA-DMAEA) demonstrates, at the same time, characteristics of BA ligands and nanogels. By taking AgNPs as fluorescence codes, the glucose-induced swelling/shrinking of p(VPBA-DMAEA) conveys the glucose concentration into optical signals thereafter regulating preloaded insulin delivery [170]. With the similar

Table 5.2 Core–shell multifunctional stimuli-responsive nanogels

Core material	Shell material	Functions	Ref.
AgNPs	Poly(*N*-isopropylacrylamide-co-acrylic acid)	Imaging for cancer cell with pH drug release control	[171]
AuNPs	Poly(2-(2-methoxyethoxy) ethyl methacrylate	Shell thickness tunable; converting temperature into optical signals	[172]
NaYF4:Yb^{3+}–Er^{3+} nanocrystals	Poly(*N*-isopropylacrylamide co *N*-acrylyl-*N*-rhodamine B acylhydrazine thiourea)	Response to multistimuli. Can be used as detector for pH, temperature, Hg^{2+} ions	[173]
Carbon nanodots	Poly(*N*-isopropylacrylamide) (PNIPAM)	Sensitive to temperature with drug delivery ability	[174]
Carbon nanodots with magnetic iron oxide nanocystals	Poly(*N*-isopropylacrylamide-co-acrylamide)	Temperature sensitive, tumor imaging with magnetic/NIR-thermally responsive drug carriers	[175]
Porphyrin	PEG-poly(ε-caprolactone) (PCL) copolymer	Imaging for hepatoma tumor with drug deliver ability	[176]
Protoporphyrin	PEG–PCL copolymer	Fluorescence imaging with thermosensitive	[177]
Graphene with doxorubicin	Hyaluronic acid	Photoluminescence with laser irradiation drug release control	[178]

design, other materials were reported to have been used for core–shell multifunctional stimuli-responsive nanogels. Some of recent reports are summarized in Table 5.2.

5.6.3 Nanogels as sensory elements of biosensors

As nanogel simultaneously possesses characteristics of hydrogel system and NP system, the injectable liquid morphology, protein resistance, responsive swelling–shrinking volume transitions, and tunable 3D nanostructure properties make it a candidate for sensory elements of biosensors.

Membranes are known to greatly affect the lifetime, sensitivity and accuracy of biosensors, posing a significant challenge in the field of biosensors development. Despite the fact that great progress has been made on membrane techniques in the recent decades, there are still many requirements to be satisfied, such as the lifetime prolongation, the further enhancement of biocompatibility and, mostly, the higher resistance to protein absorption and to cell adhesion. Scott et al. [179] developed a low-protein-absorption/low-cell-adhesion membrane made from PEG-octavinylsulfone and BSA nanogels. By testing poly(ethylene terephthalate) PET surface, this membrane exhibited higher CHO cell adhesion resistance (2.3 ± 3.2 adhered cells/mm^2) compared to air plasma modified PET (1100 ± 216 cells/mm^2). Tessler et al. [180] demonstrated that PEG/bovine serum albumin (BSA)-based nanogel membrane also has the ability to resist single molecule (SM) proteins and even DNA adsorption. Compared to BSA surface and multi-arm PEG membrane, PEG/BSA nanogel membrane absorbed only fourfold less SM proteins than did the BSA surface and twofold less SM proteins than did the multi-armed PEG membrane. Another study [181] improved Scott's research in terms of protein absorption resistance by using a clickable copper catalyzed azide/alkyne cycloaddition (CuAAC) and functional PEG (CuAAC/functional-PEG) nanogel, which escapes the risk of bulk gelation due its stability, contrary to PEG/BSA nanogels. Apart from protein/cell resistance, nanogels are also used as biosensor membranes due to their multiresponsive volume-transition property. Atta et al. [182] used epoxy-based nanogels as self-healing membranes to fill the micro- and nanocracks using the nanogels temperature-responsive swelling–shrinking capability. Sun et al. [183] developed a temperature- and ethanol-responsive nanogel membrane used on microchips. This membrane, formed by chitosan and PNIPAM nanogels in the microchannels of the chip, served as a platform of nanovalves, enabling volume shifting based on the temperature and ethanol changes. Luo et al. [184] also reported in situ fabricated PNIPAM nanogel membranes working as "gates" for the nanogel's pore sizes and they noted that the nanogel's surface properties can be controlled as the "open/close" gates in response to the temperature.

Nanogels are not only useful as part of a biosensor's membranes, but also as other elements of biosensor. Wu et al. [185] prepared NH_3 responsive nanofibers by electrospinning polyaniline/polyacrylonitrile/L-lysine-based nanogels. The prepared nanofibers exhibited highly selective response toward NH_3 at room temperature with 2.2 ppm detection limit. Ramakrishnan et al. [186] used PNIPAM nanogel as sensing medium in surface acoustic wave (SAW) devices to measure relative humidity (RH). PNIPAM nanogels exhibited unique absorption properties; the membrane mass increased as RH rose, which resulted into resonance frequency shifts. Based on the observation that the PNIPAM nanogels showed nanosecond volume transitions when passing the LCST, which is about 32°, Reese et al. [187] developed a nanosecond photonic crystal optical switching devices with PNIPAM nanogels. This device exhibited fast light transmission switches within 900 ns. By exploiting the swelling/de-swelling property of nanogels, Lee et al. [188] formed glucose sensitive artificial muscle via introducing BA nanogels into carbon multiwalled nanotube (MWNT) yarn. Given that the BA nanogels were sensitive to glucose, this artificial muscle rotated to different angles, responding accordingly to the glucose concentration.

5.7 Conclusion and future prospective

Nanogels have been explored as promising drug delivery vehicles, for both small molecule chemical drugs and for proteins/peptides. The applications of getting drugs delivered to the central nervous system and targeting cancer cells are the two hotspots of this field. Off-target effect is always a critical problem which, needs to be minimized when designing the structure and components of the nanogel drug delivery system. Regarding the safety of using metal-containing nanogels, the mechanisms of metabolism and cytotoxicity have to be investigated further. In general, the studies of nanogels with large animal models are very limited, and the registered clinical trials are even less. Therefore, nanogel translational activities have to be planned very diligently. Finally, nanogels seem to hold great promise in the field of biosensors. Future work should focus on developing specific implantable nanogel-based devices that would monitor biological reactions in vivo or even test the behavior of new drug compounds in the human body.

References

[1] Salatin S, Barar J, Barzegar-Jalali M, Adibkia K, Milani M, Jelvehgari M. Hydrogel nanoparticles and nanocomposites for nasal drug/vaccine delivery. Arch Pharm Res 2016;39:1181–92.

[2] Pedrosa SS, Pereira P, Correia A, Moreira S, Rocha H, Gama FM. Biocompatibility of a self-assembled crosslinkable hyaluronic acid nanogel. Macromol Biosci 2016;16(11):1610–20.

[3] Farhana SM, Imran-Ul-Haque Md, Arafat M, Sharmin S. An overview of nanogel drug delivery system. J Appl Pharm Sci 2013;3(8 suppl 1):95–105.

[4] Zhang YN, Poon W, Tavares AJ, McGilvray ID, Chan WC. Nanoparticle-liver interactions: cellular uptake and hepatobiliary elimination. J Control Release 2016;28(240):332–48.

[5] Nic M, Jirat J, Kosata B. Compendium of chemical terminology gold book. Int Union Pure Appl Chem 2014.

[6] Lim CK, Singh A, Heo J, Kim D, Lee KE, Jeon H, et al. Gadolinium-coordinated elastic nanogels for in vivo tumor targeting and imaging. Biomaterials 2013;34(28):6846–52.

[7] Lee J, Lee C, Kim TH, Lee ES, Shin BS, Chi SC, et al. Self-assembled glycol chitosan nanogels containing palmityl-acylated exendin-4 peptide as a longacting anti-diabetic inhalation system. J Control Release 2012;161:728–34.

[8] Makhlof A, Werle M, Tozuka Y, Takeuchi H. Nanoparticles of glycol chitosan and its thiolated derivative significantly improved the pulmonary delivery of calcitonin. Int J Pharm 2010;397:92–5.

[9] de la Fuente M, Ravina M, Paolicelli P, Sanchez A, Seijo B, Alonso M. J. Chitosan-based nanostructures: a delivery platform for ocular therapeutics. Adv Drug Deliv Rev 2010;62:100–17.

[10] Douglas KL, Piccirillo CA, Tabrizian M. Effects of alginate inclusion on the vector properties of chitosan-based nanoparticles. J Control Release 2006;115:354–61.

[11] Goycoolea FM, Lollo G, Remunan-Lopez C, Quaglia F, Alonso MJ. Chitosan-alginate blended nanoparticles as carriers for the transmucosal delivery of macromolecules. Biomacromolecules 2009;10:1736–43.

[12] Demoulins T, Bassi I, Thomann-Harwood L, Jandus C, Kaeuper P, Simon HU, et al. Alginate-coated chitosan nanogel capacity to modulate the effect of TLR ligands on blood dendritic cells. Nanomedicine 2013;9:806–17.

[13] Nasti A, Zaki NM, de Leonardis P, Ungphaiboon S, Sansongsak P, Rimoli MG, et al. Chitosan/TPP and Chitosan/TPP-hyaluronic acid nanoparticles: systematic optimisation of the preparative process and preliminary biological evaluation. Pharm Res 2009;26:1918–30.

[14] Gwak SJ, Jung JK, An SS, Kim HJ, Oh JS, Pennant WA, et al. Chitosan/TPP-hyaluronic acid nanoparticles: a new vehicle for gene delivery to the spinal cord. J Biomater Sci Polym Ed 2012;23:1437–50.

[15] Schmitt F, Lagopoulos L, Kauper P, Rossi N, Busso N, Barge J, et al. Chitosan-based nanogels for selective delivery of photosensitizers to macrophages and improved retention in and therapy of articular joints. J Control Release 2010;144:242–50.

[16] Schutz CA, Juillerat-Jeanneret L, Kauper P, Wandrey C. Cell response to the exposure to chitosan-TPP/alginate nanogels. Biomacromolecules 2011;12:4153–61.
[17] Jonassen H, Kjoniksen AL, Hiorth M. Stability of chitosan nanoparticles cross-linked with tripolyphosphate. Biomacromolecules 2012;13:3747–56.
[18] Huang Y, Lapitsky Y. Salt-assisted mechanistic analysis of chitosan/tripolyphosphate micro- and nanogel formation. Biomacromolecules 2012;13:3868–76.
[19] Jin HQ, Tan H, Zhao LL, Sun WP, Zhu LJ, Sun YG, et al. Ultrasound-triggered thrombolysis using urokinase-loaded nanogels. Int J Pharm 2012;434:384–90.
[20] Yong CP, Gan LM. Microemulsion polymerizations and reactions. Adv Polym Sci 2005;175:257–98.
[21] Saraogi GK, Gupta P, Gupta UD, Jain NK, Agrawal GP. Gelatin nanocarriers as potential vectors for effective management of tuberculosis. Int J Pharm 2010;385:143–9.
[22] Koul V, Mohamed R, Kuckling D, Adler HJP, Choudhary V. Interpenetrating polymer network (IPN) nanogels based on gelatin and poly(acrylic acid) by inverse miniemulsion technique: synthesis and characterization. Colloids Surf B 2011;83:204–13.
[23] Oh EJ, Park K, Kim KS, Kim J, Yang JA, Kong JH, et al. Target specific and long-acting delivery of protein, peptide, and nucleotide therapeutics using hyaluronic acid derivatives. J Control Release 2010;141:2–12.
[24] Choi KY, Lee S, Park K, Kim K, Park JH, Kwon IC, et al. Preparation and characterization of hyaluronic acid-based hydrogel nanoparticles. J Phys Chem Solids 2008;69:1591–5.
[25] Oyarzun-Ampuero FA, Goycoolea FM, Torres D, Alonso MJ. A new drug nanocarrier consisting of polyarginine and hyaluronic acid. Eur J Pharm Biopharm 2011;79:54–7.
[26] He Y, Cheng G, Xie L, Nie Y, He B, Gu Z. Polyethyleneimine/DNA polyplexes with reduction-sensitive hyaluronic acid derivatives shielding for targeted gene delivery. Biomaterials 2013;34:1235–45.
[27] Knowles DB, Shkel IA, Phan NM, Sternke M, Lingeman E, Cheng X, et al. Chemical interactions of polyethylene glycols (PEGs) and glycerol with protein functional groups: applications to effects of PEG and glycerol on protein processes. Biochemistry 2015;54(22):3528–42.
[28] Tamura M, Ichinohe S, Tamura A, Ikeda Y, Nagasaki Y. In vitro and in vivo characteristics of core-shell type nanogel particles: optimization of core cross-linking density and surface poly(ethylene glycol) density in PEGylated nanogels. Acta Biomater 2011;7(9):3354–61.
[29] Sigma-Aldrich <http://www.sigmaaldrich.com/materials-science/polymer-science/nipam-polymers.html>.
[30] Verma NK, Purohit MP, Equbal D, Dhiman N, Singh A, Kar AK, et al. Targeted smart pH and thermoresponsive N,O-carboxymethyl chitosan conjugated nanogels for enhanced therapeutic efficacy of doxorubicin in MCF-7 breast cancer cells. Bioconjug Chem 2016;27(11):2605–19.
[31] Zhang W, Jiang P, Chen J, Zhu C, Mao Z, Gao C. Application of melatonin-loaded poly(*N*-isopropylacrylamide) hydrogel particles to reduce the toxicity of airborne pollutes to RAW264.7 cells. J Colloid Interface Sci 2017;490:181–9.
[32] Tim JH, Lee TR. Hydrogel-templated growth of large gold nanoparticles: synthesis of thermally responsive hydrogel–nanoparticle composites. Langmuir 2007;23:6504–9.
[33] Lux J, White AG, Chan M, Anderson CJ, Almutairi A. Nanogels from metal-chelating crosslinkers as versatile platforms applied to copper-64 PET imaging of tumors and metastases. Theranostics 2015;5(3):277–88.
[34] Chan M, Lux J, Mishimura T, Akiyoshi K, Almutairi A. Long-lasting and efficient tumor imaging using a high relaxivity polysaccaride nanogel magnetic resonance imaging contrast agent. Biomacromolocules 2015;16:2964–71.

[35] Jain KK. Drug delivery systems—an overview. Methods Mol Biol 2008;437:1–50.
[36] Coelho JF, Ferreira PC, Alves P, Cordeiro R, Fonseca AC, Góis JR, et al. Drug delivery systems: advanced technologies potentially applicable in personalized treatments. EPMA J 2010;1(1):164–209.
[37] Pond SM, Tozer TN. First-pass elimination. Basic concepts and clinical consequences. Clin Pharmacokinet 1984;9(1):1–25.
[38] Chacko RT, Ventura J, Zhuang J, Thayumanavan S. Polymer nanogels: a versatile nanoscopic drug delivery platform. Adv Drug Deliv Rev 2012;64(9):836–51.
[39] Atala A, editor. Principles of regenerative medicine. : Academic Press, London, United Kingdom, 2010.
[40] Wichterle O, Lím D. Hydrophilic gels for biological use. Nature 1960;185(4706):117–8.
[41] Gupta P, Vermani K, Garg S. Hydrogels: from controlled release to pH-responsive drug delivery. Drug Discov Today 2002;7(10):569–79.
[42] Molinos M, Carvalho V, Silva DM, Gama FM. Development of a hybrid dextrin hydrogel encapsulating dextrin nanogel as protein delivery system. Biomacromolecules 2012;13(2):517–27.
[43] Kang H, Liu H, Zhang X, Yan J, Zhu Z, Peng L, et al. Photoresponsive DNA-crosslinked hydrogels for controllable release and cancer therapy. Langmuir ACS J Surf Colloids 2011;27(1):399–408.
[44] Mohd Amin MCI, Ahmad N, Halib N, Ahmad I. Synthesis and characterization of thermo- and pH-responsive bacterial cellulose/acrylic acid hydrogels for drug delivery. Carbohydr Polym 2012;88(2):465–73.
[45] Dalwadi C, Patel G. Application of nanohydrogels in drug delivery systems: recent patents review. Recent Pat Nanotechnol 2015;9(1):17–25.
[46] Blanco E, Shen H, Ferrari M. Principles of nanoparticle design for overcoming biological barriers to drug delivery. Nat Biotechnol 2015;33(9):941–51.
[47] Rolland JP, Maynor BW, Euliss LE, Exner AE, Denison GM, DeSimone JM. Direct fabrication and harvesting of monodisperse, shape-specific nanobiomaterials. J Am Chem Soc 2005;127(28):10096–100.
[48] Glangchai LC, Caldorera-Moore M, Shi L, Roy K. Nanoimprint lithography based fabrication of shape-specific, enzymatically-triggered smart nanoparticles. J Control Release Off J Control Release Soc 2008;125(3):263–72.
[49] Kersey FR, Merkel TJ, Perry JL, Napier ME, DeSimone JM. Effect of aspect ratio and deformability on nanoparticle extravasation through nanopores. Langmuir ACS J Surf Colloids 2012;28(23):8773–81.
[50] Beija M, Marty J-D, Destarac M. RAFT/MADIX polymers for the preparation of polymer/inorganic nanohybrids. Prog Polym Sci 2011;36(7):845–86.
[51] Siegwart DJ, Oh JK, Matyjaszewski K. ATRP in the design of functional materials for biomedical applications. Prog Polym Sci 2012;37(1):18–37.
[52] Maya S, Sarmento B, Nair A, Rejinold NS, Nair SV, Jayakumar R. Smart stimuli sensitive nanogels in cancer drug delivery and imaging: a review. Curr Pharm Des 2013;19(41):7203–18.
[53] Ghasemi A, Mohtashami M, Sheijani SS, Aliakbari K. Chitosan-genipin nanohydrogel as a vehicle for sustained delivery of alpha-1 antitrypsin. Res Pharm Sci 2015;10(6):523–34.
[54] Vashist A, Vashist A, Gupta YK, Ahmad S. Recent advances in hydrogel based drug delivery systems for the human body. J Mater Chem B 2014;2(2):147–66.
[55] Hamidi M, Azadi A, Rafiei P. Hydrogel nanoparticles in drug delivery. Adv Drug Deliv Rev 2008;60(15):1638–49.

[56] Vaishya R, Khurana V, Patel S, Mitra AK. Long-term delivery of protein therapeutics. Expert Opin Drug Deliv 2015;12(3):415–40.
[57] Abandansari HS, Nabid MR, Rezaei SJT, Niknejad H. pH-sensitive nanogels based on Boltorn® H40 and poly(vinylpyridine) using mini-emulsion polymerization for delivery of hydrophobic anticancer drugs. Polymer 2014;55(16):3579–90.
[58] Su S, Wang H, Liu X, Wu Y, Nie G. iRGD-coupled responsive fluorescent nanogel for targeted drug delivery. Biomaterials 2013;34(13):3523–33.
[59] Wu W, Shen J, Banerjee P, Zhou S. Core–shell hybrid nanogels for integration of optical temperature-sensing, targeted tumor cell imaging, and combined chemo-photothermal treatment. Biomaterials 2010;31(29):7555–66.
[60] Liu T, Wu T, Liu H, Ke B, Huang H, Jiang Z, et al. Ultraviolet-crosslinked hydrogel sustained-release hydrophobic antibiotics with long-term antibacterial activity and limited cytotoxicity. J Appl Polym Sci 2014;131:13.
[61] Watanabe K, Nishio Y, Makiura R, Nakahira A, Kojima C. Paclitaxel-loaded hydroxyapatite/collagen hybrid gels as drug delivery systems for metastatic cancer cells. Int J Pharm 2013;446(1–2):81–6.
[62] Nagahama K, Kawano D, Oyama N, Takemoto A, Kumano T, Kawakami J. Self-assembling polymer micelle/clay nanodisk/doxorubicin hybrid injectable gels for safe and efficient focal treatment of cancer. Biomacromolecules 2015;16(3):880–9.
[63] Kang H, Trondoli AC, Zhu G, Chen Y, Chang Y-J, Liu H, et al. Near-infrared light-responsive core–shell nanogels for targeted drug delivery. ACS Nano 2011;5(6):5094–9.
[64] Satarkar NS, Biswal D, Hilt JZ. Hydrogel nanocomposites: a review of applications as remote controlled biomaterials. Soft Matter 2010;6(11):2364.
[65] Yavuz MS, Cheng Y, Chen J, Cobley CM, Zhang Q, Rycenga M, et al. Gold nanocages covered by smart polymers for controlled release with near-infrared light. Nat Mater 2009;8(12):935–9.
[66] Jaque D, Maestro LM, del Rosal B, Haro-Gonzalez P, Benayas A, Plaza JL, et al. Nanoparticles for photothermal therapies. Nanoscale 2014;6(16):9494–530.
[67] Appel EA, Tibbitt MW, Webber MJ, Mattix BA, Veiseh O, Langer R. Self-assembled hydrogels utilizing polymer–nanoparticle interactions. Nat Commun 2015;6:6295.
[68] Dong R, Zhao X, Guo B, Ma PX. Self-healing conductive injectable hydrogels with antibacterial activity as cell delivery carrier for cardiac cell therapy. ACS Appl Mater Interfaces 2016;8(27):17138–50.
[69] Hsieh F-Y, Tseng T-C, Hsu S. Self-healing hydrogel for tissue repair in the central nervous system. Neural Regen Res 2015;10(12):1922–3.
[70] Wei Z, Yang JH, Zhou J, Xu F, Zrínyi M, Dussault PH, et al. Self-healing gels based on constitutional dynamic chemistry and their potential applications. Chem Soc Rev 2014;43(23):8114–31.
[71] Zhang Y, Tao L, Li S, Wei Y. Synthesis of multiresponsive and dynamic chitosan-based hydrogels for controlled release of bioactive molecules. Biomacromolecules 2011;12(8):2894–901.
[72] Wu H-Q, Wang C-C. Biodegradable smart nanogels: a new platform for targeting drug delivery and biomedical diagnostics. Langmuir ACS J Surf Colloids 2016;32(25):6211–25.
[73] Tirotta I, Dichiarante V, Pigliacelli C, Cavallo G, Terraneo G, Bombelli FB, et al. (19) F magnetic resonance imaging (MRI): from design of materials to clinical applications. Chem Rev 2015;115(2):1106–29.
[74] Sierra-Martin B, Fernandez-Barbero A. Multifunctional hybrid nanogels for theranostic applications. Soft Matter 2015;11(42):8205–16.

[75] Lux J, Chan M, Elst LV, Schopf E, Mahmoud E, Laurent S, et al. Metal chelating crosslinkers form nanogels with high chelation stability. J Mater Chem B 2013;1(46):6359–64.
[76] Sanchez C, de AA Soler-Illia GJ, Ribot F, Lalot T, Mayer CR, Cabuil V. Designed hybrid organic – inorganic nanocomposites from functional nanobuilding blocks. Chem Mater 2001;13(10):3061–83.
[77] Sanchez C, Julián B, Belleville P, Popall M. Applications of hybrid organic–inorganic nanocomposites. J Mater Chem 2005;15(35-36):3559–92.
[78] Yang P, Li D, Jin S, Ding J, Guo J, Shi W, et al. Stimuli-responsive biodegradable poly(methacrylic acid) based nanocapsules for ultrasound traced and triggered drug delivery system. Biomaterials 2014;35(6):2079–88.
[79] Soni KS, Desale SS, Bronich TK. Nanogels: an overview of properties, biomedical applications and obstacles to clinical translation. J Control Release 2016;240:109–26.
[80] Chen Y, Zheng X, Wang X, Wang C, Ding Y, Jiang X. Near-infrared emitting gold cluster–poly(acrylic acid) hybrid nanogels. ACS Macro Lett 2014;3(1):74–6.
[81] Nakamura T, Tamura A, Murotani H, Oishi M, Jinji Y, Matsuishi K, et al. Large payloads of gold nanoparticles into the polyamine network core of stimuli-responsive PEGylated nanogels for selective and noninvasive cancer photothermal therapy. Nanoscale 2010;2(5):739–46.
[82] Yasui H, Takeuchi R, Nagane M, Meike S, Nakamura Y, Yamamori T, et al. Radiosensitization of tumor cells through endoplasmic reticulum stress induced by PEGylated nanogel containing gold nanoparticles. Cancer Lett 2014;347(1):151–8.
[83] Rejinold NS, Ranjusha R, Balakrishnan A, Mohammed N, Jayakumar R. Gold–chitin–manganese dioxide ternary composite nanogels for radio frequency assisted cancer therapy. RSC Adv 2014;4(11):5819–25.
[84] Liang R, Wei M, Evans DG, Duan X. Inorganic nanomaterials for bioimaging, targeted drug delivery and therapeutics. Chem Commun 2014;50(91):14071–81.
[85] Chiang W-H, Ho VT, Chen H-H, Huang W-C, Huang Y-F, Lin S-C, et al. Superparamagnetic hollow hybrid nanogels as a potential guidable vehicle system of stimuli-mediated MR imaging and multiple cancer therapeutics. Langmuir ACS J Surf Colloids 2013;29(21):6434–43.
[86] Ruhland TM, Reichstein PM, Majewski AP, Walther A, Müller AHE. Superparamagnetic and fluorescent thermo-responsive core–shell–corona hybrid nanogels with a protective silica shell. J Colloid Interface Sci 2012;374(1):45–53.
[87] Shen J-M, Guan X-M, Liu X-Y, Lan J-F, Cheng T, Zhang H-X. Luminescent/magnetic hybrid nanoparticles with folate-conjugated peptide composites for tumor-targeted drug delivery. Bioconjug Chem 2012;23(5):1010–21.
[88] Bulte JWM, Kraitchman DL. Iron oxide MR contrast agents for molecular and cellular imaging. NMR Biomed 2004;17(7):484–99.
[89] Sanson C, Diou O, Thévenot J, Ibarboure E, Soum A, Brûlet A, et al. Doxorubicin loaded magnetic polymersomes: theranostic nanocarriers for MR imaging and magneto-chemotherapy. ACS Nano 2011;5(2):1122–40.
[90] Rejinold NS, Chennazhi KP, Tamura H, Nair SV, Rangasamy J. Multifunctional chitin nanogels for simultaneous drug delivery, bioimaging, and biosensing. ACS Appl Mater Interfaces 2011;3(9):3654–65.
[91] Hasegawa U, Nomura SM, Kaul SC, Hirano T, Akiyoshi K. Nanogel-quantum dot hybrid nanoparticles for live cell imaging. Biochem Biophys Res Commun 2005;331(4):917–21.
[92] Mochalin VN, Shenderova O, Ho D, Gogotsi Y. The properties and applications of nanodiamonds. Nat Nanotechnol 2011;7(1):11–23.

[93] Schrand AM, Hens SAC, Shenderova OA. Nanodiamond particles: properties and perspectives for bioapplications. Crit Rev Solid State Mater Sci 2009;34(1-2):18–74.
[94] Chow EK, Zhang X-Q, Chen M, Lam R, Robinson E, Huang H, et al. Nanodiamond therapeutic delivery agents mediate enhanced chemoresistant tumor treatment. Sci Transl Med 2011;3(73) 73ra21.
[95] Moore L, EK-H Chow, Osawa E, Bishop JM, Ho D. Diamond–lipid hybrids enhance chemotherapeutic tolerance and mediate tumor regression. Adv Mater 2013;25(26):3532–41.
[96] Lee JW. 3D nanoprinting technologies for tissue engineering applications. J Nanomater 2015:1–14.
[97] Zhao J, Swartz LA, Lin W, Schlenoff PS, Frommer J, Schlenoff JB, et al. Three-dimensional nanoprinting via scanning probe lithography-delivered layer-by-layer deposition. ACS Nano 2016;10(6):5656–62.
[98] Metri K, Bhargav H, Chowdhury P, Koka PS. Ayurveda for chemo-radiotherapy induced side effects in cancer patients. J Stem Cells 2013;8(2):115–29.
[99] Mehta NK, Moynihan KD, Irvine DJ. Engineering new approaches to cancer vaccines. Cancer Immunol Res 2015;3(8):836–43.
[100] Sathish JG, Sethu S, Bielsky M-C, de Haan L, French NS, Govindappa K, et al. Challenges and approaches for the development of safer immunomodulatory biologics. Nat Rev Drug Discov 2013;12(4):306–24.
[101] Wang H, Di J, Sun Y, Fu J, Wei Z, Matsui H, et al. Biocompatible PEG-chitosan@carbon dots hybrid nanogels for two-photon fluorescence imaging, near-infrared light/pH dual-responsive drug carrier, and synergistic therapy. Adv Funct Mater 2015;25(34): 5537–47.
[102] Yang J, Yao M-H, Wen L, Song J-T, Zhang M-Z, Zhao Y-D, et al. Multifunctional quantum dot-polypeptide hybrid nanogel for targeted imaging and drug delivery. Nanoscale 2014;6(19):11282–92.
[103] Li P, Luo Z, Liu P, Gao N, Zhang Y, Pan H, et al. Bioreducible alginate-poly(ethylenimine) nanogels as an antigen-delivery system robustly enhance vaccine-elicited humoral and cellular immune responses. J Control Release Off J Control Release Soc 2013;168(3):271–9.
[104] Nochi T, Yuki Y, Akiyoshi K, Kiyono H. Self-assembled polysaccharide nanogels for nasal delivery of biopharmaceuticals Neves J, das, Sarmento B, editors. Mucosal delivery of biopharmaceuticals. US: Springer; 2014. p. 325–32.
[105] Vaupel P, Harrison L. Tumor hypoxia: causative factors, compensatory mechanisms, and cellular response. Oncologist 2004;9(Supplement 5):4–9.
[106] Swietach P, Vaughan-Jones RD, Harris AL, Hulikova A. The chemistry, physiology and pathology of pH in cancer. Philos Trans R Soc B Biol Sci 2014;369(1638).
[107] Eckmann DM, Composto RJ, Tsourkas A, Muzykantov VR. Nanogel carrier design for targeted drug delivery. J Mater Chem B 2014;2(46):8085–97.
[108] Steinhilber D, Witting M, Zhang X, Staegemann M, Paulus F, Friess W, et al. Surfactant free preparation of biodegradable dendritic polyglycerol nanogels by inverse nanoprecipitation for encapsulation and release of pharmaceutical biomacromolecules. J Control Release Off J Control Release Soc 2013;169(3):289–95.
[109] Zhu J-Y, Lei Q, Yang B, Jia H-Z, Qiu W-X, Wang X, et al. Efficient nuclear drug translocation and improved drug efficacy mediated by acidity-responsive boronate-linked dextran/cholesterol nanoassembly. Biomaterials 2015;52:281–90.
[110] Manchun S, Dass CR, Cheewatanakornkool K, Sriamornsak P. Enhanced anti-tumor effect of pH-responsive dextrin nanogels delivering doxorubicin on colorectal cancer. Carbohydr Polym 2015;126:222–30.

[111] Manchun S, Cheewatanakornkool K, Dass CR, Sriamornsak P. Novel pH-responsive dextrin nanogels for doxorubicin delivery to cancer cells with reduced cytotoxicity to cardiomyocytes and stem cells. Carbohydr Polym 2014;114:78–86.
[112] Ju C, Mo R, Xue J, Zhang L, Zhao Z, Xue L, et al. Sequential intra-intercellular nanoparticle delivery system for deep tumor penetration. Angew Chem Int Ed 2014;53(24):6253–8.
[113] Madhusudana Rao K, Krishna Rao KSV, Ramanjaneyulu G, Ha C-S. Curcumin encapsulated pH sensitive gelatin based interpenetrating polymeric network nanogels for anti cancer drug delivery. Int J Pharm 2015;478(2):788–95.
[114] Zan M, Li J, Luo S, Ge Z. Dual pH-triggered multistage drug delivery systems based on host–guest interaction-associated polymeric nanogels. Chem Commun Camb Engl 2014;50(58):7824–7.
[115] Chatterjee DK, Diagaradjane P, Krishnan S. Nanoparticle-mediated hyperthermia in cancer therapy. Ther Deliv 2011;2(8):1001–14.
[116] Zhao X, Wang T, Liu W, Wang C, Wang D, Shang T, et al. Multifunctional Au@IPN-pNIPAAm nanogels for cancer cell imaging and combined chemo-photothermal treatment. J Mater Chem 2011;21(20):7240–7.
[117] Shirakura T, Kelson TJ, Ray A, Malyarenko AE, Kopelman R. Hydrogel nanoparticles with thermally controlled drug release. ACS Macro Lett 2014;3(7):602–6.
[118] Zhang L, Guo R, Yang M, Jiang X, Liu B. Thermo and pH dual-responsive nanoparticles for anti-cancer drug delivery. Adv Mater 2007;19(19):2988–92.
[119] Li Z, Shen J, Ma H, Lu X, Shi M, Li N, et al. Preparation and characterization of pH- and temperature-responsive hydrogels with surface-functionalized graphene oxide as the crosslinker. Soft Matter 2012;8(11):3139–45.
[120] Schmaljohann D. Thermo- and pH-responsive polymers in drug delivery. Adv Drug Deliv Rev 2006;58(15):1655–70.
[121] Xing Z, Wang C, Yan J, Zhang L, Li L, Zha L. Dual stimuli responsive hollow nanogels with IPN structure for temperature controlling drug loading and pH triggering drug release. Soft Matter 2011;7(18):7992–7.
[122] Chen Y, Ding D, Mao Z, He Y, Hu Y, Wu W, et al. Synthesis of hydroxypropylcellulose-poly(acrylic acid) particles with semi-interpenetrating polymer network structure. Biomacromolecules 2008;9(10):2609–14.
[123] Song J-Y, Cha J, Lee J, Roe J-H. Glutathione reductase and a mitochondrial thioredoxin play overlapping roles in maintaining iron–sulfur enzymes in fission yeast. Eukaryot Cell 2006;5(11):1857–65.
[124] Russo A, DeGraff W, Friedman N, Mitchell JB. Selective modulation of glutathione levels in human normal versus tumor cells and subsequent differential response to chemotherapy drugs. Cancer Res 1986;46(6):2845–8.
[125] Hastings KT, Cresswell P. Disulfide reduction in the endocytic pathway: immunological functions of gamma-interferon-inducible lysosomal thiol reductase. Antioxid Redox Signal 2011;15(3):657–68.
[126] Wu W, Yao W, Wang X, Xie C, Zhang J, Jiang X. Bioreducible heparin-based nanogel drug delivery system. Biomaterials 2015;39:260–8.
[127] Maciel D, Figueira P, Xiao S, Hu D, Shi X, Rodrigues J, et al. Redox-responsive alginate nanogels with enhanced anticancer cytotoxicity. Biomacromolecules 2013;14(9):3140–6.
[128] Chen L, Xue Y, Xia X, Song M, Huang J, Zhang H, et al. A redox stimuli-responsive superparamagnetic nanogel with chemically anchored DOX for enhanced anticancer efficacy and low systemic adverse effects. J Mater Chem B 2015;3(46):8949–62.

[129] Zhao M, Hu B, Gu Z, Joo K-I, Wang P, Tang Y. Degradable polymeric nanocapsule for efficient intracellular delivery of a high molecular weight tumor-selective protein complex. Nano Today 2013;8(1):11–20.
[130] Shi B, Zhang H, Qiao SZ, Bi J, Dai S. Intracellular microenvironment-responsive label-free autofluorescent nanogels for traceable gene delivery. Adv Healthc Mater 2014;3(11):1839–48.
[131] Yang C, Wang X, Yao X, Zhang Y, Wu W, Jiang X. Hyaluronic acid nanogels with enzyme-sensitive cross-linking group for drug delivery. J Control Release Off J Control Release Soc 2015;205:206–17.
[132] Yim H, Park S, Bae YH, Na K. Biodegradable cationic nanoparticles loaded with an anticancer drug for deep penetration of heterogeneous tumours. Biomaterials 2013;34(31):7674–82.
[133] Kim K, Bae B, Kang YJ, Nam J-M, Kang S, Ryu J-H. Natural polypeptide-based supramolecular nanogels for stable noncovalent encapsulation. Biomacromolecules 2013;14(10):3515–22.
[134] Lakshmanan S, Gupta GK, Avci P, Chandran R, Sadasivam M, Jorge AES, et al. Physical energy for drug delivery; poration, concentration and activation. Adv Drug Deliv Rev 2014;71:98–114.
[135] Shanmugam V, Selvakumar S, Yeh C-S. Near-infrared light-responsive nanomaterials in cancer therapeutics. Chem Soc Rev 2014;43(17):6254–87.
[136] Fuller KJ, Issels RD, Slosman DO, Guillet JG, Soussi T, Polla BS. Cancer and the heat shock response. Eur J Cancer Oxf Engl 1994;30A(12):1884–91.
[137] Harmon BV, Takano YS, Winterford CM, Gobé GC. The role of apoptosis in the response of cells and tumours to mild hyperthermia. Int J Radiat Biol 1991;59(2):489–501.
[138] Zha L, Banik B, Alexis F. Stimulus responsive nanogels for drug delivery. Soft Matter 2011;7(13):5908–16.
[139] Fomina N, Sankaranarayanan J, Almutairi A. Photochemical mechanisms of light-triggered release from nanocarriers. Adv Drug Deliv Rev 2012;64(11):1005–20.
[140] Wang Y, Nie J, Chang B, Sun Y, Yang W. Poly(vinylcaprolactam)-based biodegradable multiresponsive microgels for drug delivery. Biomacromolecules 2013;14(9): 3034–46.
[141] Chen W, Achazi K, Schade B, Haag R. Charge-conversional and reduction-sensitive poly(vinyl alcohol) nanogels for enhanced cell uptake and efficient intracellular doxorubicin release. J Control Release Off J Control Release Soc 2015;205:15–24.
[142] Zhang X, Achazi K, Steinhilber D, Kratz F, Dernedde J, Haag R. A facile approach for dual-responsive prodrug nanogels based on dendritic polyglycerols with minimal leaching. J Control Release Off J Control Release Soc 2014;174:209–16.
[143] Peng J, Qi T, Liao J, Chu B, Yang Q, Li W, et al. Controlled release of cisplatin from pH-thermal dual responsive nanogels. Biomaterials 2013;34(34):8726–40.
[144] Turner AP. Biosensors: Fundamentals and applications—historic book now open access. Biosens Bioelectron 2015;65:A1.
[145] Kazakov S, Kaholek M, Gazaryan I, Krasnikov B, Miller K, Levon K. Ion concentration of external solution as a characteristic of micro- and nanogel ionic reservoirs. J Phys Chem B 2006;110(31):15107–16.
[146] Weng J, Ren J. Luminescent quantum dots: a very attractive and promising tool in biomedicine. Curr Med Chem 2006;13(8):897–909.
[147] Riedinger A, Pernia Leal M, Deka SR, George C, Franchini IR, Falqui A, et al. Nanohybrids" based on pH-responsive hydrogels and inorganic nanoparticles for drug delivery and sensor applications. Nano Lett 2011;11(8):3136–41.

[148] Goswami S, Pant HJ, Biswal J, Samantray JS, Sharma VK, Dash A. Synthesis, characterization and application of Au-198 nanoparticles as radiotracer for industrial applications. Appl Radiat Isot 2016;111:18–25.
[149] Liong M, Lu J, Kovochich M, Xia T, Ruehm SG, Nel AE, et al. Multifunctional inorganic nanoparticles for imaging, targeting, and drug delivery. ACS Nano 2008;2(5):889–96.
[150] Raj L, Chauhan GS, Azmi W, Ahn JH, Manuel J. Kinetics study of invertase covalently linked to a new functional nanogel. Bioresource Technol 2011;102(3):2177–84.
[151] Dharela R, Chauhan GS. Effect of nanogel structure and reaction parameters on activity of immobilized glucose oxidase. Curr Catal 2013;2(3):225–36.
[152] Yan M, Liu Z, Lu D. Fabrication of single carbonic anhydrase nanogel against denaturation and aggregation at high temperature. Biomacromolecules 2007;8(2):560–5.
[153] Ge J, Lu D, Wang J, Yan M, Lu Y, Liu Z. Molecular fundamentals of enzyme nanogels. J Phys Chem B 2008;112(45):14319–24.
[154] Wang J, Zhao G, Li Y, Liu X, Hou P. Reversible immobilization of glucoamylase onto magnetic chitosan nanocarriers. Appl Microbiol Biotechnol 2013;97(2):681–92.
[155] Wang R, Zhang Y, Ge J, Liu J. Activation of enzyme nanogel in organic solvents by PEG-substrate joint imprinting. RSC Adv 2014;4(76):40301–4.
[156] Guo X, Zhang X, Wang S, Li S, Hu R, Li Y, et al. Sensing for intracellular thiols by water-insoluble two-photon fluorescent probe incorporating nanogel. Anal Chim Acta 2015;869:81–8.
[157] Peng HS, Stolwijk JA, Sun LN, Wegener J, Wolfbeis OS. A nanogel for ratiometric fluorescent sensing of intracellular pH values. Angew Chem 2010;122(25):4342–5.
[158] Cao L, Li X, Wang S, Li S, Li Y, Yang G. A novel nanogel-based fluorescent probe for ratiometric detection of intracellular pH values. Chem Commun 2014;50(63):8787–90.
[159] Iwasaki Y, Kondo J-I, Kuzuya A, Moriyama R. Crosslinked duplex DNA nanogels that target specified proteins. Sci Technol Adv Mater 2016;17(1):285–92.
[160] Wang H, Ke F, Mararenko A, Wei Z, Banerjee P, Zhou S. Responsive polymer–fluorescent carbon nanoparticle hybrid nanogels for optical temperature sensing, near-infrared light-responsive drug release, and tumor cell imaging. Nanoscale 2014;6(13):7443–52.
[161] Xia LW, Xie R, Ju XJ, Wang W, Chen Q, Chu LY. Nano-structured smart hydrogels with rapid response and high elasticity. Nat Commun 2013;4:2226.
[162] Sui X, Feng X, Hempenius MA, Vancso GJ. Redox active gels: synthesis, structures and applications. J Mater Chem B 2013;1(12):1658–72.
[163] Wu W, Aiello M, Zhou T, Berliner A, Banerjee P, Zhou S. In-situ immobilization of quantum dots in polysaccharide-based nanogels for integration of optical pH-sensing, tumor cell imaging, and drug delivery. Biomaterials 2010;31(11):3023–31.
[164] Asher SA, Alexeev VL, Goponenko AV, Sharma AC, Lednev IK, Wilcox CS, et al. Photonic crystal carbohydrate sensors: low ionic strength sugar sensing. J Am Chem Soc 2003;125(11):3322–9.
[165] Zhou S, Min X, Dou H, Sun K, Chen CY, Chen CT, et al. Facile fabrication of dextran-based fluorescent nanogels as potential glucose sensors. Chem Commun 2013;49(82):9473–5.
[166] Sahiner N, Ozay O, Aktas N. 4-Vinylpyridine-based smart nanoparticles with *N*-isopropylacrylamide, 2-hydroxyethyl methacrylate, acrylic acid, and methacrylic acid for potential biomedical applications. Curr Nanosci 2011;7(3):453–62.
[167] Wu W, Shen J, Banerjee P, Zhou S. Chitosan-based responsive hybrid nanogels for integration of optical pH-sensing, tumor cell imaging and controlled drug delivery. Biomaterials 2010;31(32):8371–81.

[168] Zhu H, Li Y, Qiu R, Shi L, Wu W, Zhou S. Responsive fluorescent Bi2O3@PVA hybrid nanogels for temperature-sensing, dual-modal imaging, and drug delivery. Biomaterials 2012;33(10):3058–69.
[169] Li C, Liu S. Responsive nanogel-based dual fluorescent sensors for temperature and Hg2+ ions with enhanced detection sensitivity. J Mater Chem 2010;20(47): 10716–23.
[170] Wu W, Mitra N, Yan EC, Zhou S. Multifunctional hybrid nanogel for integration of optical glucose sensing and self-regulated insulin release at physiological pH. ACS Nano 2010;4(8):4831–9.
[171] Wu W, Zhou T, Berliner A, Banerjee P, Zhou S. Smart core – shell hybrid nanogels with Ag nanoparticle core for cancer cell imaging and gel shell for pH-regulated drug delivery. Chem Mater 2010;22(6):1966–76.
[172] Guarrotxena N, Quijada-Garrido I. Optical and swelling stimuli-response of functional hybrid nanogels: feasible route to achieve tunable smart core@shell plasmonic@polymer nanomaterials. Chem Mater 2016;28(5):1402–12.
[173] Li T, Zhou W, SONG Q, Fang W. NaYF4:Yb3 +–Er3+ nanocrystals/P(NIPAM-co-RhBHA) core–shell nanogels: preparation, structure, multi stimuli-responsive behaviors and application as detector for Hg2+ ions. J Photochem Photobiol A: Chem 2015;302: 51–8.
[174] Kim Y, Lee TS. Thermoresponsive, and reversibly emissive, core–shell nanogel composed of PNIPAM and carbon nanodots. Polym Bull 2016;73:2615.
[175] Wang H, Yi J, Mukherjee S, Banerjee P, Zhou S. Magnetic/NIR-thermally responsive hybrid nanogels for optical temperature sensing, tumor cell imaging and triggered drug release. Nanoscale 2014;6(21):13001–11.
[176] Dong X, Wei C, Lu L, Liu T, Lv F. Fluorescent nanogel based on four-arm PEG–PCL copolymer with porphyrin core for bioimaging. Mater Sci Eng: C 2016;61:214–9.
[177] Dong X, Wei C, Lu L, Liu T, Lv F. Real-time fluorescence tracking of protoporphyrin incorporated thermosensitive hydrogel and its drug release in vivo. ACS Appl Mater Interfaces 2016;8(8):5104–13.
[178] Khatun Z, Nurunnabi M, Nafiujjaman M, Reeck GR, Khan HA, Cho KJ, et al. A hyaluronic acid nanogel for photo-chemo theranostics of lung cancer with simultaneous light-responsive controlled release of doxorubicin. Nanoscale 2015;7(24):10680–9.
[179] Scott EA, Nichols MD, Cordova LH, George BJ, Jun YS, Elbert DL. Protein adsorption and cell adhesion on nanoscale bioactive coatings formed from poly (ethylene glycol) and albumin microgels. Biomaterials 2008;29(34):4481–93.
[180] Tessler LA, Donahoe CD, Garcia DJ, Jun YS, Elbert DL, Mitra RD. Nanogel surface coatings for improved single-molecule imaging substrates. J R Soc Interface 2011;8(63):1400–8.
[181] Donahoe CD, Cohen TL, Li W, Nguyen PK, Fortner JD, Mitra RD, et al. Ultralow protein adsorbing coatings from clickable PEG nanogel solutions: benefits of attachment under salt-induced phase separation conditions and comparison with PEG/albumin nanogel coatings. Langmuir 2013;29(12):4128–39.
[182] Atta AM, Al-Lohedan HA, Al-Haddad KA. Epoxy coating with embedded self-healing networks formed by nanogel particles. RSC Adv 2016;6(47):41229–38.
[183] Sun YM, Wang W, Wei YY, Deng NN, Liu Z, et al. In situ fabrication of a temperature- and ethanol-responsive smart membrane in a microchip. Lab Chip 2014;14(14): 2418–27.
[184] Luo F, Xie R, Liu Z, Ju XJ, Wang W, Lin S, et al. Effects of fabrication conditions on the microstructures and performances of smart gating membranes with in situ assembled nanogels as gates. J Membr Sci 2016;519:32–44.

[185] Wu DQ, Wu LL, Cui HC, Zhang HN, Yu JY. A rapid ammonia sensor based on lysine nanogel-sensitized PANI/PAN nanofibers. J Mater Chem B 2016;4(8):1520–7.
[186] Ramakrishnan N, Vamsi T, Khan A, Nemade HB, Palathinkal RP. Humidity sensor using NIPAAm nanogel as sensing medium in SAW devices. Int J Nanosci 2011;10(01n02):259–62.
[187] Reese CE, Mikhonin AV, Kamenjicki M, Tikhonov A, Asher SA. Nanogel nanosecond photonic crystal optical switching. J Am Chem Soc 2004;126(5):1493–6.
[188] Lee J, Ko S, Kwon CH, Lima MD, Baughman RH, Kim SJ. Carbon Nanotube yarn-based glucose sensing artificial muscle. Small 2016.

Further Reading

Huang Y, Lapitsky Y. Monovalent salt enhances colloidal stability during the formation of chitosan/tripolyphosphate microgels. Langmuir 2011;27:10392–10399.
Cheng R, Feng F, Meng F, Deng C, Feijen J, Zhong Z. Glutathione-responsive nano-vehicles as a promising platform for targeted intracellular drug and gene delivery. J Control Release Off J Control Release Soc 2011;152(1):2–12.
Wan X, Liu H, Yao S, Liu T, Yao Y. A stimuli-responsive nanogel-based sensitive and selective fluorescent sensor for Cr3+ with thermo-induced tunable detection sensitivity. Macromol Rapid Commun 2014;35(3):323–9.

Lipid-based nanobiomaterials

6

Parisa Nazemi[1] *and Mehdi Razavi*[2]
[1]Isfahan University of Technology, Isfahan, Iran
[2]Stanford University, Palo Alto, CA, United States

6.1 Introduction

Nanobiomaterials are a highly developed branch of biomedicine [1–7]. Among them, nanodrug carriers including liposomes, oil-in-water (O/W) nanoemulsions, nanoparticles, nanocrystals, lipid-based nanobiomaterials, and so on, have been about to prove advantages such as enhanced drug solubility and stability, improved performance, and increased efficacy of using nanosized dosage forms for medical purposes [8–11]. In this category, liposomes are an interesting group of carriers. They were first introduced in 1970s with the purpose of reducing toxic side effects of drugs. Two main groups of these colloidal lipid-based carriers are nanostructured lipid carriers (NLCs) and solid lipid nanoparticles (SLNs). These systems substitute the oil (lipid) by solid lipid. Nanoparticles based on solid lipids (SLN, NLC) have been proposed as an alternative colloidal drug delivery system to polymeric nanoparticles, emulsions, and liposomes [12,13]. They are composed of solid lipids stabilized with an emulsifying layer in an aqueous dispersion [14]. SLNs are easily prepared nanoparticles made from inexpensive, safe, stable, and biodegradable materials. The average particle size of SLN is 10–1000 nm. They are such a desired carrier because of having all the advantages of other colloidal carriers and not having their disadvantages. These carriers are from natural or synthetic resources of solid lipids and lecithin, respectively. So, polymers, emulsions, and liposomes could be replaced by SLNs and improve the delivery system. Formerly, it was hard to find an appropriate chemical substance having high solubility or complete absorption. NLCs, which are a new generation of colloidal drug delivery system, are promising type of carriers having the most advantages needed. Recently, they have been used successfully in many fields such as dermal, topical, and so on. The base structures of NLCs are solid and liquid lipid nanoparticles dispersed in water. This aqueous mixture is stabilized with surfactants [15–17].

6.2 Applications

SLNs are such an appropriate group of carriers in drug delivery system. Basically, lipids have been brought into pharmaceutical field to be a superior alternative for liposomes, emulsions, and polymeric nanoparticles and their limitations. Some advantages of SLNs are their small size and subsequently large surface area; this large surface area gives the potential of loading high amounts of drug and more interaction of phases on the surface [18].

Nanobiomaterials Science, Development and Evaluation. DOI: http://dx.doi.org/10.1016/B978-0-08-100963-5.00006-9

These advantages are not only for drug delivery systems, but also for using in other materials, for example nutrients. Because of the lipid nature of NLCs they are potential systems to enhance skin hydration. But they have low viscosity that makes them inapplicable to topical usage. To solve this problem, NLCs should be mixed with common semisolid systems of drug delivery with higher viscosity. Accordingly, the mixture will be a more stable nanoparticle. Despite all benefits of NLCs they have defects in their structures, for example amorphous or multiple state type that results in lowering drug leakage meanwhile of storage [19]. Oral bioavailability improved by loading drugs with low solubility in water by lipid formulations [20]. Yet there are fewer studies on oral routs with NLC systems.

NLCs have advantages and limitations; some of the advantages are stability, easy to prepare, enhanced carrier system, improved release of drug, better dispersion in aqueous system, regular particle sizes, increase in skin hydration and its occlusion, and so on. Having toxicity to the nature and not being totally developed are among the most important limitations of NLCs [21,22].

6.3 Classification of SLNs

According to the nature of lipid and the active ingredients, the solubility of actives in the melted lipid, nature and concentration of surfactants, method of production, and its temperature. SLNs have 3 different types including type 1, 2, and 3. Type 1 is obtained from a solid solution of lipid and active ingredient. A solid solution can be made when SLNs are produced by the cold homogenization method. A lipid blend can be produced containing the active ingredient in a molecularly dispersed form. After solidification of this blend, it is ground in its solid state to avoid the enrichment of active molecules in different parts of the lipid nanoparticles. Type 2 can be obtained by the hot technique and the active ingredient concentration is low during the cooling process. SLN type 3 can be made by high concentration of active ingredient in the melt. Cooling down of the hot oil droplets will, in most cases, reduce the solubility of the active ingredient in the melt [23].

6.4 Classification of NLC

Depending on their structures, NLCs are divided into three types, type 1, 2, and 3. NLC type 1 has a mixture of solid and liquid lipids, this mixture leads to an amorphous structure because of differences in crystallization processes for solid and liquid. Subsequently, amorphous structures let the drugs to be placed amorphous and in the form of clusters on NLC, which is undesired. Because of higher solubility of drugs in liquid lipids than solid form, these particles are produced in liquid form first, and then crystalized into solid form. In high amounts of lipids (solid and liquid mixture), solubility gap might occur during crystallization step. This gap increases the possibility of separation of two phases and precipitation of nanocomponents. Type 2 consists

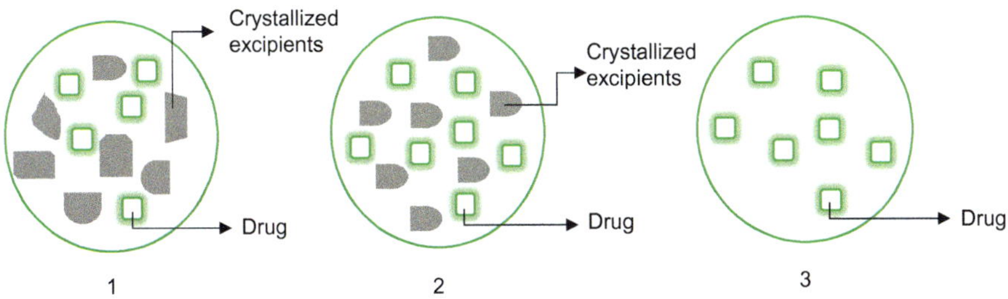

Figure 6.1 Different types of NLCs, type 1, 2, and 3.

of mixed oil-fat water, so, at low solubility, the drug is more able to be set in solid part(Fig. 6.1).

As solubility increases, drug placing is shifted to the oily parts. Like NLC type 1, miscibility gap occurs at high oil concentrations, leading to separation between the phases and precipitation of oily components. Type 3 is an enhanced one, in which the mixture of them is in such a way that they can't be crystallized. Also, this type has an amorphous lipid matrix in solid phase. Preventing from crystallization avoids drug release during it. To accommodate the drugs, based on the drug's hydrophilic or lipophilic characteristics, different particles can be used. Lipid-based particles are potentially suitable for lipophilic drugs, and hydrophilic drugs can be incorporated with peptides and proteins [16,24,25].

6.5 Preparation methods

Several techniques have been developed for synthesis of carriers based on their sensitivities about stability, solubility, and so on, the most important methods are high-pressure homogenization, microemulsion technique, solvent emulsification-evaporation technique, solvent emulsification-diffusion technique, phase inversion temperature (PIT) method [26], melting dispersion method, ultrasonication technique, solvent displacement technique, and double emulsion technique [15,17,23,26–39].

6.5.1 High-pressure homogenization (HPH) method

This technique is a promising method for preparing different types of lipid-based particles most likely for SLNs, NLCs, and lipid drug conjugate (LDC). The procedure is to pushing lipids through a narrow gap in order to decrease their size by a high pressure about 100–200 bars. This pressure results in shear stress and cavitation that makes the particles to minify into submicron range. One of the most important advantages of this technique is being capable of large-scale production. Two types of production by this method are hot and cold homogenization techniques. In both the mentioned techniques, drug should be dissolved in the melting lipid at temperatures about 5–10°C higher than the melting point [40–42].

In hot high-pressure homogenization (HPH) method, the drug and lipid are melted at a temperature 10°C higher than the lipids melting point and then mixed with a surfactant solution at the same temperature. Consequently, a hot preemulsion forms by the use of a high-speed stirrer. In the next step, this hot preemulsion is processed in a temperature-controlled high-pressure homogenization under 500 bar. The final nanoemulsion cools down to room temperature and crystals of SLN, NLC, or LDC forms [27].

Cold HPH is appropriate for drugs that are heat liable or hydrophilic. The drug is melted with lipid simultaneously and quickly cooled by liquid nitrogen leading to a solid lipid microparticle, which is a presuspension and is then homogenized at or below room temperature and forming SLN, NLC, or LDC. Both hot and cold HPH techniques yield narrow particle size distributions; they both are also suitable for processing lipid concentrations up to 40%. Besides, cold homogenization minimizes the thermal exposure of the sample [28].

6.5.2 Microemulsion method

In this technique, the lipids containing fatty acids or glycosides are liquefied and simultaneously the drug is added to liquefied lipid. These lipids will then be added to a mixture of water, cosurfactant(s), and the surface-active agent, which is heated to a similar temperature under a moderate stirring till the lipid softens. Now a microemulsion is formed, which is a clear, thermodynamically stable system with the particular ratios of components. This microemulsion has the needed properties for the formation of nanoparticles with a desired size. The microemulsion is then spread in a very cold liquid medium with moderate mixing of hot microemulsion with water during a quantitative relation in the range of 1:25–1:50. This dispersion in cold liquid medium results in fast recrystallization of the oil droplets [29].

6.5.3 Solvent emulsification-evaporation or diffusion technique

In this method, the hydrophobic drug and lipophilic material are dissolved in a water-immiscible organic solvent such as cyclohexane, dichloromethane, toluene, chloroform, and so on, and then it turns into an emulsified mixture in an aqueous phase using high-speed homogenizer. To improve the efficiency of fine emulsification, the coarse emulsion is immediately passed through the microfluidizer. This organic solvent is evaporated by stirring at room temperature and reduced pressure leaving lipid precipitates of SLNs. In this technique, the final particle size depends on the concentration of lipid in organic phase. Very small particle size could be obtained with low lipid load (5%) related to organic solvent. One of the advantages of this method is the avoidance of heat during the process, which makes it suitable for the incorporation of highly thermolabile drugs. However, some problems may arise due to solvent residues in the final dispersion [26]. These dispersions are commonly dilute, because of the low solubility of lipid in the organic material. Normally, lipid concentrations in the final SLN dispersion range around 0.1 g/L; therefore, the particle concentration has to be increased by means of, for example ultrafiltration or evaporation.

In the solvent-diffusion technique, partially water-miscible solvents (e.g., benzyl alcohol, ethyl formate) are used. First, they are saturated with water to ensure initial thermodynamic equilibrium of both liquids. Then, the lipid is dissolved in the water-saturated solvent and subsequently emulsified with solvent-saturated aqueous surfactant solution at elevated temperatures. The SLN precipitate after the addition of excess water (typical ratio: 1:5–1:10) due to the diffusion of the organic solvent from the emulsion droplets to the continuous phase. Similar to the production of SLN via microemulsions, the dispersion is fairly dilute and needs to be concentrated by means of ultrafiltration or lyophilization. Average particle sizes of 100 nm and very low particle size distributions can be achieved by both solvent evaporation methods [43].

6.5.4 Solvent emulsification-diffusion technique

Solvent emulsification-diffusion technique can be done in both aqueous phase and oil, so the solvent that is used for this method should be partially miscible with water. Methyl acetate, ethyl acetate, isopropyl acetate, butyl lactate, and benzyl alcohol are some of these solvents. For being sure of thermodynamic equilibrium of solvent and water, they are saturated mutually. If there is a need of heating to solubilize the lipid, the saturation step should be done at that temperature. In the next step, the lipid and drug are dissolved in water-saturated solvent and this organic phase (internal phase) is emulsified with solvent-saturated aqueous solution-containing stabilizer (dispersed phase) using stirrer. After the formation of O/W emulsion, water (dilution medium) in the usual ratio ranges from 1:5 to 1:10, are added to the system in order to allow solvent diffusion into the continuous phase, thus forming aggregation of the lipid in the nanoparticles. Then, both phases are maintained at equal higher temperatures and the diffusion step is done at room temperature or at the temperature under which the lipid is dissolved. At the end, the diffused solvent should be removed, and it can be done by vacuum distillation or lyophilization [34,44].

6.5.5 Melting dispersion method

In melting dispersion method, drug and solid lipid are melted in an organic solvent regarded as oil phase, and simultaneously water phase is also heated to the same temperature as oil phase. Subsequently, the oil phase is added to a small volume of water phase and the resulting emulsion is stirred at high speed for few hours. Finally, it is cooled down to room temperature to yield nanoparticles [31].

6.5.6 Phase inversion temperature (PIT) method

PIT is one of the most well-known methods for production of microemulsions stabilized with nonionic surfactants, and involves phase inversion of O/W to water-in-oil (W/O) emulsions and vice versa induced by temperature. The technique is based on the change in the properties of polyoxyethylated surfactants at different temperatures. At 25 °C the hydrophilic parts of the saccharide (SAC) molecules are hydrated to a certain extent; at this temperature, the hydrophilic–lipophilic balance (HLB) value of surfactants defined by Griffin is valid. An increase in the temperature causes dehydration of the ethoxy groups. Subsequently, the lipophilicity of the molecules of the SAC increases with corresponding decrease in HLB value. At a specific temperature the SAC is equally dependent on the aqueous and lipid phases. This temperature is defined as the PIT. This special state is known by very low surface tension and the presence of complex structures in the system. If the temperature is further increased, the SAC's dependence to the lipid phase becomes high enough to stabilize emulsions of the W/O type [30,45].

6.5.7 High-shear homogenization or ultrasonication technique

Ultrasonication is based on the cavitation mechanism. In the first step, the drug is added to previously melted solid lipid. Then, aqueous phase that has been heated to the same temperature is added to the melted lipid. This mixture can be emulsified in three ways: by probe sonication, by using high-speed stirrer, or aqueous phase added to lipid phase drop by drop followed by magnetic stirring. The obtained preemulsion is ultrasonicated using probe sonicator with water bath at 0 °C. The production temperature keeps at least 5 °C above the lipid melting point to prevent recrystallization during the process [32].

6.5.8 Solvent displacement technique

This technique involves a rapid solvent distribution in water (solvents such as dimethyl sulfoxide (DMSO) or ethanol). In the first step the lipid is dissolved in the solvent. By using a needle it is quickly injected into an aqueous solution of surfactants. The solvent migrates rapidly in the water and the lipid particles precipitate in the aqueous solution. Small particle sizes are affected by the high velocity of distribution processes. The more lipophilic, the solvents give larger particles that may cause problems, for example physical instability. The advantages of this method are low temperatures, easy handling, and the equipment are easily available. But, the main disadvantage is the use of organic solvents [33].

6.5.9 Double emulsion technique

Double emulsion is a novel technique in which the drug is dissolved in aqueous solution, and further emulsified in melted lipid. The primary emulsion is stabilized by adding stabilizer that is dispersed in aqueous phase containing hydrophilic emulsifier, which is followed by stirring and filtration. Double emulsion technique avoids the necessity to melt the lipid for the preparation of peptide-loaded lipid nanoparticles and the surface of the nanoparticles could be modified in order to sterically stabilize them by means of the incorporation of lipid-PEG (polyethylene glycol) derivatives, This technique has been used for the preparation of sodium cromoglycate-containing SLN [34,46,47].

6.6 Conclusion

Lipid-based nanobiomaterials are one of the new and innovative therapeutic delivery systems, which have a high potential to enhance the bioavailability of drugs with low solubility and also target the site of action. This can be the key point in delivery system for critical drugs like the drugs for different cancers. The nanocarriers, especially SLNs and NLCs, are the drug delivery systems that reach the targeted site in the body with desired concentration and in the appropriate time. The NLCs as the new form of carriers have more flexibility in drug loading, drug release and enhanced performance in producing final dosage forms such as injectable, tablets, creams, and capsules. Being capable of large-scale production helps these materials to take an important role in pharmaceutical world in the near future. The investigations on lipid-based nanobiomaterials should extend to find alternative routes and to treat more diseases with them.

References

[1] Razavi M, Salahinejad E, Fahmy M, Nowman A, Jazayeri H, Shah P, et al. Nanobiomaterials in periodontal tissue engineering. Nanobiomaterials in Hard Tissue Engineering: Applications of Nanobiomaterials 2016:323.

[2] Razavi M, Salahinejad E, Fahmy M, Yazdimamaghani M, Vashaee D, Tayebi L. Green chemical and biological synthesis of nanoparticles and their biomedical applications Green Processes for Nanotechnology. Springer; 2015. p. 207–35.

[3] Heidari F, Razavi M, Bahrololoom ME, Bazargan-Lari R, Vashaee D, Kotturi H, et al. Mechanical properties of natural chitosan/hydroxyapatite/magnetite nanocomposites for tissue engineering applications. Materials Science and Engineering: C. 2016;65:338–44.

[4] Razavi M, Fathi M, Savabi O, Vashaee D, Tayebi L. In vivo study of nanostructured akermanite/PEO coating on biodegradable magnesium alloy for biomedical applications. Journal of Biomedical Materials Research Part A. 2015;103(5):1798–808.

[5] Razavi M, Fathi M, Savabi O, Vashaee D, Tayebi L. Improvement of biodegradability, bioactivity, mechanical integrity and cytocompatibility behavior of biodegradable Mg based orthopedic implants using nanostructured bredigite (Ca7MgSi4O16) bioceramic coated via ASD/EPD technique. Annals of biomedical engineering 2014;42(12):2537–50.

[6] Razavi M, Fathi M, Savabi O, Vashaee D, Tayebi L. In vivo biocompatibility of Mg implants surface modified by nanostructured merwinite/PEO. Journal of Materials Science: Materials in Medicine 2015;26(5):1–7.

[7] Razavi M, Fathi M, Savabi O, Vashaee D, Tayebi L. Regenerative influence of nanostructured bredigite (Ca 7 MgSi 4 O 16)/anodic spark coating on biodegradable AZ91 magnesium alloy implants for bone healing. Materials Letters 2015;155:97–101.

[8] Al Khouri Fallouh N, Roblot-Treupel L, Fessi H, Devissaguet JP, Puisieux F. Development of a new process for the manufacture of polyisobutylcyanoacrylate nanocapsules. International Journal of Pharmaceutics 1986;28(2):125–32.

[9] Moghimi SM, Hunter AC, Murray JC. Nanomedicine: current status and future prospects. The FASEB journal 2005;19(3):311–30.

[10] Mura S, Nicolas J, Couvreur P. Stimuli-responsive nanocarriers for drug delivery. Nat Mater 2013;12(11):991–1003.

[11] Sahoo SK, Labhasetwar V. Nanotech approaches to drug delivery and imaging. Drug discovery today 2003;8(24):1112–20.
[12] Müller R, Mehnert W, Lucks J-S, Schwarz C, Zur Mühlen A, Meyhers H, et al. Solid lipid nanoparticles (SLN): an alternative colloidal carrier system for controlled drug delivery. European Journal of Pharmaceutics and Biopharmaceutics 1995;41(1):62–9.
[13] Muller R. Extended patent on the basis of (11). PCT application PCT/EP00/04112. 2000.
[14] Varshosaz J, Eskandari S, Tabbakhian M. Freeze-drying of nanostructure lipid carriers by different carbohydrate polymers used as cryoprotectants. Carbohydrate polymers 2012;88(4):1157–63.
[15] zur Mühlen A, Schwarz C, Mehnert W. Solid lipid nanoparticles (SLN) for controlled drug delivery–drug release and release mechanism. European journal of pharmaceutics and biopharmaceutics 1998;45(2):149–55.
[16] Zhuang C-Y, Li N, Wang M, Zhang X-N, Pan W-S, Peng J-J, et al. Preparation and characterization of vinpocetine loaded nanostructured lipid carriers (NLC) for improved oral bioavailability. International journal of pharmaceutics 2010;394(1):179–85.
[17] Sivaramakrishnan R, Nakamura C, Mehnert W, Korting H, Kramer K, Schäfer-Korting M. Glucocorticoid entrapment into lipid carriers—characterisation by parelectric spectroscopy and influence on dermal uptake. Journal of controlled release 2004;97(3):493–502.
[18] Araújo J, Gonzalez E, Egea MA, Garcia ML, Souto EB. Nanomedicines for ocular NSAIDs: safety on drug delivery. Nanomedicine: Nanotechnology, Biology and Medicine 2009;5(4):394–401.
[19] Müller RH, Radtke M, Wissing SA. Solid lipid nanoparticles (SLN) and nanostructured lipid carriers (NLC) in cosmetic and dermatological preparations. Advanced drug delivery reviews 2002;54:S131–55.
[20] Mukherjee S, Ray S, Thakur R. Solid lipid nanoparticles: a modern formulation approach in drug delivery system. Indian journal of pharmaceutical sciences 2009;71(4):349.
[21] Schäfer-Korting M, Mehnert W, Korting H-C. Lipid nanoparticles for improved topical application of drugs for skin diseases. Advanced drug delivery reviews 2007;59(6):427–43.
[22] Bunjes H, Westesen K, Koch MH. Crystallization tendency and polymorphic transitions in triglyceride nanoparticles. International journal of pharmaceutics 1996;129(1):159–73.
[23] Jenning V, Thünemann AF, Gohla SH. Characterisation of a novel solid lipid nanoparticle carrier system based on binary mixtures of liquid and solid lipids. International Journal of Pharmaceutics 2000;199(2):167–77.
[24] Karunakar G, Patel NP, Kamal SS. Nano structured lipid carrier based drug delivery system. Journal of Chemical and Pharmaceutical Research 2016;8(2):627–43.
[25] Vitorino C, Almeida J, Gonçalves L, Almeida A, Sousa J, Pais A. Co-encapsulating nanostructured lipid carriers for transdermal application: from experimental design to the molecular detail. Journal of Controlled Release 2013;167(3):301–14.
[26] Trotta M, Cavalli R, Carlotti M, Battaglia L, Debernardi F. Solid lipid micro-particles carrying insulin formed by solvent-in-water emulsion–diffusion technique. International journal of pharmaceutics 2005;288(2):281–8.
[27] Gasco MR. Method for producing solid lipid microspheres having a narrow size distribution. Google Patents; 1993.
[28] Moulik S, Paul B. Structure, dynamics and transport properties of microemulsions. Advances in Colloid and Interface science 1998;78(2):99–195.
[29] Zhang D, Tan T, Gao L. Preparation of oridonin-loaded solid lipid nanoparticles and studies on them in vitro and in vivo. Nanotechnology 2006;17(23):5821.
[30] Reithmeier H, Herrmann J, Göpferich A. Lipid microparticles as a parenteral controlled release device for peptides. Journal of Controlled Release 2001;73(2):339–50.

[31] Eldem T, Speiser P, Hincal A. Optimization of spray-dried and-congealed lipid micropellets and characterization of their surface morphology by scanning electron microscopy. Pharmaceutical research 1991;8(1):47–54.
[32] Schubert M, Müller-Goymann C. Solvent injection as a new approach for manufacturing lipid nanoparticles–evaluation of the method and process parameters. European journal of pharmaceutics and biopharmaceutics 2003;55(1):125–31.
[33] Date AA, Joshi MD, Patravale VB. Parasitic diseases: liposomes and polymeric nanoparticles versus lipid nanoparticles. Advanced drug delivery reviews 2007;59(6):505–21.
[34] Trotta M, Debernardi F, Caputo O. Preparation of solid lipid nanoparticles by a solvent emulsification–diffusion technique. International journal of pharmaceutics 2003;257(1):153–60.
[35] ISO13321 I. Methods for determination of particle size distribution part 8: Photon correlation spectroscopy. International Organisation for Standardisation (ISO). 1996.
[36] Nogueiras-Nieto L, Sobarzo-Sánchez E, Gómez-Amoza JL, Otero-Espinar FJ. Competitive displacement of drugs from cyclodextrin inclusion complex by polypseudorotaxane formation with poloxamer: implications in drug solubilization and delivery. European Journal of Pharmaceutics and Biopharmaceutics 2012;80(3):585–95.
[37] Jain SK, Agrawal GP, Jain NK. A novel calcium silicate based microspheres of repaglinide: in vivo investigations. Journal of controlled release 2006;113(2):111–6.
[38] Date AA, Vador N, Jagtap A, Nagarsenker MS. Lipid nanocarriers (GeluPearl) containing amphiphilic lipid Gelucire 50/13 as a novel stabilizer: fabrication, characterization and evaluation for oral drug deliveryIndian patent application number 2167/MUM/2008. Nanotechnology 2011;22(27):275102.
[39] Doktorovova S, Souto EB. Nanostructured lipid carrier-based hydrogel formulations for drug delivery: a comprehensive review. Expert opinion on drug delivery 2009;6(2):165–76.
[40] Schwarz C, Mehnert W, Lucks J, Müller R. Solid lipid nanoparticles (SLN) for controlled drug delivery. I. Production, characterization and sterilization. Journal of Controlled Release 1994;30(1):83–96.
[41] Muller R, Lucks J. Azneistoffträger aus festen Lipidteilchen feste Lipid Nanosphären (SLN) European Patent 0605497. CIT0052. 1996.
[42] Lim S-J, Kim C-K. Formulation parameters determining the physicochemical characteristics of solid lipid nanoparticles loaded with all-trans retinoic acid. International journal of pharmaceutics 2002;243(1):135–46.
[43] Kasongo KW, Pardeike J, Müller RH, Walker RB. Selection and characterization of suitable lipid excipients for use in the manufacture of didanosine-loaded solid lipid nanoparticles and nanostructured lipid carriers. Journal of pharmaceutical sciences 2011;100(12):5185–96.
[44] Hu F, Yuan H, Zhang H, Fang M. Preparation of solid lipid nanoparticles with clobetasol propionate by a novel solvent diffusion method in aqueous system and physicochemical characterization. International journal of pharmaceutics 2002;239(1):121–8.
[45] Montenegro L, Sarpietro M, Ottimo S, Puglisi G, Castelli F. Differential scanning calorimetry studies on sunscreen loaded solid lipid nanoparticles prepared by the phase inversion temperature method. International journal of pharmaceutics 2011;415(1):301–6.
[46] Kakar S, Singh R. Preparation of magnetic microspheres of mesalamine by phase separation emulsion polymerisation technique. African journal of pharmacy and pharmacology 2014;8(9):246–58.
[47] Cortesi R, Esposito E, Luca G, Nastruzzi C. Production of lipospheres as carriers for bioactive compounds. Biomaterials 2002;23(11):2283–94.

Peptide-based nanobiomaterials

7

Yasemin Budama-Kilinc, Burak Ozdemir and Kubra Gozutok
Yildiz Technical University, Istanbul, Turkey

7.1 Introduction

Nanotechnology involves the use of nanostructures with a size of 1–100 nm and nanoparticles, which are described as small structures that act as a whole unit with regard to their transports and properties [1–3]. In the formation of hybrid structures, peptides and proteins can be used as patterns for nanobiomaterials [4,5]. Besides, they can be considered as functional nanoscale biomaterials. It has been shown that various peptides and their derivatives have molecular architectures such as tubes, fibers, planes, ribbons, nanospheres, gels, and three-dimensional (3D) networks [3]. Peptide nanomaterials have been prominently used in applications such as bioengineering, drug delivery, regenerative medicine, tissue engineering, and molecular devices, because of their advantageous properties, including their biocompatibility, structural diversity, and biological functionality [6]. In recent years, bionanocomposites have been considered hybrid materials derived from natural and synthetic biodegradable polymers and organic/inorganic fillers [7].

7.2 Peptides

Peptides are composed of two or three to hundreds of amino acid residues covalently connected through amide bonds called peptide bonds. Two amino acids combine through a peptide bond to form a dipeptide. The peptide bond is formed by dehydration between the α-carboxyl group of an amino acid and the α-amino group of another amino acid. Peptide bond formation is an example of the condensation reaction, the main reaction class of living cells. Three amino acids connected by two peptide bonds form a tripeptide, and tetrapeptides and pentapeptides occur similarly by connection of amino acids. In this way, a structure formed by the connection of a small number of amino acids are called oligopeptide, and a structure formed by connection of large number of amino acids is called polypeptide [8–11].

7.3 Peptide nanomaterials

Peptide-based nanomaterials are formed from small peptide sequences that have the flexibility to develop desired biophysical characteristics by connection with various nanomaterials or through self-assembly [12–14]. A structure of peptide-based nanomaterials, which comprises single peptides, can affect another peptide by noncovalent

Nanobiomaterials Science, Development and Evaluation. DOI: http://dx.doi.org/10.1016/B978-0-08-100963-5.00007-0

interactions, such as ionic, hydrophobic, and hydrogen bonding. Desired supramolecular structures can be formed by including a large number of these building blocks [15].

In recent years, there has been increasing research interest in peptide nanomaterials because of their biocompatibility and structural diversity. Peptide nanomaterials are used in drug delivery systems and tissue engineering as contrast agents, gene transfer tools, and gene therapy agents [16].

For example, Chilkoti et al. showed that artificial recombinant chimeric polypeptides that conjugated with hydrophobic chemotherapeutics can self-assemble into nanoparticles. Drugs, imaging agents, and targeting moieties can thus self-assemble into multifunctional nanoparticles [17].

7.4 Advantages of peptide-based nanomaterials

Peptide-based nanomaterials have several advantages, depending on the areas of usage. They show excellent properties such as high biological activity, biofunctionality, easy modifiability, injectability, biodegradability, and biocompatibility. These important advantages increase the biomedical applications of peptide-based nanomaterials [16,18,19]. These advantages also provide several resources for studies based on drug targeting and regenerative medicine. Peptide-based nanomaterials are more stable and have superior activity per mass unit. They also have long-term storage and easy manipulation capacities because of their small size. For that matter, decorated nanocarriers cannot be easily modified on the basis of physicochemical properties. Peptides are lightly modified by some functional groups because of their chemical properties, and this increases their biological activity [16,20]. The most important feature of peptides is that they can generate several nanostructures by themselves with the help of the peptide self-assembly process. Their synthesis and purification methods are very simple because of automated solid-phase synthesis methods and standard high-performance liquid chromatography (HPLC). Peptides serve as building blocks to create complex 3D structures that can be used to manipulate various nanostructures and provide many features to nanomaterials. Consequently, these peptide-based nanomaterials have wide application areas because of these properties, when compared to other nanomaterials [18,21–24]. One of the most remarkable properties of peptide-based nanomaterials is self-assembly. When choosing the self-assembly method for producing peptide-based nanomaterials, there are several benefits, for instance, peptides can generate different nanostructures such as nanofibers, nanoparticles, nanotapes, gels, and nanorods [25]. Because of these properties, peptide-based nanomaterials can be used in widespread applications areas such as regenerative medicine, drug targeting, cosmetics, and vaccines [24–26].

7.5 Applications of peptide-based nanomaterials

Peptide-based nanomaterials have significant and widespread applications because of their features such as injectability, biodegradability, and biocompatibility. One of the major application fields of peptide-based nanomaterials is delivery systems, and peptide-based nanomaterials serve as drug carriers in this field. These nanocarriers have specific ligands for releasing the drug to a target area of the body [27,28]. Peptide-based nanomaterials have been used as agents for regenerating and repairing tissue in tissue engineering [29]; as a vaccine because of several advantages of peptide-based nanosized vaccines such as easy uptake by cells owing to their small size and protection of enzymatic degradation [30]; and as an antiaging agent in cosmetic [31]. All these application fields will be described in the following text.

7.5.1 Tissue engineering

Tissue engineering has developed rapidly in the last few decades after the development of bioengineering technologies and the appearance of stem cell therapies [32–34]. In tissue engineering studies, scaffolds are key components that can provide a well-defined biomimetic environment surrounding the cells [35,36]. These scaffolds can support cell adhesion, cell proliferation, and infiltration to prove the success of tissue engineering [37]. Thus, scaffolds exhibit significant applications for tissue engineering [38]. Self-assembling peptide nanofibrous scaffolds (SAPNF) have been used to regenerate tissues such as nerve, cartilage, and bone [39].

Since bone and cartilage are very dynamic tissues and respond to changes in the applied mechanical forces by growth or matrix modification, damage to cartilage and bone is common [40,41]. Therefore, repair and regeneration of cartilage and bone have critical importance in the development of modern regenerative medicine. Peptide nanotechnology has been used to promote cartilage regeneration [16]. To understand the function of TATVHL (Thr-Ala-Thr-Val-His-Leu) peptide-grafted scaffolds, bovine knee cartilages were cultured in these scaffolds, and it was found that the surface of the TATVHL peptides increases the adhesion of the bovine knee chondrocytes to the scaffolds. The surface of the TATVHL peptides effectively promotes the amount of cartilage components as well as accelerates the proliferation of bovine knee chondrocytes. Peptide-based nanocarriers can stimulate cartilage regeneration by delivering growth factor to the deficient sides [42].

Stupp et al. chose self-assembled peptide amphiphile (PA) molecules to form nanofibers. They bound the growth factor β-1 (TGFβ-1) with PA nanofibers. Results of their in vitro experiments have shown that these nanofibers can induce human mesenchymal cells to undergo chondrogenic differentiation. Their in vivo experiments have also shown that the peptide-TGFβ-1 complexes substantially increase the regeneration of microfracture-treated chondral defects [43]. The peptide KLD12 including the Ac-KLDLKLDLKLDL-NH2 sequence was modified with Substance P (SP). Polylactic acid and beta tricalcium phosphate were used to fabricate KLD12/KLD12-SP, which enhance bone regeneration. The results of in vitro and in vivo experiments have shown that KLD12/KLD12-SP have several advantages, such as accelerated formation of bone tissue and repair of bone deficiencies [44]. An important aspect of the bone tissue growth is the mineralization of scaffolds that can be controlled by calcium phosphate and short peptides. Nonoyama et al. showed that polyethylene glycol (PEG)-conjugated (leucine-glutamate) peptide molecules can be arranged antiparallel to each other in a mica surface [45].

Nerve injury or damage may be due to a variety of human diseases or health problems [46,47]. Thus, there has been an increasing focus on nerve regeneration [48]. Self-assembling peptide nanotechnology is also used for nerve healing. Tekinay et al. designed and synthesized four PA molecules, namely heparan-sulfate-mimicking PA (HSM-PA), laminin epitope carrier PA (IKVAV-PA), Glu-PA, and Lys-PA. These PAs were self-assembled into nanofibers and mimicked neural extracellular matrices (ECMs). All of these PAs exhibit the same hydrophobic alkyl tails and VVAG peptide sequence constituting β-sheet. After the cells were cultured with scaffolds, results showed that the PA scaffolds promote PC-12 cell neurite growth compared to scaffolds having only laminin-derived signals [49].

Three specific motifs, arginine–glycine–aspartic acid (RGD), bone marrow homing peptide 1 (BMHP1), and bone marrow homing peptide 2 (BMHP2), were used to modify the self-assembling peptide by Cunha et al., and then, this self-assembling peptide was modified again depending on a 16-residue peptide-RADA16. RADA16-RGD, RADA16-BMHP1, and RADA16-BMHP2 were made functional after they were self-assembled into scaffolds for the use of a 3D culture of adult neural stem cells (NSCs). These self-assembling peptides provide stimulative 3D microenvironment effects for different cell types, and promote proliferation and differentiation of adult NSCs. Various peptide-based nanomaterials can induce cell proliferation and neuro-regeneration as explained above, but they have some function in extensive loss of cerebral parenchyma [50]. Through experiments, Wu et al. showed that injured nerve tissue can be regenerated with the help of the self-assembling peptide nanofibers. Nanofiber scaffolds were prepared using peptide self-assembly of Ac-RADARADARADARADA-CONH2 (RADA16-I), and the results revealed that seriously injured brain might be reconstructed using peptide nanofiber scaffolds. Several experiments confirmed that self-assembling peptide nanomaterials are invaluable in the healing of nerve disease [51].

7.5.2 Delivery systems

Targeted drug delivery has been commonly used for increasing the efficiency of drugs and for decreasing the adverse effects with canalizing drugs to specific areas of body [52]. This excellent mechanism enables the drug carriers to identify molecular targets that are on cell surface or nuclear membranes by means of specific targeting ligands. Performing surface modification of the drug carrier is another way to induce the active drug targeting, especially in nanocarriers, for effective targeted moieties of cells. Polymeric nanoparticles, liposomes, micelles, polymer-drug conjugates, peptides, proteins, and antibodies are identified as nanosized drug carrier systems and are widely used in this ever-developing field [53]. Nanosized drug carrier molecules can identify and bind to target antigens or receptors that are overexpressed or selectively expressed via cells or tissue components [52].

The high specificity (depends on complex) and strong molecular identification are the main characteristic properties of nanosized drug carriers, which have several interconnection areas with targets such as peptides and proteins. Usage of peptide-based targeting is more advantageous than the other targeting molecules since peptides and proteins show great affinities and specificities for other biomolecules [52].

The peptide-based delivery molecules have several advantages. When compared to antibodies or proteins and conventional drugs, peptides have more efficient penetration capacity and more specificity to the tissue because of their small size [54]. Peptides are inexpensive when considered chemically, they do not have immunogenic effect, and they can be used various times on the same individual [55]. Further, peptides do not accumulate in tissues because of their short half-life and rapid clearance, and this avoids possible metabolite formation. For these several advantages, peptide-based delivery molecules have several applications such as delivery of small molecule drugs and genes [52].

Amphiphilic peptides (APs), which are a type of self-assembling peptides, have been widely used in the delivery of small molecule drugs [56]. APs have a hydrophilic head and hydrophobic tail [57]. The interaction of the hydrophobic alkyl tails, hydrogen bonding, and electrostatic repulsions are three major forces that affect AP self-assembly systems [58,59]. Zhang's research has shown that AP includes the sequences KKGRGDS and VVVVVV that could self-assemble into micelles. Doxorubicin (DOX) is known as an antitumor drug, and it is trapped to these micelles. Zhang then performed experiments delivering these DOX-loaded micelles to human cervical cancer Hela and monkey kidney COS7 cells. At the end of the experiments, the antitumor drug was released from the micelles with intracellular uptake and was efficiently delivered into the Hela cells. This is because of the RGD sequence as revealed by the research results. Integrins are well-known as heterodimeric cell receptors that are overexpressed in the blood vessel of solid tumors. Integrins promote tumor cell migration and tumor growth because of mediating the adhesion and ECM. High binding affinity for Arg–Gly–Asp (RGD) sequences is a characteristic property of integrins, and this makes RGD peptides the most popular tool for drug delivery systems and imaging agents [60].

Gene delivery or gene therapy is another outstanding research field for treatment of human diseases. Gene delivery has shown promising potential treatment methods for various diseases such as cancer and cardiovascular disease [61,62]. Target gene and delivery vectors are the main factor for the therapeutic efficiency of gene delivery [63]. The delivery efficiency is also related to protein coatings, DNA complexes, and interactions among cells [64]. Many molecules have been used as delivery vectors for gene delivery. Peptides are one of these molecules, and recent researches have shown that peptide-based nanomaterials can be used for gene-targeting delivery systems [65].

Zhang et al. used APs for targeted gene delivery systems. They produced two types of biocompatible BolA-like APs. These BolA-like APs have dual ligands, of which one is the tumor-targeting peptide Arg-Gly-Asp RGD and another is a cell-penetrating peptide. These two molecules can bind DNA easily, because they include the RGD motif, which has some advantages for gene delivery such as transporting DNA through cell membranes easily andits essential sequence for cell attachment. BolA-like APs induce cervical cancer Hela cell arrest and tumor suppression and also regulates the gene expression property [66].

7.5.3 Vaccines

Nanovaccines comprise of nanosized particles attached or formulated with components that can stimulate the immune response. Nanovaccines can stimulate the immune system to prohibit or kill infections and prevent the spread of diseases [67]. Nanovaccines have attracted attention in recent years owing to their remarkable advantages such as low toxicity, wide surface area, low dosage, and stable dosage forms [68,69]. Nanomaterials that will be used for vaccine development can be produced from polymers, lipids, peptides, or inorganic components.

Peptide-based vaccines have several advantages such as safety, stability, and ease of production, and because of these properties, they have been considered to be promising for the development of therapeutic vaccines [70]. Peptide-based nanovaccines are produced by the use of antigenic peptides that cause the pathogenesis of viruses, parasites, and bacteria [70]. These vaccines show better effect on the immune system, are resistant to enzymes, and do not require additional adjuvant [70–72].

Peptide-based nanovaccines can be produced in several forms: with polymer nanoparticles by encapsulation or attaching peptide antigen to the surface of polymer nanoparticles, by lipidation of peptides that can self-assemble into nanoparticles and induce strong immune responses, by self-assembly of peptides that are biodegradable, biocompatible, and can induce both cellular and humoral immune responses without the help of an adjuvant, and with inorganic nanoparticles and nanotubes that can serve as carriers for peptide-based vaccines. These forms can induce immune responses and often have optimal efficacy [30].

7.5.4 Diagnosis

The capabilities of peptide-based diagnostics in recognition of specific viral or bacterial infections have been demonstrated through several studies. Peptide-based diagnostics have been used in the determination of antibodies [73–75]. Results have shown 96.7% sensitivity and 100% specificity by an enzyme-linked immunosorbent assay (ELISA) using an 18-amino acid (AA) peptide from the glycoprotein of virus [76]. It has also been reported that peptide-based diagnostics have 100% sensitivity and 99% specificity for bacterial pathogens by peptide-based ELISA and are not just limited to viral pathogens [77]. Therefore, peptide-based diagnostics have a significant role in serological identification of a variety of infectious diseases.

In a study on the use of peptides in diagnosis, Navalkar et al. showed that peptide epitopes have higher sensitivity and specificity compared to random peptide sequences [78].

In recent years, brain natriuretic peptide (BNP), which is 32 AA peptide synthesized from ventricles, has gained importance for use in the diagnosis of heart failure for patients admitted to the emergency services [79].

Another peptide sequence that has been used in diagnosis is C-peptide. Insulin is synthesized as a pro-peptide and released into circulation with C-peptide, and therefore, exogenous insulin lacks C-peptide [80]. Peripheral C-peptide concentrations have been used for detection of beta cell secretory activity because C-peptide is secreted from the beta cell in equimolar concentration with insulin. Plasma C-peptide has thus been used in control of insulin secretion in patients with insulin antibodies for type 1 diabetes and investigation of patients with hypoglycemic disorders [81].

Shen et al. aimed at developing rapid diagnostic tests for tuberculosis using three immunodominants antigens (Ag85B, BfrB, and TrxC), which are obtained from TB patients. The researchers selected synthetic peptides from these immunodominant proteins. The result of their study revealed that these peptides exhibit the potential for producing rapid diagnostic kits [82].

Mukherjee et al. aimed at producing freeze-dried kits for PET imaging of neuroendocrine tumors using ^{68}Ga-labeled 1,4,7,10-tetraazacyclododecane-N,N′,N″,N‴-tetraacetic acid (DOTA) peptides. They successfully produced vial kits that are available and useful for using PET imaging of neuroendocrine tumors [83].

OspC is a peptide antigen in *Borrelia burgdorferi*, which causes Lyme disease. Arnolbaldi et al. used OspC peptides for detecting Lyme disease using ELISA. Their results showed that OspC peptides have the potential for rapid diagnosis of Lyme disease [84].

Fachiroh et al. aimed at developing rapid diagnostic kits for detecting nasopharyngeal carcinoma. They used a combination of Epstein–Barr Virus (EBV) EBNA1- and viral capsid antigen-p18-derived synthetic peptides. In addition, they used IgA and IgG for ELISA. Their study proved that the combined IgA EBNA1 + VCA-p18 ELISA is a potential tool for primary diagnosis of nasopharyngeal carcinoma [85].

Protein 85 (OMP85) is a highly conserved outer membrane protein of Neisseria meningitidis. This protein was used by Reddy for the rapid diagnosis of bacterial meningitis. In that study, the peptide sequence between 720 and 745 residues was chosen, which is the unique region of Neisseria meningitidis. Polyclonal antibodies against this peptide sequence were also prepared. Subsequently, OMP85 was conjugated with colloidal gold nanoparticles. The results revealed that GNP-OMP85 is a promising material for rapid diagnosis of Neisseira meningitidis at low concentration of bacterial and protein antigens [86].

In another study, M2e and hemagglutinin peptides are used for developing ELISA method against Influenza. The result showed that the antibody response was high against both M2e and hemagglutinin peptides [87].

7.5.5 Cosmetics

Several researches have been carried out on peptides and proteins that have cosmetic properties such as promoting skin and hair health and on their potential role as hair conditioning agents in following years and at the beginning of the 1960s. The functionalities of peptides can be controlled through the production process. For example, the hydrophobicity of peptides influences their cosmetic properties (substantivity to hair and skin, tenside binding capacity, foaming and emulsifying performance, interaction with radical species, and solubility) [82].

In the market, peptides can be counted as cosmetic components consisting of short-chain amino acid sequences such as 6–7 amino acids, but there are also exceptions to this rule (8– and 20– peptides have been found).

Various studies have shown that peptides and amino acids can reverse the effects of aging on the skin, and this property has been utilized in wound-healing research [83].

Various studies have shown that peptides may upregulate cellular growth factors, and they may heal skin by mimicry of angiogenesis and granulation tissue and new collagen synthesis. Peptides have been therefore been considered as cosmetic agents.

7.6 Conclusion and future trends

In recent years, application fields of peptide-based materials have been consistently developing. These materials are nonimmunogenic, biocompatible, biodegradable, and easily modifiable. Peptide-based nanomaterials are therefore an extremely interesting research area for the development of new delivery systems.

Regenerative medicine, which involves tissue engineering and 3D cell culture for repair and treatment of defective tissue, is one of the most outstanding applications of peptide-based nanomaterials. Scaffolds produced from peptide-based nanomaterials can mimic the ECM environment.

Peptide-based nanomaterials are useful for drug delivery systems, another field that has become attractive for researches. In particular, peptide-based nanocarriers are very suitable for carrying antitumor and imaging agent to the relative tissue or area of body because they have some advantages such as easy modifiability, injectability, biodegradability, and biocompatibility. The main problems in vaccines are the efficacy of vaccine preparations, distribution, and availability of the vaccine. Developing nanotechnology can be used to solve these problems with peptide-based nanovaccines. These materials can be injectable, biodegradable, exhibit high bioactivities and stability. They will be very useful for developing new cancer, Alzheimer, and allergy vaccines in the future.

Rapid diagnosis is crucial in treating disease and decreasing morbidity and mortality. In particular, a peptide-based strip test is very useful for rapid diagnosis of several diseases. Developing molecular biology and genetics enables production of synthetic peptides that are unique, highly conserved, and immunodominant for bacterial causes of disease. These developments enable treatment of incurable diseases in the future.

Cosmeceuticals are important, and this industry is growing rapidly every year. This growth leads to the necessity of new products. Researchers are therefore searching for new molecules that can be used in the cosmetic industry. Peptide-based nanomaterials are one of these new molecules in cosmetics. They serve as signal, carrier, and neurotransmitter-affecting molecules [88–89], which are useful for wound healing and antiaging. Searching new peptide-based materials will be collaterally developed with this growing cosmetic industry.

To sum up, peptide-based nanomaterials are a topic of increasing interest for researchers.

Acknowledgment

The authors thank the Scientific and Technological Research Council of Turkey for their support with the "Development of a Rapid Diagnostic Kit with an Immunochromatographic Method Depending on the IgY Antibody Specific for the (M2e) Peptide for the Diagnosis of Influenza A Infection" study (Project No. 115S132).

References

[1] Torchilin VP. Nanoparticulates as Drug Carriers. Imperial College Press; 2006.
[2] Schwarz JA, Contescu CI, Putyera K. Dekker Encyclopedia of Nanoscience and Nanotechnology. M. Dekker; 2004.
[3] Lee J-H, et al. Protein/peptide based nanomaterials for energy application. Curr Opin Biotechnol 2013;24(4):599–605.
[4] Ruso JM, Piñeiro Á. Proteins in Solution and at Interfaces: Methods and Applications in Biotechnology and Materials Science. Wiley; 2013.
[5] Leonida MD, Kumar I. Bionanomaterials for Skin Regeneration. Springer International Publishing; 2016.
[6] Renliang H, et al. Peptide Based Nanomaterials and Their Technological Applications. Prog Chem 2010;22(12):2328–37.
[7] Hule RA, Pochan DJ. Polymer nanocomposites for biomedical applications. Mrs Bull 2007;32(04):354–8.
[8] Nelson DL, Cox MM. Lehninger Principles of Biochemistry. W.H. Freeman; 2013.
[9] Petsko GA, Ringe D. Protein Structure and Function. New Science Press; 2004.
[10] Champe PC, Harvey RA, Ferrier DR. Biochemistry. Lippincott/Williams & Wilkins; 2005.
[11] Reid R. Peptide and Protein Drug Analysis. CRC Press; 1999.
[12] Fraysse-Ailhas C, et al. Peptide nanoparticles for drug delivery applications. Eur Cell Mater 2007;14:115.
[13] Raman S, et al. Structure-based design of peptides that self-assemble into regular polyhedral nanoparticles. Nanomedicine 2006;2(2):95–102.
[14] Avti, P.K., S.C. Patel, and B. Sitharaman, *Nanobiomaterials: Current Status and Future Prospects*. 2011.
[15] Ulijn RV, Smith AM. Designing peptide based nanomaterials. Chem Soc Rev 2008;37(4):664–75.
[16] Yu C-Y, et al. Progress in Self-assembling Peptide-based Nanomaterials for Biomedical Applications. Curr Top Med Chem 2016;16(3):281–90.
[17] Zelzer M, Ulijn RV. Next-generation peptide nanomaterials: molecular networks, interfaces and supramolecular functionality. Chem Soc Rev 2010;39(9):3351–7.
[18] Nicolas J, et al. Design, functionalization strategies and biomedical applications of targeted biodegradable/biocompatible polymer-based nanocarriers for drug delivery. Chem Soc Rev 2013;42(3):1147–235.
[19] Gong C, et al. Target delivery of a gene into the brain using the RVG29-oligoarginine peptide. Biomaterials 2012;33(12):3456–63.
[20] Pérez CMR, et al. The powerful functions of peptide-based bioactive matrices for regenerative medicine. Ann Biomed Eng 2015;43(3):501–14.
[21] Doles T, et al. Functional self-assembling polypeptide bionanomaterials. Biochem Soc Trans 2012;40(4):629–34.
[22] Gilead S, Gazit E. Self-organization of short peptide fragments: from amyloid fibrils to nanoscale supramolecular assemblies. Supramol Chem 2005;17(1–2):87–92.
[23] Ladner RC, et al. Phage display-derived peptides as therapeutic alternatives to antibodies. Drug Discov Today 2004;9(12):525–9.
[24] Koo H, et al. In vivo targeted delivery of nanoparticles for theranosis. Acc Chem Res 2011;44(10):1018–28.
[25] Castillo-León J, Svendsen W. Micro and Nanofabrication Using Self-Assembled Biological Nanostructures. Elsevier Science; 2014.

[26] Deming T. Peptide-Based Materials. Springer Berlin Heidelberg; 2012.
[27] Ben-Yedidia T, Arnon R. Design of peptide and polypeptide vaccines. Curr Opin Biotechnol 1997;8(4):442–8.
[28] Alemán C, Bianco A, Venanzi M. Peptide Materials: From Nanostuctures to Applications. John Wiley & Sons; 2013.
[29] Holmes TC. Novel peptide-based biomaterial scaffolds for tissue engineering. Trends Biotechnol 2002;20(1):16–21.
[30] Skwarczynski M, Toth I. Recent advances in peptide-based subunit nanovaccines. Nanomedicine 2014;9(17):2657–69.
[31] Sadick NS, et al. Cosmeceutical Science in Clinical Practice. CRC Press; 2010.
[32] Watts RA, et al. Oxford Textbook of Rheumatology. OUP Oxford; 2013.
[33] Kamolz LP, et al. Handbook of Burns Volume 2: Reconstruction and Rehabilitation. Vienna: Springer; 2012.
[34] Steinhoff G. Regenerative Medicine - from Protocol to Patient: 3. Tissue Engineering, Biomaterials and Nanotechnology. Springer International Publishing; 2016.
[35] Mishra AK. Nanomedicine for Drug Delivery and Therapeutics. Wiley; 2013.
[36] Gaharwar AK, et al. Nanomaterials in Tissue Engineering: Fabrication and Applications. : Elsevier Science; 2013.
[37] Engineering, T. and R.M.I. Society, *Tissue Engineering*. 2008: Mary Ann Liebert, Incorporated.
[38] Ma PX. Biomimetic materials for tissue engineering. Adv Drug Deliv Rev 2008;60(2):184–98.
[39] Nune M, et al. Self-assembling peptide nanofibrous scaffolds for tissue engineering: novel approaches and strategies for effective functional regeneration. Curr Protein Pept Sci 2013;14(1):70–84.
[40] Sathananthan PAH. Human Cell and Tissue Fine Structure for Teaching and Research In Stem Cells. CSIRO; 2015.
[41] Royce PM, Steinmann B. Connective Tissue and Its Heritable Disorders: Molecular, Genetic, and Medical Aspects. Wiley; 2003.
[42] Kuo Y-C, Wang C-C. Cartilage regeneration by culturing chondrocytes in scaffolds grafted with TATVHL peptide. Colloids Surf B 2012;93:235–40.
[43] Hartgerink JD, Beniash E, Stupp SI. Self-assembly and mineralization of peptide-amphiphile nanofibers. Science 2001;294(5547):1684–8.
[44] Kim JE, et al. Effect of self-assembled peptide–mesenchymal stem cell complex on the progression of osteoarthritis in a rat model. Int J Nanomedicine 2014;9(Suppl 1):141.
[45] Nonoyama T, et al. Morphology control of calcium phosphate by mineralization on the β-sheet peptide template. Chem Commun 2010;46(37):6983–5.
[46] Tubbs RS, et al. Nerves and Nerve Injuries: Vol 1: History, Embryology, Anatomy, Imaging, and Diagnostics. Elsevier Science; 2015.
[47] Cousins MJ. Cousins and Bridenbaugh's Neural Blockade in Clinical Anesthesia and Pain Medicine. Wolters Kluwer Health; 2012.
[48] Copulsky W. Practical Sales Forecasting. : American Management Association; 1970.
[49] Mammadov B, et al. Cooperative effect of heparan sulfate and laminin mimetic peptide nanofibers on the promotion of neurite outgrowth. Acta Biomater 2012;8(6):2077–86.
[50] Cunha C, et al. 3D culture of adult mouse neural stem cells within functionalized self-assembling peptide scaffolds. Int J Nanomedicine 2011;6:943–55.
[51] Guo J, et al. Self-assembling peptide nanofiber scaffold promotes the reconstruction of acutely injured brain. Nanomedicine 2009;5(3):345–51.
[52] Webster TJ. Nanomedicine: Technologies and Applications. : Elsevier Science; 2012.

[53] Vasir JK, Reddy MK, Labhasetwar VD. Nanosystems in drug targeting: opportunities and challenges. Curr Nanosci 2005;1(1):47–64.
[54] Laakkonen P, Zhang L, Ruoslahti E. Peptide targeting of tumor lymph vessels. Ann N Y Acad Sci 2008;1131(1):37–43.
[55] Laakkonen P, Vuorinen K. Homing peptides as targeted delivery vehicles. Integr Biol 2010;2(7–8):326–37.
[56] Lebl M. Peptides Across the Pacific: Proceedings of the 23rd American Peptide Symposium and the 6th International Peptide Symposium. Prompt Scientific Publishing; 2013.
[57] Wang J-X, et al. Controlled Arrays of Self-Assembled Peptide Nanostructures in Solution and at Interface. Langmuir 2013;29(23):6996–7004.
[58] Castillo J, Sasso L, Svendsen WE. Self-Assembled Peptide Nanostructures: Advances and Applications in Nanobiotechnology. Pan Stanford Publishing; 2012.
[59] Subramani K, Ahmed W. Emerging Nanotechnologies in Dentistry: Materials, Processes, and Applications. Elsevier/William Andrew; 2012.
[60] Liang J, et al. pH Responsive micelle self-assembled from a new amphiphilic peptide as anti-tumor drug carrier. Colloids Surf B 2014;114:398–403.
[61] Fishbein I, Chorny M, Levy RJ. Site-specific gene therapy for cardiovascular disease. Curr Opin Drug Discov Devel 2010;13(2):203.
[62] Chen J, et al. Production and clinical development of nanoparticles for gene delivery. Mol Ther Methods Clin Dev 2016;3:16023.
[63] Doelle, H.W., J.S. Rokem, and M. Berovic, BIOTECHNOLOGY - Volume XI: Fundamentals in Biotechnology. 2009.
[64] Templeton NS, Lasic DD. Gene Therapy: Therapeutic Mechanisms And Strategies. Taylor & Francis; 2000.
[65] Amiji MM. Polymeric Gene Delivery: Principles and Applications. CRC Press; 2004.
[66] Zhang H, et al. Biocompatible pillararene-assembly-based carriers for dual bioimaging. ACS Nano 2013;7(9):7853–63.
[67] Zaman M, Good MF, Toth I. Nanovaccines and their mode of action. Methods 2013;60(3):226–31.
[68] Skwarczynski M, Toth I. Peptide-based subunit nanovaccines. Curr Drug Deliv 2011;8(3):282–9.
[69] Bachmann MF, Jennings GT. Vaccine delivery: a matter of size, geometry, kinetics and molecular patterns. Nat Rev Immunol 2010;10(11):787–96.
[70] Liu T-Y, et al. Advances in peptide-based human papillomavirus therapeutic vaccines. Curr Top Med Chem 2012;12(14):1581–92.
[71] Dudek NL, et al. Epitope discovery and their use in peptide based vaccines. Curr Pharm Des 2010;16(28):3149–57.
[72] Yamada A, et al. Next-generation peptide vaccines for advanced cancer. Cancer Sci 2013;104(1):15–21.
[73] Shin SY, et al. The use of multiple antigenic peptide (MAP) in the immunodiagnosis of human immunodeficiency virus infection. IUBMB Life 1997;43(4):713–21.
[74] Gnann JW, et al. Synthetic peptide immunoassay distinguishes HIV type 1 and HIV type 2 infections. Science 1987;237(4820):1346–9.
[75] Porstmann T, et al. Two-colour combination enzyme-linked immunosorbent assay for the simultaneous detection of HBV and HIV infection. J Immunol Methods 1993;158(1): 95–106.
[76] Oladepo D, Klapper P, Marsden H. Peptide based enzyme-linked immunoassays for detection of anti-HSV-2 IgG in human sera. J Virol Methods 2000;87(1):63–70.

[77] Liang FT, et al. Sensitive and specific serodiagnosis of Lyme disease by enzyme-linked immunosorbent assay with a peptide based on an immunodominant conserved region of Borrelia burgdorferi VlsE. J Clin Microbiol 1999;37(12):3990–6.

[78] Navalkar KA, Johnston SA, Stafford P. Peptide based diagnostics: Are random-sequence peptides more useful than tiling proteome sequences? J Immunol Methods 2015;417:10–21.

[79] NEDiR, B., ACÎL SERVISTE BEYÎN NATRÍÜRETÍK FAKTOR (BNP) KULLANIMI.

[80] Mughal R, et al. Cellular mechanisms by which proinsulin C-peptide prevents insulin-induced neointima formation in human saphenous vein. Diabetologia 2010;53(8):1761–71.

[81] Polonsky KS, Rubenstein AH. C-peptide as a measure of the secretion and hepatic extraction of insulin. Pitfalls and limitations. Diabetes 1984;33(5):486–94.

[82] Shen G, et al. Peptide-based antibody detection for tuberculosis diagnosis. Clin Vaccine Immunol 2009;16(1):49–54.

[83] Mukherjee A, et al. Development of single vial kits for preparation of 68Ga-labelled peptides for PET imaging of neuroendocrine tumours. Mol Imaging Biol 2014;16(4):550–7.

[84] Arnaboldi PM, et al. Outer surface protein C peptide derived from Borrelia burgdorferi sensu stricto as a target for serodiagnosis of early Lyme disease. Clin Vaccine Immunol 2013;20(4):474–81.

[85] Fachiroh J, et al. Single-assay combination of Epstein-Barr Virus (EBV) EBNA1-and viral capsid antigen-p18-derived synthetic peptides for measuring anti-EBV immunoglobulin G (IgG) and IgA antibody levels in sera from nasopharyngeal carcinoma patients: options for field screening. J Clin Microbiol 2006;44(4):1459–67.

[86] Reddy BRS. A novel gold nanoparticle-based approach for the rapid diagnosis of meningococcal infection. Melbourne: RMIT University; 2008.

[87] Kılınç YB, Koç RÇ, Badur S. The development of a universally conserved M2e and hemagglutinin peptide-based ELISA method against Influenza A. J Clin Anal Med 2016;7(7).

[88] Kecel-Gunduz S, Celik S, Ozel AE, Akyuz S. The conformational and vibrational behavior of the inhibitory neuropeptide derived from beta-endorphin. J Biomol Struct Dyn 2016:1–18.

[89] Kecel S, Ozel AE, Akyuz S, Celik S, Agaeva G. Conformational analysis and vibrational spectroscopic investigation of l-proline–tyrosine (l-Pro–Tyr) dipeptide. J Mol Struct 2011;993(1):349–56.

Nanoparticles hybridization to engineer biomaterials for drug delivery

8

M. Rezaa Mohammadi[1], *Wenchao Sun*[1,2], *Mohammed Inayathullah*[1,2] *and Jayakumar Rajadas*[1,2]
[1]Biomaterials and Advanced Drug Delivery Laboratory, Stanford University School of Medicine, Palo Alto, CA, United States
[2]Cardiovascular Pharmacology Division, Cardiovascular Institute, Stanford University School of Medicine, Stanford, CA, United States

8.1 Introduction

A new era of disease diagnosis and therapy is dawning as a result of knowledge advancements in biology, materials science, chemistry, and medicine. Cooperation between scientists of these areas is inevitable with the development of personalized medicines and advanced biomaterials. Drug delivery is one such area that requires multidisciplinary expertise. Medicinal chemists have devoted their efforts to synthesize therapeutic moieties with superior properties such as improved potency and bioavailability. Bioengineers and pharmacologists focused on developing materials that have minimal undesired in vivo interactions. Immunologists have studied and intervened in the foreign body response against the biomaterials. Materials scientists, through incorporation of materials of different sizes, shapes, compositions, and chemistries are creating novel materials with higher therapeutic indices. In this respect, widespread classes of materials have been designed to enhance the efficacy and decrease the toxicity, through controlled and targeted delivery of the therapeutics [1–5].

One notable active area in drug delivery is targeted cancer therapy with the goal to reduce the side effects associated with regular chemotherapy. It is now evident that efficient in vivo drug uptake into cancer cells requires drug carriers with small and tailored sizes (10–100 nm) to avoid rapid clearance as well as capitalize on the enhance permeability and retention (EPR) effect. This is where nanotechnology comes into play. Through employment of various classes of nanoparticles (NPs) for drug delivery, it is now possible to design a nanotherapy for a particular target or disease. The properties of NPs can be fine-tuned by altering their sizes, geometry, chemistry, and many other factors. Despite the immense efforts to apply nanotechnology to drug delivery, in vivo uptake of synthetic NPs still lacks desired efficiency [6]. Lack of specificity is another challenge in developing targeted drug delivery, and various strategies such as using targeting peptides and antibodies have not demonstrated promising effects [7]. It is reported that on average only 0.7% of the administered therapeutic agents would eventually be delivered to the solid tumor [7], and the remaining would be delivered to

Nanobiomaterials Science, Development and Evaluation. DOI: http://dx.doi.org/10.1016/B978-0-08-100963-5.00008-2

undesired targets (known as off-target delivery) and body clearance system. This has a deleterious impact on nanomaterials-based translational medicine from the efficiency point of view, as well as from the toxicity and potential side effects perspectives.

As mentioned earlier, close collaboration between multiple branches of science is required for further advancements in nanotherapeutics. For instance, biologists and pharmacologist need a source of materials with low toxicity, which could preserve drug's activity and efficiently target the relevant receptors. They also prefer materials that are capable of integrating with the target tissue, are responsive to stimuli, and possess drug release capability of desired doses and time frame. Delivery of drugs to specific targets (i.e., organ, tissue, wound, or even cells) in the human body using bio- and/or synthetic materials-based drug carriers has revolutionized biomedical research for the past few decades. Among various proposed carriers, liposomes [1], NPs [2], polymersomes [3], dendrimers [4], nanotubes [8], and hydrogels [5] have demonstrated to be cost-effective with decreased toxicity and minimum side effects. In addition to targeting capabilities, the material component of the drug delivery systems are desired to possess properties including but not limited to biocompatibility, biodegradability, and minimum immunogenicity. However, single-component materials that can meet the requirement of multiple characteristics are scarce, if any. Therefore, intensive research has been focused on engineering materials through hybridization of two or more components, with each playing specific and vital roles. The term *hybridization* is usually used for interpenetration of materials at the nanometer (less than 1 μm) or molecular level. International Union of Pure and Applied Chemistry (IUPAC) has defined hybrid materials as "material composed of an intimate mixture of inorganic components, organic components, or both types of components" [9]. Here, we refer to the engineered NPs (with more than one component present together), a hybrid structure. We also utilize the term *hybridization* to refer to the process of making these NPs composite.

8.2 Nanoparticles hybridization techniques

Fabrication of a hybridized structure on the nanometer scale requires extensive information on functional groups, conjugation chemistries, and physical behavior of materials. A stable hybrid nanomaterial consists of different components, which are complexed together properly. It should be noted that while in some instances very stable bonding is essential between the components, in others controlled degradable hybrids are of interest. Contrast enhancement NP is an example of the former, and controlled release nanohybrids the latter. Generally, three methods are known for conjugation of the materials on the nanoscale: (1) chemical bonding through electron sharing between the components, (2) physical bonding (other than self-assembly), and (3) self-assembly, where materials arrange together desirably. Here the first two methods are discussed.

8.2.1 Physically conjugated hybrid nanoparticles

Generally, chemisorption or physisorption approaches could be applied to stabilize NPs with polymers, in which NPs are covalently or physically linked to the polymer, respectively [10,11]. Physically attached hybrids are more sensitive to the surrounding media, pH, and temperature, whereas chemically bonded NPs (also known as covalently bonded) are more stable. The most important benefit of physisorption technique over the chemisorption is that chemical reactions between the moieties of US Food and Drug Administration (FDA) approved materials can impact their original FDA approval [12], while physical interactions are generally known to be safe and do not lead to further FDA assessments. In other words, physically bonded nanohybrid formulation usually face less regulatory barriers in the translational process.

The interbonding between physisorbed hybrid NPs are due to physical interactions, including hydrogen bonding or other types of electrostatic interactions. Thermodynamically, the bonding energy of physisorbed hybrids are lower than chemisorbed systems—the adsorption enthalpy is between 5 and 40 kJ/mol for physical bonds and 40 and 800 kJ/mol for covalent bonds, although polarity and molecular mass can influence this range [13]. In physiological media, competitive exchange between proteins and polymer-core NP interbond may culminate in NPs fast aggregation [14]. However, physisorption strategy may offer an advantage in other cases. Compared to core–shell hybrids with chemisorbed polymeric shell, water molecules have better accessibility to the core of hybrids with a shell structure consisting of a physisorbed polymeric corona. In the case of iron oxide NPs (IONPs), for example, this accessibility provides enhanced relaxivity rate [15] through faster exchange rate of water molecules within the first hydration layer of IONPs, which is a crucial characteristic for magnetic resonance imaging (MRI) applications. It should be noted that commercial IONPs are generally taking advantage of physisorbed coating of dextran around IONPs mainly for this purpose.

In drug-loaded physisorbed hybrid NPs, physical forces between absorbed polymer and NP core determine the loading efficiency of the drug. Cheng et al. incorporated amino-functionalized silicon phthalocyanine, which is a photodynamic therapy (PDT) compound, into polyethylene glycol (PEG)-coated gold NPs through hydrophobic interactions [16]. They reported that PEG acts as a physical cage around NPs, allowing delivery of hydrophobic drug to the target. They reported that the net negative charge from anion adsorption on the gold NPs surface interacts with the protonated amine of the PDT compound to further promote drug loading and stabilize the hybrid NPs. Kim et al. also reported that hydrophobic drug loading on gold NPs dramatically increases when a moiety containing amine group (tamoxifen) presents on the surface of NPs [17]. Thus, physical coating is a promising method to load hydrophobic drugs onto the surface of NPs.

Although the physical bondings in these examples are known to be inherently weak, thus limiting their application in intravenous drug delivery [15], physical interaction between avidin and biotin molecules is the strongest known noncovalent interaction ($K_d = 10^{-15}$ M). This bonding is now widely used in nanomedicine. Once the bond forms between biotin and avidin it is insensitive to extreme conditions of pH, ionic strength, and temperature, offering a promising nanomaterials hybridization method for biomedical applications. Biotinylation, owing to its mild nature, is one of the most popular methods to conjugate different moieties to cells without compromising their viability or biological activity [18]. Ma et al. developed a multifunctional hybrid structure for a targeted drug and gene codelivery system [19]. They achieved the joining of two biotinylated moieties by taking advantage of avidin's tetravalency for biotin binding. Doxorubicin (DOX)-conjugated polyion complex (D-PIC) was prepared using poly(L-aspartic acid) and poly(2-(2-aminoethylamino) ethyl methacrylate). Plasmid DNA (pDNA) was added to generate D-PIC-pDNA NPs with positively charged surfaces. Then, the negatively charged macromolecule avidin/ biotin–PEG-co-poly(L-glutamate acid) was coated onto D-PIC-pDNA NPs. Finally, biotinylated transferrin was attached to the surface of the complexes as a targeting agent. The complexes protected pDNA against nuclease degradation, minimized interference from blood proteins, facilitated tumor cell uptake, and delivered both doxorubicin (DOX) and the gene payload. In vitro cell tests indicated that their hybrid had increased transfection efficiency in the presence of serum in HeLa and HepG2 cells. This multifunctional ternary complex proved to be an efficient carrier for the targeted release of anticancer drugs and genes [19].

8.2.2 Chemically conjugated hybrid nanoparticles

To form strong bonds between various moieties, chemical conjugation techniques can be applied, where moieties are connected via one or more covalent bonds. Every chemical modification process requires the reaction of two functional groups with each other, leading to the formation of a covalent bond. One important benefit of this technique is the strong bonding between the moieties, which can be engineered to survive harsh environment. Some of the most utilized chemistries are described below to provide some insights into the chemical hybridization.

8.2.2.1 Amine reactions

Functional groups capable of reacting with amine-containing moieties are the most common groups for chemical cross-linking. In an amine, one or more hydrogen atoms from ammonia are replaced by organic substituents such as alkyl (alkane chain) and aryl (aromatic ring) groups.

Amine functional group has been introduced to afford various drug delivery benefits, even though some limitations have been argued as well. For instance, presence of amine group in the backbone of phenyl boronic acid hydrogels enhances the formation of complexes, which enables tuning of insulin release from the hydrogel matrix [20]. Amine-coupling process can be applied to conjugate almost all proteins and peptides. Here, we briefly introduce isothiocyanate and N-hydroxysuccinimide (NHS) ester chemistries.

The reactions between amine-functionalized NPs and isothiocyanate or NHS functionalized compounds are shown in Fig. 8.1. These chemistries are frequently used for generating fluorescently labeled NPs. NPs functionalized with amine groups react with available fluorescence dyes, such as fluorescein isothiocyanate, rhodamine B isothiocyanate, and Cy5.5 NHS ester (Fig. 8.1).

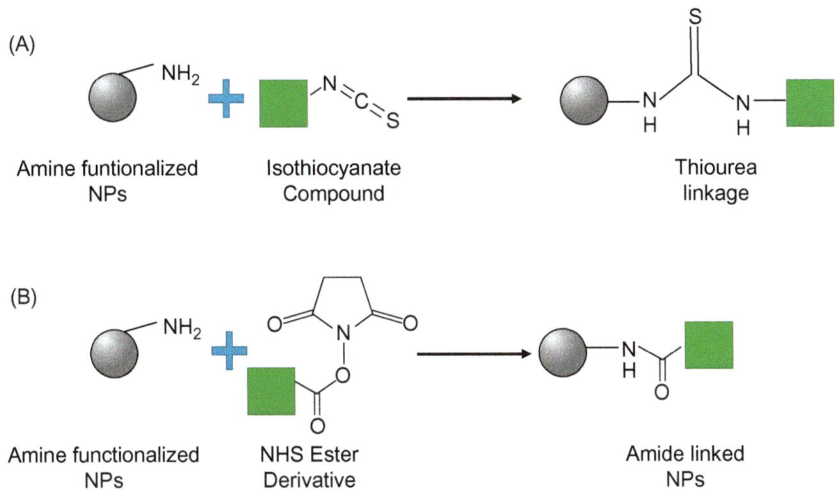

Figure 8.1 Chemical reactions based on amine-functionalized nanoparticles. (A) Isothiocyanate functional group reaction leads to formation of isothiourea. (B) NHS ester reaction forms amide bond.

However, some limitations are associated with introducing amine groups. Excessive unconjugated primary amines are, biologically, highly active and may result in unwanted in vivo interactions.

8.2.2.2 Sulfonyl chlorides

Sulfonyl chlorides are highly reactive derivatives of sulfonic acid and have analogous properties and reactivity to acid chlorides of carboxylates. Their reaction with nucleophiles including amines necessitates alkaline conditions (pH 9–10) and undergoes the formation of a penta-valent transition state, which is unstable. The reaction with amines proceeds with better yield when conducted in organic solvents because hydrolysis is a major competing reaction in water. Sulfonyl chlorides have played a vital role in bioconjugation chemistry, as sulfonic acids can be simply converted into sulfonyl chlorides via phosphorus pentachloride in nonaqueous conditions.

8.2.2.3 Thiol reactions

Another common bioconjugation chemistry is the thiol reactions, in which reactive groups are able to couple with sulfhydryl-containing molecules. Thiols, which are also called mercaptans, are analogous to alcohols. They are named in a similar fashion as alcohols except the suffix-*thiol* is used in place of-*ol*. By itself the -SH group is called a mercapto group. It generally refers to the reaction of compounds containing thiol with "enes," with very high conversion rate [12]. This chemistry is very common among biologists due to its high reaction kinetic in biological media. Generally,

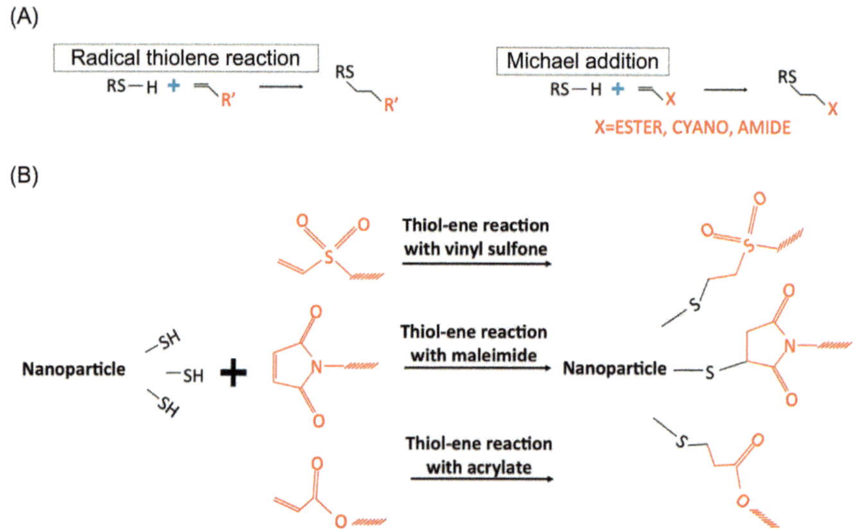

Figure 8.2 Two widely used thiol reaction chemistries. (A) Thiols react with alkenes through two mechanisms: Michael-type addition, or radical-mediated reaction. (B) Thiol-functionalized nanomaterials can further be conjugated with variable molecules, including vinyl sulfone, maleimide, and acrylate groups.

thiols react with alkenes through two mechanisms: Michael-type addition, or radical-mediated reaction as shown in Fig. 8.2. In the former, generally a base abstracts a proton from a thiol, forming a thiolate anion, which performs as a nucleophile. Then, thiolate anion attacks the electrophilic β-carbon on alkene to form carbon-centered anion. This intermediate then abstracts a proton from conjugate acid to give rise to the Michael addition.

Thiol–disulfide exchange reaction is also widely used. The stability of disulfide bond in various biological milieu needs to be carefully examined to prevent premature degradation or cargo release.

8.2.2.4 Carboxylate reactions

Carboxylate functionality demonstrates a low nucleophilicity in aqueous solution, which makes it unreactive with many nucleophilic-based bioconjugate reagents. Carboxylic acid derivatives such as esters, anhydrides, and acid halides react well with good nucleophiles. Carbodiimides have been successfully developed, and function as zero-length cross-linking agents. Carbodiimides activate a carboxylate group for coupling with primary amines, without becoming part of the final product. For instance, Cho et al. used 1-ethyl-3-(3-dimethylaminopropyl)carbodiimide (EDC) chemistry to conjugate acid-capped gold NPs to daunorubicin [21].

8.3 Polymer–biomacromolecule hybrid

Providing biological characteristics for synthetic polymers was always of great interest among polymer scientists. In doing so, polymer–biomacromolecule hybrid conjugates were first introduced by Ringsdorf in 1975 [28]. Since then, diverse polymer–biomacromolecule hybrids have been established and implemented in a vast range of areas including bioseparations, drug/siRNA delivery, enzymatic catalytic processes, diagnostics and biosensing, cell culture processes, and DNA motors. Generally, three methods are applied to generate polymer–biomacromolecule NPs: (1) The "grafting-to" approach involves the covalent or physical attachment of a synthetic polymer to a biomacromolecule by reactive or affinity coupling (Fig. 8.3a). In this method, a preexisting polymer containing a functional end-group reacts with a complementary functional group on the biomacromolecule, resulting in the coupling of biomacromolecule and polymer. (2) In the "grafting from" method, the biomacromolecule is functionalized with a specific moiety (Fig. 8.3b). Polymerization initiates from this precise site on the biomacromolecule capable of generating radicals (initiator or chain transfer agent) and initiates polymerization of monomers. (3) In the "grafting-through" approach, the biomacromolecule is primarily attached to monomers, followed by polymerization (Fig. 8.3c). This technique, therefore, may culminate in hybrids with manifold biological species attached along the polymer backbones [29].

8.3.1 Polymer–protein hybrid

The field of protein–polymer conjugation is of utmost interest in bioengineering, as the properties of protein could be remarkably improved after modification with polymers. Polymeric NPs have much medical promise with a large number of products presently in clinical trials or approved for clinical use [22]. It has been shown that attaching polymers significantly enhances protein solubility, stability, pharmacokinetics (blood half-life), and biodistribution, while decreasing immunogenicity [23,24]. Advances in protein–polymer hybridization have focused on developing the ability to attach the polymer to protein in a site-specific manner. Site-specific control over the location of the polymer attachment on the protein prevents heterogeneity and preserves the activity or the structure of the protein. Grafting the polymer from the protein prevents the steric problems associated with coupling two large molecules of differing properties; it greatly simplifies purification of the new protein–polymer hybrid because the low molecular weight residual monomer can be easily removed. Protein–hydrophobic polymer conjugates are expected to have interesting functionalities due to their amphiphilic molecular structures. Zare group reported a successful hybridization of bovine serum albumin with poly(methyl methacrylate) to fabricate self-assembled NPs with an encapsulated anticancer drug, camptothecin [25]. NPs were given intravenously into mice with subcutaneously injected colon cancer cells. They observed a significant decrease in the size of the tumor through delivering the drug via NPs, rather than naked drug [25].

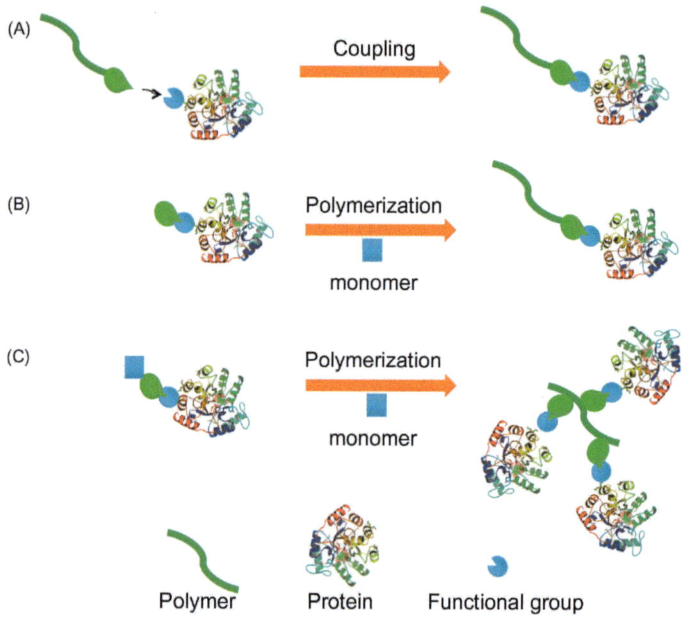

Figure 8.3 Primary synthesize methods of polymer bioconjugates through controlled radical polymerization. (A) Grafting to, (B) grafting from, (C) and grafting through approaches.

8.3.2 Polymer-RNA hybrid

Expression of oncogenes can be inhibited by small double-stranded interfering RNA (siRNA) molecules, which are able to mediate the cleavage of complementary mRNA sequence [26]. Since siRNA molecules possess inherent negative charge, their transportation across the cell membrane is limited. Therefore, some attempts have been made to take advantage of hybridization of siRNA. Jung et al. reported siRNA–quantum dot hybrid construct, which successfully inhibited epidermal growth factor receptor variant III (EGFRvIII) expression in human U87 glioblastoma [27].

8.4 Bioinspired hybrid

Nature has long been the inspiring source for scientists from various disciplines and will definitely keep playing a vital role in future science and technology advancements. Owing to its natural origin, biomimetic materials have attracted much attention in the field of biomaterials to address the difficulties in drug delivery. As an illustration, biotechnological experience demonstrates that delivery of drugs has remained a challenge, as poor membrane crossing, low solubility, toxicity, and poor stability of drugs limit their in vivo benefits. Among various strategies, hybridizing drugs with engineered bacteria, viruses, and various cells such as macrophages has shown to be highly effective to address the above-mentioned issues [30]. For instance, pathogens attack immune system and induce interactions with target cells. By taking advantage of viruses and bacteria as biomimetic carriers, these pathogens can be used to deliver drugs (or therapeutic moiety) to the desired target in efficient dose and favorable time frame. However, lack of functionality is the major drawback of biomimetic NPs. Therefore, some studies attempted to hybridize biomimetic materials to create functional biomimetic platforms. In one study, Wang et al. employed eukaryotic cell-like hybrid platform (EukaCell) for encapsulation of theranostic agents (DOX and indocyanine green). Their hybrid vesicle, EukaCell, contains fullerene (C60), mesoporous silica, and phospholipid (1,2-dihexadecanoyl-sn-glycero-3-phosphocholine (DPPC)). Using this hybrid platform, they reported a 58- and 21-fold enhancement in encapsulation efficiency and loading content, respectively, in comparison with conventional silica NPs. They also reported that release of the encapsulated drug can be precisely controlled via near infrared laser irradiation. Interestingly, the irradiation-induced release was attributed to the disruption of the interactions between DOX–fullerene–silica hybrid [31].

One of the vital platforms in biomimetic drug delivery systems is based on bioengineered bacteria. This area has gained a lot of attention during the past few years, especially, for the targeted drug delivery to tumors [32], as some strains of bacteria are revealed to possess inherent tumor homing nature. For instance, *Bifidobacterium bifidum* and *Salmonella typhimurium*—have a natural tumor-targeting behavior and they specifically colonize in tumor tissues [33]. In this respect, bioengineered bacteria offer a promising platform for targeted therapeutic delivery to tumors.

Through advancements in genetic engineering it is now possible to encode a protein within the bacteria (recombinant bacteria). Since bacteria possess RNA polymerases, plasmid vectors can encode any protein (antibody, cytokine, and enzyme) within the bacteria to produce the desired protein in the preferred target. For instance, bacteria has been engineered to secrete human immunodeficiency virus type 1 (HIV-1) prototypic virucidal compound cyanovirin-N, which potently inhibits HIV-1 infection. However, both cytotoxicity and immunogenicity issues have hampered the translation of this protein into a viable therapeutic agent. Chen et al., demonstrated that PEGylation of cyanovirin-N significantly enhances its anti-HIV-1 activity with attenuated cytotoxicity [34].

What makes bacteria promising for drug delivery is the feasibility of bacteria bioconjugation. This is achieved mainly by taking advantage of the strong biotin–streptavidin interaction for attachment of cargo to benign bacteria [32]. Three main domains may be classified within bacteria-based targeted drug delivery: (1) recombinant bacteria, (2) tumor-targeting bacteria, and (3) NP–bacteria hybrid structure (Fig. 8.4). All these classes have been developed by utilizing the hybridization techniques.

Hybridization of NPs with bacteria is an interesting platform that greatly enhances the efficiency of drug delivery systems. For example, Akin et al. fabricated a hybrid delivery system comprising a bioluminescence reporter gene loaded into NPs, which was carried on the bacteria surface. When incubated with cells, the cargo-carrying bacteria (they named it as "microbots") were internalized by the cells, and the genes released from the NPs were expressed in the cells. Mice injected with microbots also expressed the genes in different organs. Their approach offers a possibility to deliver

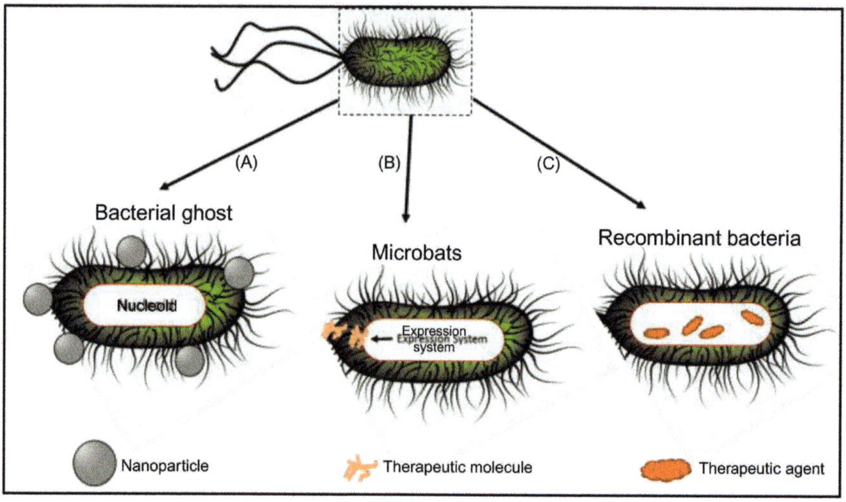

Figure 8.4 Engineering methods for bacteria-based drug delivery. In bacterial ghosts, plasma components including genetic materials are eliminated (A). Microbots are hybridized with nanoparticles on their surface (B). Recombinant bacteria are genetically modified by expression systems that encode antigens, cytokines, and other biologically active proteins (C).

different classes of moieties to live animals (in vivo) and a variety of cells (in vitro) without complicated genetic manipulations [32].

8.5 NPs hybridization to overcome biological barriers

Efficient accumulation of nanotherapeutics at diseased sites is often impeded by biological barriers. Many research efforts have been devoted to hybridize multiple functionalities and moieties within the overall NP design. Targeted delivery of therapeutics will remain unachievable unless NPs be engineered with consideration of the biological barriers they are likely to encounter. To overcome these barriers, novel hybrid design features can be rationally added to create a new generation of nanotherapeutics [35].

The main difficulty that limits the site-specific delivery of nanotherapeutics is their nonspecific and unfavorable uptake by healthy organs. Immediately after being injected, mononuclear phagocyte system (MPS) sequesters NPs and clear them from circulation. MPS system consists of phagocytic cells, which are mostly resident macrophages in the spleen [35]. Following administration of NPs into the biological media, proteins get adsorbed onto the surface of NPs, forming a protein corona. This corona leads NPs to attach to specific receptors on the surface of phagocytes, and go through phagocytosis [36].

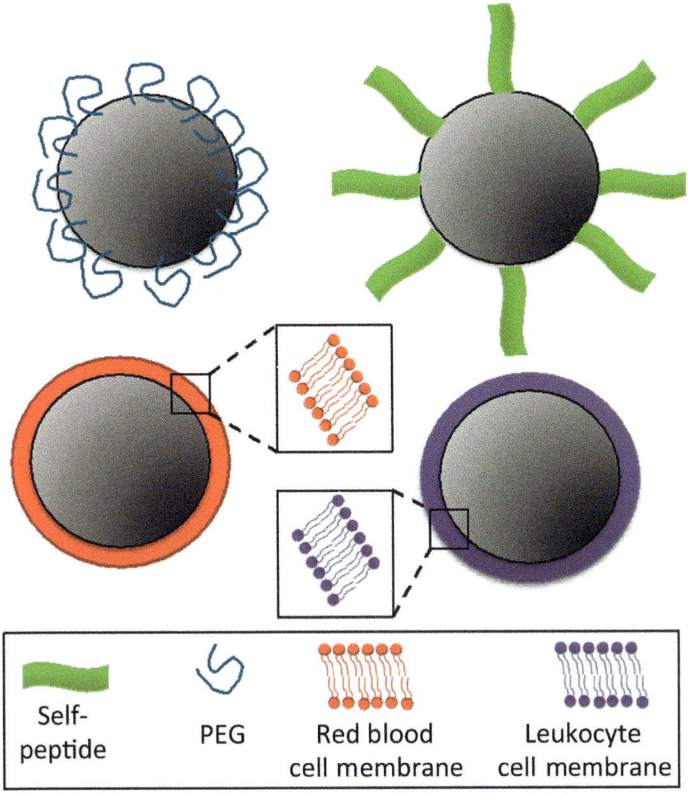

Figure 8.5 Surface coating of NPs is a well-established approach to limit their clearance by MPS. As soon as NPs contact the biological media, proteins adsorbed onto their surface to form a protein corona, leading to NPs attachment to specific receptors on the surface of phagocytes. PEG, for instance, limits this phenomenon through forming a hydration layer and conformational cloud around NPs. CD47 is a "don't eat me" peptide and limits the NPs recognition by MPS for phagocytosis. The last but not the least approach is to "camouflage" NPs with biomimetic coatings such as cell membranes extracted from autologous leukocytes and red blood cells which provides a longer blood half-life.

Fig. 8.5 demonstrates different methods to circumvent the nonspecific uptake of NPs with the focus on surface engineering of NPs. For instance, hybridizing the surface of NPs with PEG is an established strategy to overcome the short half-life in blood circulation. PEG has highly flexible hydrocarbon chains, with a large number of plausible conformations. This behavior leads to the formation of a conformational "cloud" around the NPs [37]. PEG also consists of oxygen atom (ether group) in every repeating unit of the polymer, which creates tight conjunction with the surrounding water molecules, thus forming a hydration layer around NPs, making them invisible for the MPS system. Indeed, water molecules can readily adsorb to the PEGylated NPs with hydrophilic surfaces, leading to NPs with enhanced blood half-lives [38].

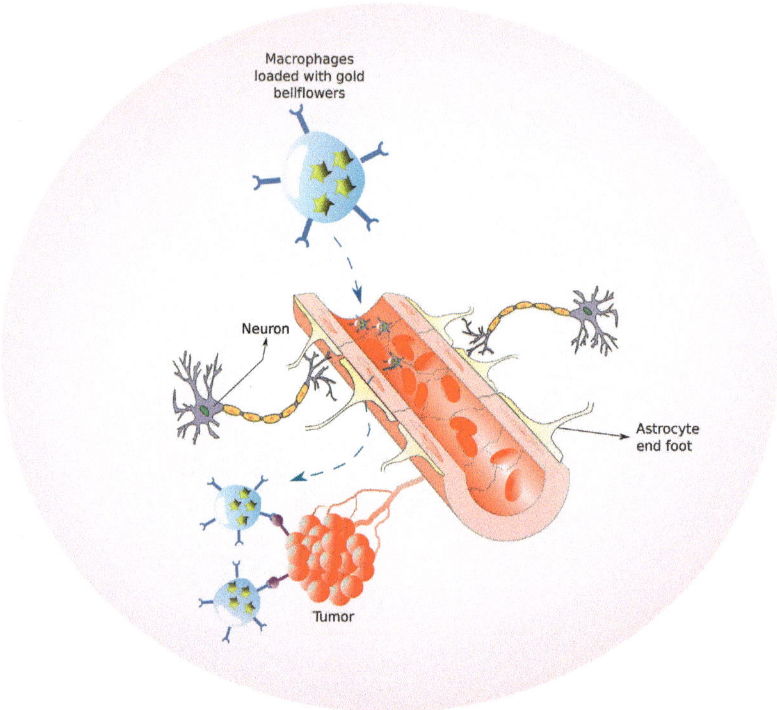

Figure 8.6 Macrophages carrying gold bellflowers for photothermal therapy, which can be decorated with neuron-specific or tumor-specific ligands [43]. Macrophages enter the brain parenchyma via paracellular and transcellular pathways. Both macrophages and exosomes are known to be capable of delivering cargo directly into the cytosol of the target cells independent of endosomes. The blood–brain barrier (BBB): brain capillary endothelial cells with unfenestrated tight junctions are primarily responsible for maintaining the integrity of the BBB. Additional components of the BBB are astrocytes, pericytes, neurons, and perivascular macrophages. One mechanism of cell-mediated transcytosis to cross BBB is normally used by monocytes/macrophages and probably by exosomes.

Although PEG has been used in several clinical products, the recent anti-PEG immunological responses has led researchers to find other stealth-coating alternatives [37]. Another recently emerged area in biomimetic hybridization is the coating of synthetic NPs with biological moieties such as cell membrane, which combines the functionalities of membranes with the versatile synthetic NPs for enhanced targeted drug delivery [39]. For instance, Ren et al. embedded IONPs within the red blood cells and showed a significant circulation time enhancement-24 h after intravenous injection, 10% of the NPs were still in the circulation [40]. In another study, the membrane of cancer cells of the human estrogen-independent breast carcinoma model was used as a coating to target tumors of the same origin [41]. Poly lactic-co-glycolic (PLGA) polymer was then fused into the cell membrane. As control samples, PLGA itself as well as red blood cell coated PLGA NPs were also studied for uptake efficiencies. Through quantification with flow cytometry assay, they reported that cancer cell membrane-camouflaged PLGA NPs demonstrated 20- and 40-fold increase in uptake comparing to PLGA NPs and red blood cell coated PLGA NPs, respectively.

One promising example of overcoming the biological barriers is to hybridize NPs to cross the blood–brain barrier (BBB). Every year many new drugs are being developed for central nervous system (CNS) disorders; yet, few reach the market. The brain capillary endothelial cells are the major barriers, limiting the transfer of most drugs [2]. The delivery of drugs and other molecules across the intact BBB to the CNS is an ongoing challenge in drug delivery research. BBB provides a tight regulating gate, which controls the influx and efflux transport to the brain. To pass this barrier, hybridization of NPs offers a possibility of CNS drug delivery. Recently, Huang et al. incorporated macrophages with various cargos and gold bellflower inside hyaluronic acid NPs for photothermal therapy [42] (Fig. 8.6).

8.6 Conclusion

Very few single-type NPs-based biomaterials are available that are having all the attributes such as nonimmunogenicity, biocompatibility, and biodegradability. Physical conjugation methods such as nanoscale layering and nanoencapsulation, and various types of chemical conjugations of different materials would result in nanomaterials with enormous prospects and opportunities. Such a combination of NPs with different formulation process can be tailored to have greater efficacy with less systemic toxicity. Therefore, multifunctional hybrid nanomaterials are the natural choice for the better application of the biomaterials.

References

[1] Allen TM, Cullis PR. Liposomal drug delivery systems: From concept to clinical applications. Advanced Drug Delivery Reviews 2013;65(1):36–48.
[2] Wohlfart S, Gelperina S, Kreuter J. Transport of drugs across the blood–brain barrier by nanoparticles. Journal of Controlled Release 2012;161:264–73.
[3] Lee JS, Feijen J. Polymersomes for drug delivery: Design, formation and characterization. Journal of Controlled Release 2012;161(2):473–83.
[4] Kesharwani P, Jain K, Jain NK. Dendrimer as nanocarrier for drug delivery. Progress in Polymer Science 2014;39(2):268–307.
[5] Wu W, et al. Chitosan-based responsive hybrid nanogels for integration of optical pH-sensing, tumor cell imaging and controlled drug delivery. Biomaterials 2010;31(32):8371–81.
[6] Conde J, et al. Local triple-combination therapy results in tumour regression and prevents recurrence in a colon cancer model. Nat Mater 2016 advance online publication.
[7] Wilhelm S, et al. Analysis of nanoparticle delivery to tumours. Nature Reviews Materials 2016;1(16014).
[8] Peng L, et al. Long-Term Small Molecule and Protein Elution from TiO(2) Nanotubes. Nano Letter 2009;9(5):1932–6.

[9] PAC, Definitions of terms relating to the structure and processing of sols, gels, networks, and inorganic-organic hybrid materials (IUPAC Recommendations 2007), in IUPAC God Book. 2007.
[10] Larsen EKU, et al. Accumulation of magnetic iron oxide nanoparticles coated with variably sized polyethylene glycol in murine tumors. Nanoscale 2012;4:2352–61.
[11] Barrera C, Herrera AP, Rinaldi C. Colloidal dispersions of monodisperse magnetite nanoparticles modified with poly(ethylene glycol). Journal of Colloid and Interface Science 2009;329:107–13.
[12] Kharkar PM, et al. Thiol–ene Click Hydrogels for Therapeutic Delivery. ACS Biomaterials Science & Engineering 2016;2(2):165–79.
[13] Guo Z, Tan L. Fundamentals and applications of nanomaterials. MA, USA: Artech house; 2009.
[14] Moore TL, et al. Nanoparticle colloidal stability in cell culture media and impact on cellular interactions.pdf. Chemical Society Review 2015;44:6285–305.
[15] Amstad E, Textor M, Reimhult E. Stabilization and functionalization of iron oxide nanoparticles for biomedical applications. Nanoscale 2011;3:2819–43.
[16] Cheng Y, et al. Highly efficient drug delivery with gold nanoparticle vectors for in vivo photodynamic therapy of cancer. Journal of American Chemical Society 2008;130(32):10643–7.
[17] Kim CK, et al. Entrapment of Hydrophobic Drugs in Nanoparticle Monolayers with Efficient Release into Cancer Cells. Journal of American Chemical Society 2009;131(4):1360–1.
[18] Su Y, et al. Design Strategies and Applications of Circulating Cell-Mediated Drug Delivery Systems. ACS Biomaterials Science & Engineering 2015;1(14):201–17.
[19] Ma M, et al. A facile preparation of novel multifunctional vectors by non-covalent bonds for co-delivery of doxorubicin and gene. Acta Biomaterialia 2012;8(2):599–607.
[20] Peppas NA. Devices based on intelligent biopolymers for oral protein delivery. International Journal of Pharmaceutics 2004;277(1–2):11–17.
[21] Cho H, Jung J, Chung BH. Scanometric analysis of DMA microarrays using DNA intercalator-conjugated gold nanoparticles. Chemical Communications 2012;48:7601–3.
[22] Farokhzad OC, Langer R. Impact of Nanotechnology on Drug Delivery. ACS Nano 2009;3(1):16–20.
[23] Pisal DS, Kosloski MP, Balu-Iyer SV. Delivery of therapeutic proteins. Jounal of Pharmaceutical Sciences 2010;99(6):2557–75.
[24] Larson N, Ghandehari H. Polymeric conjugates for drug delivery. Chemistry of Materials 2012;24(5):840–53.
[25] Ge J, et al. Protein–Polymer Hybrid Nanoparticles for Drug Delivery. Small 2012;8(23):3573–8.
[26] Rozhkova EA. Nanoscale Materials for Tackling Brain Cancer: Recent Progress and Outlook. Advanced Healthcare Materials 2011;23:136–50.
[27] Jung, J., et al., Angewante Chemistry, 2010. 49: p. 103.
[28] Ringsdorf H. Structure and properties of pharmacologically active polymers. Journal of Polymer Science: Polymer Symposia 1975;51:135–53.
[29] Cobo I, et al. Smart hybrid materials by conjugation of responsive polymers to biomacromolecules. Nature Materials 2015;14:143–59.
[30] Yoo J-W, et al. Bio-inspired, bioengineered and biomimetic drug delivery carriers. Nature Reviews Drug Discovery 2011;10:521–35.
[31] Wang H, et al. A biomimetic hybrid nanoplatform for encapsulation and precisely controlled delivery of theranostic agents. Nature Communication 2015;6(10081):1–12.

[32] Akin D, et al. Bacteria-mediated delivery of nanoparticles and cargo into cells. Nature Nanotechnology 2007;2:441–9.
[33] Pawelek Dr John M, Low KB, Bermudes D. Bacteria as tumour-targeting vectors. The Lancet Oncology 2003;4(11):658.
[34] Chen J, et al. Linker-Extended Native Cyanovirin-N Facilitates PEGylation and Potently Inhibits HIV-1 by Targeting the Glycan Ligand. Plos One 2014;9(1).
[35] Blanco E, Shen H, Ferrari M. Principles of nanoparticle design for overcoming biological barriers to drug delivery. Nature Biotechnology 2015;33:941–51.
[36] Sahay G, Alakhova DY, Kabanov AV. Endocytosis of nanomedicines. Journal of Controlled Release 2010;145(3):182–95.
[37] Katrin Knop Poly(ethylene glycol) in Drug Delivery: Pros and Cons as Well as Potential Alternatives. Angewandte Chemie International Edition 2010;49(36):6288–308.
[38] Gref R, et al. The controlled intravenous delivery of drugs using PEG-coated sterically stabilized nanospheres. Advanced Drug Delivery Reviews 1995;16(2–3):215–33.
[39] Luk BT, Zhang L. Cell membrane-camouflaged nanoparticles for drug delivery. Journal of Controlled Release 2015;220:600–7.
[40] Ren X, et al. Red blood cell membrane camouflaged magnetic nanoclusters for imaging-guided photothermal therapy. Biomaterials 2016;92:13–24.
[41] Fang RH, et al. Cancer Cell Membrane-Coated Nanoparticles for Anticancer Vaccination and Drug Delivery. Nano Letter 2014;14(4):2181–8.
[42] Huang P, et al. Triphase Interface Synthesis of Plasmonic Gold Bellflowers as NearInfrared Light Mediated Acoustic and Thermal Theranostics. Journal of American Chemical Society 2014;136:8307–13.
[43] Ali IU, Chen X. Penetrating the Blood–Brain Barrier: Promise of Novel Nanoplatforms and Delivery Vehicles. ACS Nano 2015;9(10):9470–4.

Nanotherapeutics in the management of infections and cancer

9

Madalina Elena Grigore[1], *Alina Maria Holban*[2] *and Alexandru Mihai Grumezescu*[1]
[1]University Politehnica of Bucharest, Bucharest, Romania
[2]Department of Microbiology and Immunology, Faculty of Biology and Research Institute of the University of Bucharest, University of Bucharest, Bucharest, Romania

9.1 Introduction

In the last two decades, researchers have focused on achieving controlled release systems that have the ability to target and treat the diseased area. Nanotherapeutics represents a rapidly growing field and involves the design, manufacture, and applications of such nanosized drugs. These systems have demonstrated a number of advantages, such as biocompatibility and improved pharmacokinetics, being considered promising for future personalized therapies.

For example, in the case of cancer treatment, conventional chemotherapeutic agents are spread throughout the body affecting both healthy and cancer cells and producing a high toxicity [1,2]. Nanosized drug-containing agents are considered ideal agents in cancer therapy, ensuring a controlled and targeted release [3].

One of the most important advantage of nanoparticles refers on the enhanced permeability and retention effect (EPR), which is based on the fact that the permeability of tumor vessels is much higher, allowing the entry of antitumor agents [4]. Another advantage of using nanotherapeutics refers to the possibility of magnetic nanoparticles to induce a therapeutic response through hyperthermia. This method involves injecting the magnetic nanoparticles; the patient is then placed in a magnetic field that changes the direction thousands of times each second. Magnetic nanoparticles are moved by magnetic force and begin to heat up, destroying cancerous tissue [5,6]. Also, some nanoparticles, especially metals have been studied due to their antimicrobial properties. Starting with silver, which is known for its antimicrobial properties since ancient times, numerous organic, inorganic, and complex, mixed nanoparticles have been developed and studied for their antimicrobial properties in the last 20 years [7]. Owing to their efficiency and great versatility, nanostructures could be considered a new and feasible alternative to overcome the current world crisis of antibiotics, by being able to fight against resistant microorganisms.

Nanobiomaterials Science, Development and Evaluation. DOI: http://dx.doi.org/10.1016/B978-0-08-100963-5.00009-4

9.2 Nanotherapeutics with antimicrobial properties

Given that a large diversity of bacteria is resistant to antibiotics, severe infections are becoming again a major threat to the world. A recent worldwide study reveals over 300 million cases of severe illness due to bacterial infection [8], most of them being caused by resistant bugs. Currently, antimicrobial agents that are used in hospitals are inefficient due to their weak antimicrobial activities. As an alternative, clinicians increased the dose of administered antibiotics and developed mixed therapies by combining two or more antibiotics to treat difficult infections. However, their effect is still not sufficient to cure most of those infections and, moreover, numerous side effects related to the high dosing and untargeted activity is systematically reported. Antibiotics are used to treat infections, but they show numerous disadvantages such as bacterial resistance to antibiotics and the fact that they may have various side effects. A solution for this problem could refer to the use of nanoparticles, which proved to be able to improve the efficiency of active antimicrobial agents and ensure their targeted transport and controlled release, even when utilized at low doses [9]. The main benefit of nanoparticles with antimicrobial properties is that they can specifically penetrate and modulate the behavior of target bacterial cells. Owing to these advantages, recently, numerous systems based on nanoparticles with antimicrobial properties have been developed and tested [8,10].

9.2.1 Inorganic nanotherapeutics

Metal oxide nanoparticles such as iron oxide (Fe_3O_4), silver (Ag), copper oxide (CuO), titanium dioxide (TiO_2), and zinc oxide (ZnO) were studied with interest due their antimicrobial properties. In literature, metal oxides are divided into two categories depending on their antimicrobial mechanism. These mechanisms are presented in Fig. 9.1.

The first mechanism refers to the activity reported for the metal oxide nanoparticles (TiO_2, Ag, CuO, ZnO, MgO, CaO) that have the capacity to destroy the cell wall of bacteria through the oxidation reactions and liberation of reactive oxygen species (ROS). It has been shown that the result of this mechanism (free oxygen radical) can be harmful not only to the bacteria cells but also eukaryotes, including the human body. The second mechanism involves metal oxide nanoparticles (CeO_2, Al_2O_3, Y_2O_3) that act as radical scavengers [9,11,12]. In Table 9.1, the main applications of these nanoparticles with proved antimicrobial effect are presented.

9.2.1.1 TiO_2 nanoparticles

TiO_2 is ideal for the environment and for use in medical applications due to its characteristics such as biocompatibility, low cost, and high stability. It is a metal oxide that is found in three stable polymorphic forms: anatase, brookite, and rutile [28]. It was demonstrated that TiO_2 nanoparticles are ideal for antimicrobial applications, as they present a high efficiency against a variety of bacteria, including *Bacillus* sp., which is one of the most naturally resistant organism [9,29].

It has been demonstrated that ROS are generated when TiO_2 is photoactivated by ultraviolet (UV) light. The mechanism of killing bacteria is not fully understood, it is

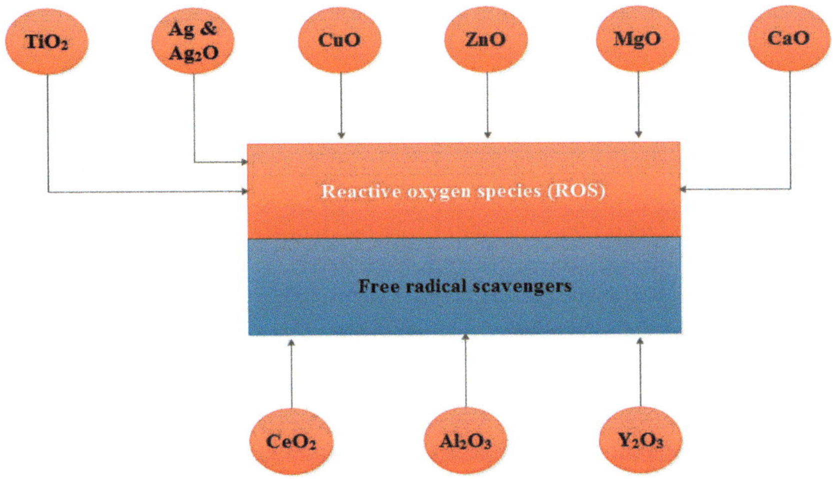

Figure 9.1 The main mechanisms to explain antimicrobial effects of nanomaterials.
Source: Image adapted from Parham, S., Wicaksono, D.H., Bagherbaigi, S., Lee, S.L. & Nur, H. 2016. Antimicrobial Treatment of Different Metal Oxide Nanoparticles: A Critical Review. Journal of the Chinese Chemical Society, 63, 385-393.

Table 9.1 **The main applications of inorganic nanoparticles with antimicrobial activity**

Materials	Applications	References
TiO_2 nanoparticles	Antimicrobial, UV protection, photo-catalyst, solar cell	Parham et al. [11,13–15]
Ag and Ag_2O nanoparticles	Antimicrobial, UV protection, disinfectant	Zhang et al. [11,16]
CuO nanoparticles	Antimicrobial, water purification, electrical conductive	Sharmila et al. [17–19]
ZnO nanoparticles	Antimicrobial, photo catalyst	Sarwar et al. [20,21]
MgO nanoparticles	Antimicrobial, photo catalyst	Bindhu et al. [22,23]
CaO nanoparticles	Antimicrobial	Marquis et al. [24]
CeO_2 nanoparticles	Antimicrobial, UV protection	Lu et al. [25]
Al_2O_3 nanoparticles	Antimicrobial	Ahmed, Nadeem [26]
Y_2O_3 nanoparticles	Antimicrobial, photoluminescence	Prasannakumar et al. [27]

assumed that ROS have the ability to destroy cell membranes and other vital cellular components, including the DNA [10,12].

Sunada et al. had tried to explain the mechanism of killing *Escherichia coli* using irradiated TiO_2. This mechanism involves three steps: the first step refers to partial decomposition of the membrane wall, resulting in permeability changes that facilitate the easy penetration of the nanoparticles in the cell and the release of ROS. In the second step, because the membrane is attacked by the released ROS, peroxidation processes of membrane lipids rapidly occur, which culminate with cell death [30].

Further studies revealed that the use of TiO_2 nanoparticles under UV light causes destruction of various types of cells, including human cells. An ideal alternative to this problem is doping the TiO_2 nanoparticles with metal ions to ensure a more specific action [11].

Dizaj et al. reported that TiO_2 nanoparticles have a real success in the inhibition of the development of bacterial biofilms, which can develop on the surface of medical devices [31]. These highly organized multicellular structures called biofilms are communities of microorganisms, which are very different from their counterparts and are very resistant to any known antimicrobial agent, including the host immune system. Thomas and Venkataramana used microorganisms isolated from patients to demonstrate the antibacterial effect of TiO_2 nanoparticles. These results were reported to control microbial growth in a dose- and time-dependent manner. The minimum inhibitory concentration results proved that bacterial growth is inhibited at concentrations higher than 15 mg/mL TiO_2 nanoparticles [32]. Another study was realized to see the antimicrobial activity of TiO_2 nanoparticles (with dimensions less than 25 nm) against *E. coli* laboratory strains. It was observed that the minimum amount of TiO_2 nanoparticles that inhibit bacteria growth was 200 μg/mL [33].

9.2.1.2 Ag and Ag_2O nanoparticles

Ag nanoparticles are used in antimicrobial applications because of their specific properties and because they can be produced by a variety of techniques in different dimensions and forms, such as photocatalysis, photochemical, biological synthesis, and so on [11,34].

The mechanism by which Ag nanoparticles act against bacteria is explained by the release of ions that destroy the cellular membrane resulting in cell death. The major disadvantage is that ions generate free radicals, they disseminate through the bloodstream, and can affect host biomolecules [12]. Also, it was reported that the dimension of Ag nanoparticles for this mechanism are imported because the nanoparticles with dimensions under 20 nm attaches to cellular membranes and proteins that contain sulfur and offer a high permeability [10]. Ag nanoparticles were intensively studied because of their antimicrobial properties. Salari et al. had synthesized Ag nanoparticles using bioreduction of Ag ions. The antimicrobial properties of Ag nanoparticles were tested against *Staphylococcus aureus*, *Salmonella typhimurium*, *Listeria monocytogenes*, and *Klebsiella* sp. It was observed that, for all tested bacteria species, a minimum concentration of 1 mg/mL is efficient to kill all inoculated cells in less than 24 h, Ag nanoparticles being very efficient [35]. Another study investigated the minimal inhibitory concentration (MIC) of using Ag nanoparticles with dimensions between 30 and 40 nm, obtained by chemical synthesis and laser ablation. It was observed that MIC for *Salmonella sp.*, *S. aureus*, and *E. coli* was 2.81 μg/mL, 4.37 μg/mL, and 2.8 μg/mL respectively, when nanoparticles were obtained by chemical synthesis, while for laser ablation method, the obtained nanoparticles proved MIC values of 2.68 μg/mL, 2.36 μg/mL, and 2.10 μg/mL, respectively [36].

Abd-Elnaby et al. had synthesized Ag nanoparticles to investigate the antimicrobial properties in combinations with antibiotic substances. It was observed that the presence of Ag nanoparticles increase the area of inhibition of *Vibrio fluvialis* compared to control plain antibiotic (without nanoparticles) [37]. Another recent study refers to Ag nanoparticles obtained from reducing and stabilizing a polysaccharide. In this research, nanoparticles with dimensions between 20 and 90 nm were obtained, and they were tested for their antimicrobial activity against *E. coli*, with great antimicrobial results [38]. Ag nanoparticles with dimension of approximately 20 nm and spherical shape were obtained by electrochemical method and tested against *E. coli*, *Pseudomonas aeruginosa*, and *S. aureus*. It was observed that the Gram positive strain of *S. aureus* had a higher resistance to the prepared nanoparticles, as compared with Gram negative rods, *E. coli* and *P. aeruginosa* [39].

9.2.1.3 CuO nanoparticles

CuO nanoparticles have attracted the attention of researchers and health care professionals because of their physical, chemical, high temperature, and photocatalytic properties, but mostly because of their antimicrobial properties [31]. Ravishankar Rai and Jamuna Baihad reported that CuO nanoparticles can be used in killing the bacteria in hospitals, but for this a high concentration of CuO nanoparticles is necessary [10]. However, the mechanism of killing bacteria by using CuO nanoparticles is not clearly understood. It is considered that CuO nanoparticles can easily enter the cell membrane and destroy exposed bacteria cells [11].

Naika et al. had synthesized CuO nanoparticles with dimensions between 5 and 10 nm by solution combustion method. They proved the antimicrobial efficiency of these nanoparticles against various microbial species, such as *Klebsiella sp.*, *E. coli, and S. aureus*, when utilized at concentrations ranging 500–1000 μg. It was observed that, at this concentration, CuO nanoparticles were more efficient against *Klebsiella sp.*, and *E. coli* than against *S. aureus* [40]. CuO nanoparticles were also efficient against *Enterococcus faecalis* infections [41].

Das et al. obtained CuO nanoparticles by thermal decomposition methods and tested their antimicrobial activity against *E. coli* and *P. aeruginosa*. Also, for these nanoparticles, an antioxidant activity by free radical scavenging was observed. The antimicrobial activity showed an increase in bacterial inhibition after 3 h at a concentration of 4 mg/mL in *E. coli* and an increase in bacterial inhibition after 4 h at a concentration of 4 mg/mL in *P. aeruginosa* [42]. Another study, which is the antimicrobial activity of these nanoparticles, was carried out by Khashan et al. who synthesized CuO nanoparticles in spherical shape and dimensions between 3 and 40 nm by laser ablation. The antimicrobial activity of CuO nanoparticles was very high, and nanotherapeutics was proposed as an efficient treatment for the therapy of severe infections produced by *E. coli* [43].

Pandey et al. had synthesized CuO nanoparticles by electrochemical routes for studying their bactericidal potential against *Bacillus anthracis*. It was observed that after 1 h a concentration of CuO nanoparticles of 1 mg/mL killed approximately 92.17% of the inoculated *B. anthracis* cells, these results being very promising for a new therapy in destroying this deadly bacillus [44].

9.2.1.4 ZnO nanoparticles

ZnO is a material utilized very often in biomedical applications because of its unique properties, such as electric conductivity, optical, and piezoelectric properties [45,46]. The mechanism of killing bacteria using ZnO nanoparticles was described by Beyth et al. as having two paths of action. The first involves the penetration of cell wall and the second involves the generation of ROS [9].

Xie et al. had demonstrated that ZnO nanoparticles with approximately 20 nm diameter, are very efficient in killing *Campylobacter jejuni*. After the treatment with a concentration of ZnO nanoparticles of 0.05 mg/mL, significant inhibition of cell growth was observed. The MIC of these nanoparticles was determined to be 0.025 mg/mL for *C. jejuni* [47]. In another study, the antimicrobial activity of ZnO nanoparticles against *E. coli* was investigated. Authors used ZnO nanoparticles with dimensions of approximately 70 nm and different concentrations, and demonstrated that the inhibition of cell growth is directly proportional to the increasing concentration of these nanotherapeutics [48].

Gunalan et al. had compared the antimicrobial activity of ZnO nanoparticles obtained by green synthesis with the ZnO nanoparticles obtained by chemical synthesis against *S. aureus, Serratia marcescens*, and *Citrobacter freundii.* It was observed that green ZnO nanoparticles possess a greater antimicrobial activity than chemical ZnO nanoparticles. The authors had reported that the green ZnO nanoparticles can be successfully used in applications such as medicine and food safety [49].

9.2.1.5 MgO nanoparticles

These nanoparticles can be synthesized by different methods (i.e., sol-gel, hydrothermal) at a low price. The mechanism of killing bacteria using MgO nanoparticles is similar to other metal oxide nanomaterials [50,51].

Sundrarajan et al. had synthesized MgO nanoparticles by chemical method using different temperatures and tested their antimicrobial activity against *S. aureus* and *E. coli.* It was observed that the inhibition zone was greater in the case of *S. aureus*, as compared with E. *coli*, grown in the presence of the same concentration of nanoparticles. Also, it was observed that the antimicrobial activity of MgO nanoparticles is higher when the calcination temperature is low [52]. In another study, the antimicrobial properties of MgO nanoparticles with average diameter of 20 nm was tested against *C. jejuni, E. coli*, and *Salmonella sp.* It was determined that for a 10^4 CFU/mL microbial inocula, the MIC was 0.5 mg/mL for *C. jejuni*, 1 mg/mL for *E. coli*, and 1 mg/mL for *Salmonella sp.* Also, the MIC for 10^{8-9} CFU/mL bacterial inocula was studied after 4 h of treatment with MgO nanoparticles and the MIC was 2 mg/mL for *C. jejuni*, and 8 mg/mL for *E. coli* and *Salmonella sp.* He et al. [53], Jin and He compared the antimicrobial activity of MgO nanoparticles against *E. coli* and *Salmonella sp.* with the antimicrobial activity of MgO nanoparticles utilized in combination with ZnO nanoparticles. It was observed that by adding ZnO nanoparticles the antimicrobial activity of MgO is not improved [54].

9.2.1.6 CaO nanoparticles

The antimicrobial activity of CaO nanoparticles (with dimensions between 14 and 24 nm) was studied against *P. aeruginosa*, *Staphylococcus epidermidis*, *Candida tropicalis*, and the highest inhibition was observed in *P. aeruginosa* and *S. epidermidis* [55]. Marquis et al. studied the antimicrobial activity of CaO nanoparticles with diameter of about 58 nm against different bacterial strains. It was observed that the greatest inhibition occurred against *E. coli* tested strain [24].

9.2.1.7 CeO_2 nanoparticles

Cerium oxide (CeO_2) nanoparticles are tolerated both in vitro and in vivo by human cells, this property making them suitable for medical applications. For this reason, the antimicrobial effect of CeO_2 nanoparticles was extremely studied. Das et al. had synthesized CeO_2 nanoparticles with average diameter of 37.6 nm by chemical method and tested their antimicrobial activity against *S. aureus*. The same mechanism of inhibition of the bacteria was previously observed for most of the above-mentioned nanoparticles; CeO_2 nanoparticles attached to the cell wall, penetrated the wall and subsequently produced the inhibition of RNA and DNA [56]. Also, dos Santos et al. had reported that the mechanism of CeO_2 to kill occurs also by producing ROS [57].

Cuahtecontzi-Delint et al. had studied the antimicrobial activity of CeO_2 nanoparticles in the presence of different surfactants (Triton X-100, polyvinyl pyrrolidone (PVP), and Tween 80) against *E. coli*. The MIC of such CeO_2 nanoparticles was 3 mg/mL^{-1}, while in the case where surfactants were utilized the best MIC was observed in the presence of Tween 80 (0.150 mg mL^{-1}) [58].

9.2.1.8 Al_2O_3 nanoparticles

Ansari et al. had studied the antimicrobial activity of aluminum oxide (Al_2O_3) nanoparticles against *S. aureus*. The MIC value of these nanoparticles was at 1700 µg/mL. It was observed by scanning electron microscopy (SEM) that cells were significantly affected by the presence of such nanoparticles. The membrane was damaged and nanoparticles caused cell death by entering inside cells [59]. Also, Al_2O_3 nanoparticles were tested against *P. aeruginosa* and the MIC was found to be 1,600 µg/mL. It was observed that at a concentration of 2,000 µg/mL results in total inhibition of bacterial activity [60].

9.2.2 Organic nanotherapeutics

The most investigated organic nanotherapeutics relies on polymeric nanoparticles. These can kill bacteria by two mechanisms: cationic surfaces or by releasing antimicrobial agents, antibiotics, and so on. Organic antimicrobial materials are considered less stable at high temperature than inorganic antimicrobial materials [9].

9.2.2.1 Chitosan nanoparticles

Chitosan is a natural polymer with great applications in medicine due to its properties such as biodegradability, biocompatibility, and nontoxicity [61,62]. The antimicrobial effect of chitosan nanoparticles with various molecular weights was tested against *Streptococcus mutans*. It was observed that the cell membrane was destroyed when bacteria cells were treated with chitosan nanoparticles. Also, a low antimicrobial activity was observed for chitosan nanoparticles with high molecular weights (20 to 25% of total amount of microbial cells were killed) and a high antimicrobial activity for chitosan nanoparticles with low molecular weights (>95% of total amount of microbial cells were killed) [63]. In another study, the antimicrobial properties of chitosan nanoparticles with dimensions of approximately 36 nm were tested against *E. coli* and *S. aureus*. It was observed that the antibacterial activity increases with the concentration of nanoparticles. For example, for a concentration of 5 mg/mL for *E. coli* the antibacterial rate was 95%, while at the same concentration for *S. aureus* the antibacterial rate was 81% [64].

Mohammadi et al. had studied the antimicrobial activity of chitosan nanoparticles and chitosan microparticles against *P. fluorescens*, *Erwinia carotovora*, and *E. coli*. The MIC and the minimum bactericidal concentration (killing dose) was investigated and it was observed that chitosan nanoparticles present a better antimicrobial activity as compared with chitosan microparticles [65].

Piras et al. wanted to increase the antimicrobial activity of chitosan nanoparticles and reduce their toxicity, so they tried to encapsulate temporin B into chitosan nanoparticles. These systems were tested against *Staphylococcus epidermidis* for 4 days and the tests demonstrated a significant antimicrobial effect. It was reported that the gradual release ensures a long-lasting antimicrobial activity [66]. In another study, the antifungal activity of chitosan nanoparticles functionalized with different molecular weight drugs against *Candida albicans*, *Fusarium solani*, and *Aspergillus niger* was tested. The MIC tests revealed that the chitosan nanoparticles with low molecular weight were very efficient in inhibiting the growth of these microfungi, being more efficient as compared with chitosan nanoparticles with high molecular weight. However, in the case of *Aspergillus niger*, a resistance to chitosan nanoparticles with low molecular weight was observed, but this exception was not observed in the case of chitosan nanoparticles with high molecular weight [61].

9.2.2.2 Poly-ε-lysine

This homopolymer is used in medical applications owing to its properties such as biocompatibility, biodegradability, solubility, nontoxic, and stable at high temperatures [67]. It had been declared that poly-ε-lysine has strong antimicrobial effects, being efficient against fungi, bacteria, and even a few types of viruses [68].

Shi et al. had reported the antimicrobial effect of poly-ε-lysine in combination with citral against *E. coli* strains. The antimicrobial properties of poly-ε-lysine was studied by the MIC. MIC of poly-ε-lysine was 2–4 μg/mL and in combination with citral was 0.5–1 μg/mL [69].

Abd-Elnaby et al. had produced poly-ε-lysine by marine *Bacillus subtilis* and investigated its antimicrobial activity against Gram negative and Gram positive bacteria after 24h incubation at 37°C (figure 5). The inhibition for all bacteria, except for *S. aureus*, was observed [37]. Also, Shima et al. had reported that poly-ε-lysine possess antimicrobial effect against Gram negative and Gram positive bacteria at a concentration of 1–8 μg/mL [70].

9.2.2.3 Polysiloxanes

Quaternary ammonium compounds are widely used because of their antimicrobial activity. Majumdar et al. had studied the antimicrobial effect of polysiloxane coating containing quaternary ammonium against *E. coli*, *S. aureus*, and *C. albicans*. It was observed that this complex composition is able to induce the microbial inhibition [71].

In another study, the antimicrobial activity of polysiloxane quaternary ammonium salts containing epoxy group against *E. coli* and *S. aureus* was evaluated. The MBC, in the case of *E. coli* was 1.5×10^{-5} mol/L, while in the case of *S. aureus* it was 2.8×10^{-5} mol/L [72]. Lin et al. had tested the antimicrobial properties of polysiloxane containing quaternary ammonium salts against *E. coli*, *S. aureus*, *R. solani*, and *Fusarium oxysporum f. sp. cubenserace*. It was observed that the complex had a very good antimicrobial activity toward *E. coli* and *F. oxysporum f. sp. cubenserace* [73].

9.2.2.4 Triclosan

Triclosan is already used in oral products owing to its antibacterial effects. About the mechanism of action of triclosan, it was initially considered that at sublethal concentrations it can inhibit a specific bacterial target, but in the last decade because of the multiple studies, it was observed that its activity is nonspecific at sublethal concentrations [74].

Suller and Russell had studied the antibacterial effect of triclosan against *S. aureus* strains. It was observed that the MIC was 0.025–1 mg/L [75].

Also, Braid and Wale had investigated the antimicrobial activity of triclosan-impregnated plastic against *S. aureus*, *E. coli*, *P. aeruginosa*, *B. cereus*, and *S. putrefaciens* at different temperatures. It was observed that the inhibitions of bacteria occurred at 22°C and 30°C, but at 4°C no inhibition was observed [76]. In another study, the MIC of triclosan against *S. aureus* was established to be 0.25 μg/mL [77].

9.2.2.5 Peptides

Most of the peptides considered for biomedical applications are cationic and amphipathic peptides. The mechanism of action consists in disintegration of the lipid bilayer structure. Also, it was reported that some peptides have a different mechanism that does not destroy the cellular membrane. It acts by binding to the DNA and RNA and inhibits replication [78,79] [80].

Guilhelmelli et al. reported that the antimicrobial activity of peptides depends on size, conformation, charge (anionic/cationic), structure, and hydrophobicity. In Table 9.2, the advantages and the disadvantages of peptides used as single therapeutic

Table 9.2 Advantages and disadvantages of peptides used as single therapeutic antimicrobial agents [81]

Advantage	Antiviral, antibacterial, and antifungal activity Quick action Antiinflammatory activities
Disadvantages	Expensive Local toxicity Pharmacodynamic and pharmacokinetic issues

Table 9.3 Nanoparticle-based drugs used in various types of cancer [87]

Product	Nanomaterials	Dimension (nm)	Application	Administration	Phase
Combidex	Iron oxide nanoparticle	20	Tumor imaging	Intravenous	Not available
Biovant	Nanosized calcium phosphate	Not available	Vaccine component	Intramuscular	Phase I
Bioconjugated nanoparticles	Luminescent quantum dots	15	Cancer imaging	Subcutaneous	Preclinical
Abraxane	Albumin-bound paclitaxel particles	130	Breast cancer	Intravenous	Approved

antimicrobial agents are presented [81]. Also, the resistance of microorganisms to antimicrobial peptides is debatable, for example *Porphiromonas gingivalis* secrete digestive proteases that destroy peptides [82].

9.3 Nanotherapeutics with antitumor properties

Anticancer drugs pose problems due to high types affecting both normal cells and tumor cells [83]. Considering that in the 21st century the complete treatment for cancerous disease remained undiscovered, the researchers concluded that the therapeutic treatment route by using nanoparticles, could bring a huge step forward in the therapy of this deadly disease [84,85]. Moreover, along with their impact in the development of cancer nanotherapeutics, nanoparticles can be used in the detection, diagnosis, and treatment of various types of cancer [85].

The use of nanotherapeutics in medicine has numerous advantages, such as targeted release, stability and solubility of drugs, lower toxicity, and a higher specificity. Also, another advantage of nanoparticles is that they present a high permeability at tumor

Table 9.4 **Types of inorganic nanoparticles for cancer therapy [88]**

Type of nanoparticles	Dimension (nm)	Advantages	Disadvantages	Applications
Metallic (silver, gold nanoparticles)	<50	Large surface area, safe	Low biocompatibility	Targeted release of drugs, diagnosis
Magnetic (supermagnetic iron oxide particles)	5–100	Biocompatible, nontoxic, stable, allow controlling the distribution	Forming aggregates	In vivo imaging (photoacoustic tomography)
Nanoshells	10–300	Therapeutic potential	Relatively large dimensions	In vivo imaging (photoacoustic tomography)
Ceramic (titanium dioxide, aluminum oxide nanoparticles)	<100	Stability, easy to prepare, water soluble	–	Carriage of drugs, proteins, etc.
Carbon nanotubes	1.5–5000 (length) × 0.5–20 (diameter)	Thermal conductivity, can reach to target	Cytotoxicity, release active compounds	Targeted delivery of drugs, thermotherapy of tumors

vessels allowing the entry of tumor agents, compared with healthy vessels [86]. In Table 9.3, some nanomaterials used in the various stages of cancer are presented [87].

9.3.1 Inorganic nanotherapeutics

Various types of inorganic nanoparticles have been developed for cancer applications, including diagnosis, therapy, and imaging. In Table 9.4, a few examples of inorganic nanoparticles, their advantages and disadvantages, and their applications are presented [88].

9.3.1.1 Silver nanoparticles

In the field of nanomedicine, Ag nanoparticles are highly used due to their unique properties. After extensive research, it was found that Ag nanoparticles have biological effects on human cells [89]. For example, Jeyaraj et al. had investigated the development of anticancer agents by studying the cytotoxic effects of Ag nanoparticles with dimensions of approximately 22 nm against human breast cancer cells. By the reduction of tetrazolium salt assay (MTT) and Hochest assay, the cytotoxic effect of Ag nanoparticles against human breast cancer cells was confirmed [90]. Lalitha had studied the cytomorphological changes in human breast cancer cells by using MTT assay. The anticancer effect of Ag nanoparticles was with the anticancer effect of cisplatin and it was observed that Ag nanoparticles have a superior activity. The complete cell inhibition in the case of Ag nanoparticles was obtained with 25 μg/mL, while in the case of cisplatin it was obtained with 30 μg/mL [91]. Also, Gurunathan et al. had reported that Ag nanoparticles can be suitable candidates for human breast cancer therapy [92].

In another study, peripheral blood mononuclear cells were used and the safe concentration by using Ag nanoparticles was investigated. It was found that a concentration of less than 39 μg/mL is considered nontoxic and the inhibition percent of tumor cells at this concentration was 60% [89].

9.3.1.2 Gold nanoparticles

Gold nanoparticles are used because of their biocompatibility and optoelectronic properties and because of the availability of different synthesis methods (biological, physical, and chemical). Also, in literature it was reported that gold nanoparticles have antitumor properties [87]. Gold nanoparticles present a good tendency to accumulate in tumor sites [93]. Gold nanoparticles can use different mechanisms of killing tumor cells, such as drug delivery systems for anticancer agents, mechanical damage, or by photothermal ablation [94]. Kumar et al. obtained gold nanoparticles with dimension of 2 nm, which had been functionalized with therapeutic peptide and a targeted peptide (CRGDK). It was observed that the targeted peptide has increased intracellular uptake of gold nanoparticles. Another remark was that, because of the presence of this complex targeted peptide, the delivery of the therapeutic peptide was better inside the targeted cells. Also, it was reported that this complex peptide can be successfully used in cancer treatments [95].

The properties of gold nanoparticles make them usable as contrast agents. For example, gold nanoparticles with dimensions of 1.9 nm were intravenously injected in vivo and a longer retention time and a superior contrast was obtained [93]. In another study, gold–gold sulfide nanoparticles with diameters of less than 25 nm, obtained by the reduction of chloroauric acid ($HAuCl_4$), were usedIt was observed that these nanoparticles produce two peaks and one is in the near infrared (NIR) region. Kennedy et al. had reported that these gold nanoparticles can be used in ablative therapy because of their absorbance in the NIR region [96].

In connection with the toxicity of gold nanoparticles are two contradictory opinions. In some studies, it was reported that gold nanoparticles do not show cellular toxicity. For example, Hainfeld et al. reported that a single dose of gold nanoparticles (2.7 g Au/kg body weight) do not produce toxicity against mice bearing subcutaneous EMT-6 mammary carcinomas. It was also observed that nanoparticles were excreted by urine and feces [97].

On the other hand, it was reported that because of the presence of gold nanoparticles ROS were generated, and also a massive cytokine release, apoptosis, necrosis or mitochondrial toxicity was observed [93]. Kennedy et al. reported that the toxicity of gold nanoparticles depends on their size and their coating and contained agent [96].

9.3.1.3 Supermagnetic iron oxide nanoparticles

These nanoparticles have unique properties such as high magnetization, contrast enhancement for imaging of affected tissue/cell and targeted release of drugs. The properties and the fact that supermagnetic Fe_3O_4 nanoparticles can be synthetized by various techniques (Table 9.5) make them able for to be used for cancer treatment [99]. Also, supermagnetic Fe_3O_4 nanoparticles can be used for the detection of cancer in four different stages. The first mechanism involves the detection of the receptor on the surface of cancer cells; the second involves detection of unusual angiogenesis in the tumor microenvironment; the third mechanism involves detection of circulating tumor cells and the last mechanism involves the detection of soluble tumor biomarkers [100].

To eliminate the opsonization of supermagnetic Fe_3O_4 nanoparticles surfactants such as polyethylene glycol (PEG), poloxamers, and so on, are used. The most used surfactant to coat these nanoparticles is PEG that improves the biocompatibility, solubility, stability, and allows loading of therapeutic agents. Peng et al. have reported the synthesis of supermagnetic Fe_3O_4 nanoparticles with dimensions between 5 and 30 nm and the coating of these nanoparticles with amphiphilic triblock polymers that allows the introduction of several functional groups [101].

Quinto et al. obtained supermagnetic Fe_3O_4 nanoparticles with average diameter of 14 nm by thermal decomposition technique and coated these nanoparticles with phospholipid-PEG. After that, doxorubicin was loaded into the supermagnetic Fe_3O_4 nanoparticles. It was observed that this complex presented a sustained of doxorubicin release over 72 h, the local produced temperature was about 43°C, and the nanosystem was capable to determine the death of cancer cells [102].

9.3.1.4 Nanoshells

Nanoshells are represented by nanoparticles which consisting of two parts. The first part is represented by a dielectric core and the second part is represented by a metallic shell who covering the shell (gold nanoshell) [103]. The gold nanoshell can be prepared by two methods. The first method involves the formation of Ag shell on the surface of silica nanoparticles and the second mechanism involves the formation of gold nanoshell by the galvanic replacement of a metallic core [104].

Table 9.5 Various techniques for synthesis of supermagnetic iron oxide nanoparticles [98]

Synthesis methods	Advantages	Disadvantages
Hydrothermal	The ability to control the dimension of nanoparticles	High reaction time
Microemulsion	The ability to control the dimension of nanoparticles	The use large quantities of solvent
Coprecipitation	Rapid synthesis	Oxidation

Also, the surface plasmon resonance wavelength of nanoshells can be changed from NIR to visible depending on the ratio of core size and thickness of the surface [105].

In vivo studies confirmed the efficiency of nanoshells against various tumor cells. Also, in comparison with free drug, the nanoshells showed a much lower toxicity [106]. Morton et al. had investigated the effect of nanoshell with PEG layer on mice subcutaneously injected with CT26 colon carcinoma tumor cells. The treatment began in the moment when the diameter of tumor had between 3 and 5.5 mm. After 10 days it was observed the complete resorption of the tumors. The treatment continued for 90 days and no trace of tumor was observed after complete treatment [105].

9.3.1.5 Titanium dioxide nanoparticles

TiO_2 has many applications in industry, such as paints, toothpastes, skincare products, and cosmetics. Recently, TiO_2 was proposed by the International Agency for Research on Cancer as "possibly carcinogenic to humans." Also, there are studies in which it was reported that TiO_2 nanoparticles can cause respiratory tract cancer [107].

Fujiwara et al. had used CT26 and LL2 mouse cancer to study the effect of TiO_2 nanoparticles on cancerous cells. First time, the cells were treated with 6 nm anatase TiO_2 nanoparticles without UV irradiation. It had been observed that induction of inflammatory cytokines and oxidative stress had started to grow. Also, when CT26 cells were treated with TiO_2 nanoparticles with dimensions between 10 to 70 nm, it was observed that the smaller nanoparticles had produced more oxidative stress and inflammatory cytokines than in the first case. As a solution, in order to minimize the toxicity and to avoid the diffusion of TiO_2 nanoparticles (10 nm), these nanoparticles were suspended in a collagen gel inserted into a subcutaneous tumor in a CT26 mouse. It was observed that this complex can be successfully applied for the local treatment of tumors [108].

You et al. synthetized hydrophilized TiO_2 nanoparticle and administered the obtained nanotherapeutics to tumor-induced mice. After that, it was observed that nanoparticles arrived to the SCC7 tumor with the help of the enhanced permeation and retention effect. Also, when the ultrasound treatment began, it was observed that the presence of ROS and tumor growth was stopped at least 15 times compared to control (mice without ultrasound treatments) [109]. Sungkaworn et al. studied the changing morphologies of TiO_2 nanoparticles against human cervical carcinoma (HeLa) cells. It was observed that in comparison with the control, the sizes, the circularity, and the diameters of colonies formed by HeLa cells were smaller when treated with TiO_2 nanoparticles [110].

9.3.1.6 Aluminum oxide nanoparticles

The toxicity of Al_2O_3 nanoparticles had been extensively studied both in vitro and in vivo since 1990 [111]. Also, it was reported in many cases that Al_2O_3 nanoparticles are toxic both to the cancerous cell lines and normal cell lines [112]. For example, Di Virgilio et al. reported that on Chinese hamster ovary cells the Al_2O_3 nanoparticles induced genotoxic and cytotoxic effects [113].

Lin et al. had compared the cytotoxicity of Al_2O_3 nanoparticles with dimensions of 13 and 22 nm in cultured human bronchoalveolar carcinoma (A549) with positive control (CeO_2 nanoparticles with dimensions of 20 nm) and with negative control (TiO_2 nanoparticles with dimensions of 40 nm). In the case of Al_2O_3 nanoparticles, it was observed that the cytotoxicity was lower than positive control and higher than negative control [111]. Sun et al. had reported that the Al_2O_3 nanoparticles may be a potential adjuvant for antitumor immunotherapy. They studied the cytotoxicity of Al_2O_3 in combination with tumor cell vaccine and observed a higher cytotoxicity against the H22 liver cancer cells, in comparison with the control (untreated BALB/c mice). Also, tumor necrosis was observed in the case of Al_2O_3 in combination with tumor cell vaccine [114].

9.3.1.7 Quantum dots

Quantum dots are semiconductor nanocrystals resistant to chemical degradation, high thermal stability, and optical properties (high brightness) [115]. Also, it was reported that because of their unique optical properties quantum dots can be successfully used in cancer imaging applications and cellular tracking [116,117].

Xing and Rao have reported two mechanisms for the accumulation of quantum dots at tumor sites. The first mechanism is called the active targeting and involves antibodies and the second mechanism is called the passive targeting, which refers to the enhanced permeability and retention effect [118].

Chen et al. had developed a new detection method for breast cancer, an analysis system compound from quantum dots–based immunofluorescence technology. It was reported that compared with other techniques, the quantum dots-based immunofluorescence technology is more precisely, sensitive and cheaper [119].

9.3.2 Organic nanotherapeutics

Over time, many systems have been developed for the treatment of cancer. Each system presents advantages and disadvantages for a particular type of application [88].

9.3.2.1 Polymers

The delivery systems consisting of polymer have the advantage that they are biocompatible, biodegradable, nontoxic, and hydrophilic. These systems are successfully used in cancer therapy [120,121]. Some examples of polymeric delivery systems are presented below.

9.3.2.2 Chitosan nanoparticles

Besides the good properties of chitosan, the most important advantage that makes it suitable for applications targeted release is that it can form polyelectrolyte complexes with DNA [120]. Arya et al. had studied the efficiency of a system that consists of Herceptin, gemcitabine, and chitosan nanoparticles against Mia Paca 2, PANC 1, and HEK293 cells. The system was prepared by ionic gelation method, and nanoparticles with dimension between 150 and 250 nm were obtained. It was observed that this system presents an increased efficiency, which is influenced by the presence of gemcitabine. Also, in the case of the tested system in vitro it was observed that it induces decreased DNA synthesis and apoptosis [122].

Park et al. obtained nanoparticles of glycol chitosan with different molecular weights and tested them to analyze the difference. From in vitro tests, it was reported that there was no difference between the three samples. From in vivo tests (SCC7 tumor-bearing mice), it was observed that the glycol chitosan nanoparticles with the biggest molecular weight are circulating in the body for a longer time [123]. Also, Zhang et al. prepared oleoyl-chitosan nanoparticles loaded with doxorubicin with different degrees of substitution (5, 11, and 27%). The in vitro drug release showed that the high release of doxorubicin was achieved in the case of nanoparticles with a degree of substitution of 5%. The in vivo tests showed a low cytotoxicity to hemolysis rates and no toxicity for mouse embryo fibroblasts [124].

In another study, Kumar et al. had used mice (with lung inflammation) injected intravenously with chitosan nanoparticles loaded with Sertoli cells and an antiinflammatory compound. After 24 h, it was observed that this system was targeted delivery, because 90% of the antiinflammatory compound was found in the lungs [125]. Ekinci et al. had synthetized a system for breast cancer diagnosis. They obtained these system methotrexate-chitosan nanoparticles by ionotropic gelation. After that these systems were radiolabeled with Technetium-99m, and their absorption in human breast cancer and human keratinocyte cell lines was studied. It was observed that Technetium-99m–methotrexate-chitosan nanoparticles present a high absorption in the cancer cell lines studied and in the case of the normal cells it was observed that these system produce minimum negative effects [126].

9.3.2.3 Poly ε-caprolactone nanoparticles

It is a class of polymers that shows both biocompatibility and biodegradability and this class can be successfully used for cancer therapy [120]. For applications of colon cancer, Ortiz et al. produced a system compound of 5-fluorouracil-loaded poly (ε-caprolactone) nanoparticles and gene E. This system was tested to observe the potential therapeutic against the SW480 human cancer cell line. The inhibition of proliferation by 40 times was observed, compared to the control (the nonincorporated drug alone) and induction of apoptosis in SW480 cells [127].

In another study, Chawla and Amiji wanted to increase the local concentration of tamoxifen for breast cancer applications. They prepared poly ε-caprolactone nanoparticles with dimensions between 250 and 300 nm by solvent displacement method and loaded them with tamoxifen. It was observed that the maximum drugloading efficiency was 64% and it was obtained with 50 mg of tamoxifen [128]. Mei et al. had reported that the system formed from docetaxel, poly (ε-caprolactone) and Pluronic F68 can be successfully used for the treatment of breast cancer [129].

9.3.2.4 Polyhydroxyalkanoates

Polyhydroxyalkanoates are polyesters that are synthesized by various bacteria under limited conditions (in the absence of oxygen, nutrients, etc.), but in the presence of carbon sources [130]. The polyhydroxyalkanoates properties such as biocompatibility, biodegradability, and the fact that kinetics of drug release can be controlled by engineering makes these materials suitable for cancer applications [131].

For example, Choiniere and his coworkers had created a delivery system based on polyhydroxyalkanoates for breast cancer applications, which can be easily modified to incorporate a targeting molecule. In this case, folic acid was used, which improves the selectivity for cancerous tissues and helps to improve the efficiency of encapsulation of anticancer drug, paclitaxel. Since polyhydroxyalkanoates nanoparticles are biocompatible and biodegradable, in this case the toxicity relate to the anticancer drug that is trapped inside the nanoparticles [132].

9.3.2.5 Carbon nanotubes

For cancer therapy, a candidate that draws attention for many years are carbon nanotubes (CNTs). The CNTs are cylindrical molecules of carbon with physicochemical properties that make them ideal as carriers for drugs, proteins, peptides, and so on [133,134]. The CNTs can be of two main types, made of a single sheet (single-walled carbon nanotubes—SWNT) or of several sheets (multiwalled carbon nanotubes—MWCNT) [135].

On the market, CNTs can be functionalized to minimize the toxicity and increase their biocompatibility. Some of the techniques used to functionalize these CNTs are presented in Table 9.6 [136].

Liu et al. had studied the effect of CNTs–paclitaxel conjugate in comparison with clinical Taxol against a murine 4T1 breast-cancer model. It was observed that CNTs–paclitaxel inhibit the tumor growth and was concluded that the enhanced permeability and retention effect had an essential role in offering a higher effective. Also, this system showed no toxicity, being released via biliary pathway [134]. In another study were used cancer cells (human Panc1 and HeLa) for investigating the anticancer activity of CNTs, etoposide and the system consisting of CNTs and etoposide. It was observed that the largest anticancer activity was obtained in the case of the system CNT + etoposide [137].

Also, Wang et al. had studied the anticancer effect of CNTs against PC3 cell line and against in a murine S180 cancer model. For in vitro tests, they tested the single-walled carbon nanotube conjugate with docetaxel (SWNT-DTX) in the first case, and

Table 9.6 The techniques used for functionalizing carbon nanotubes for biomedical applications [136]

CNT	Functionalization	Technique	Duration
MWCNT	2.8 M HNO_3	Refluxing of MWCNT nitric acid	72 h
MWCNT	14 M HNO_3	Refluxed	18 h
MWCNT	20 mL HNO_3	Sonication	1 min
SWCNT	HNO_3/H_2SO_4	Sonication	4 h
SWCNT	2.5 M of HNO_3	Refluxed	2–36 h
SWCNT	2 mg/L PL-PEG-NH_2	Sonication	1 h

in the second case the single-walled carbon nanotube conjugate with docetaxel and linked with NGR peptide (SWNT-NGR-DTX) was tested. It was observed that in PC3 cells at 48 h there was no difference between control (docetaxel), SWNT-DTX, and SWNT-NGR-DTX, but at 72 h a high difference was observed between SWNT-NGR-DTX and the control. In the case of in vivo tests, it was observed that compared to control (in this case was normal saline) the SWNT-DTX and SWNT-NGR-DTX produce the inhibition of tumor growth. It was concluded that SWNT-NGR-DTX does not produce side effects and may be promising for cancer treatment [138].

9.3.2.6 Dendrimers

Dendrimers are branched polymeric macromolecules that can be synthesized by two methods: convergent and divergent. They are composed of core molecule, branches, and surface molecules [139].

Padilla De Jesús et al. had produced a dendritic nanoformulation by covalent attachment of doxorubicin to the three-arm poly-(ethylene oxide)-polyester dendrons (G2). It was observed that the drug release depends on pH, the release was faster at a pH lower than 6. The cytotoxicity of the system on different cancer lines was reduced compared to the free drug, and to determine the biodistribution mice were used for the in vivo tests. It was observed that in the vital organs a very low accumulation was found [140]. Bhadra et al. had realized an extended release system of anticancer drug (based on 5-fluorouracil) using non-PEGylated and PEGylated (PAMAM) dendrimers. It was observed by in vitro studies that the PEGylation of the systems offers a higher load capacity and an extended drug release in comparison with the non-PEGylated dendrimers [141]. In another study, Shi et al. had reported that dendrimer-entrapped gold nanoparticles can be successfully used for the imaging of cancer. Thus, they created a system of dendrimer-entrapped gold nanoparticles linked with folic acid and fluorescein isothiocyanate molecules, which have been successfully bound to a human epithelial carcinoma cell line [142].

9.3.2.7 Liposomes

One of the advantages of using liposomes for cancer treatment, besides their properties (biocompatibility, biodegradability, and stability in colloidal solutions), is that the cytotoxic drugs can be delivered successfully in high concentrations at the tumor site [143,144]. Their mechanism of action against tumors is very simple, because the use of liposomes in cancer applications presents two advantages. In the first place, it has been demonstrated that, owing to the high temperature of the tumor, a local agglomeration of liposomes occurs. In the second place, liposomes are designed to be stable at 37°C, but become unstable at higher temperatures (39°C–42°C) [143].

Cortes et al. reported that the system consisting of irinotecan hydrochloride and oxaliplatin coloaded liposomes showed a higher cytotoxicity in vitro (HCT-116 and CT-26 cells) and an in vivo antitumor activity (CT-26 bearing BALB/c mice) compared to the single encapsulated drugs [145]. Also, Sriraman et al. had obtained a system consisting of PEGylated doxorubicin-loaded liposomes targeted with different receptors (transferrin, folic acid, and transferrin-folic acid). It was observed by in vitro tests that the system that contained transferrin-folic acid showed the higher cytotoxicity against HeLa cells and A2780-ADR ovarian carcinoma cell monolayers, compared with the systems that contained transferrin or folic acid.

The in vivo tests carried out on HeLa xenograft model in nude mice showed for the system doxorubicin-loaded liposomes a tumor growth inhibition of 42%, while the system that contained transferrin-folic showed a tumor growth inhibition of 79% [146].

9.4 Conclusions

Nanotherapeutics can be synthesized by various methods depending on the applications where they are intended to be used. A wide variety of inorganic and organic nanoparticles has been investigated for their antimicrobial and antitumoral properties, which are the main and the most investigated applications in the current medical field. It was observed that the antimicrobial and antitumoral activities of such nanotherapeutics depend on their particularities, such as dimensions, shape, mechanism of action, and cytotoxicity. Even though impressive advances have been made recently, the wide use in the current clinical practice of most nanotherapeutics remains restricted, main concerns referring not only to their long-term safety for the patient, but also to ecological and toxicological aspects.

Acknowledgment

This work has been funded by University Politehnica of Bucharest, through the "Excellence Research Grants" Program, UPB—GEX. Identifier: UPB–EXCELENȚĂ–2016 Research project "Suprafete nanobiostructurate antimicrobiene utilizate pentru stimularea fixarii la interfata os-implant", Contract number: 554.

References

[1] Hu C-MJ, Aryal S, Zhang L. Nanoparticle-assisted combination therapies for effective cancer treatment. Therapeutic Delivery 2010;1:323–34.

[2] Knežević NŽ, Durand JO. Targeted treatment of cancer with nanotherapeutics based on mesoporous silica nanoparticles. ChemPlusChem 2015;80:26–36.

[3] Liu Z, Robinson JT, Tabakman SM, Yang K, Dai H. Carbon materials for drug delivery & cancer therapy. Materials Today 2011;14:316–23.

[4] Cho K, Wang X, Nie S, Shin DM. Therapeutic nanoparticles for drug delivery in cancer. Clinical Cancer Research 2008;14:1310–6.

[5] Faunce TA. Nanotherapeutics: new challenges for safety and cost-effectiveness regulation in Australia. Medical Journal of Australia 2007;186:189.

[6] Kievit FM, Zhang M. Surface engineering of iron oxide nanoparticles for targeted cancer therapy. Accounts of Chemical Research 2011;44:853–62.

[7] Wani IA, Khatoon S, Ganguly A, Ahmed J, Ahmad T. Structural characterization and antimicrobial properties of silver nanoparticles prepared by inverse microemulsion method. Colloids and Surfaces B: Biointerfaces 2013;101:243–50.

[8] Gupta A, Landis RF, Rotello VM. Nanoparticle-Based Antimicrobials: Surface Functionality is Critical. F1000Research 2016;5.

[9] Beyth N, Houri-Haddad Y, Domb A, Khan W, Hazan R. Alternative antimicrobial approach: nano-antimicrobial materials. Evidence-Based Complementary and Alternative Medicine 2015 2015.

[10] Ravishankar Rai V, Jamuna Bai A. Nanoparticles and their potential application as antimicrobials Science against microbial pathogens, communicating current research and technological advances. Badajoz: Formatex; 2011. p. 197–209.

[11] Parham S, Wicaksono DH, Bagherbaigi S, Lee SL, Nur H. Antimicrobial Treatment of Different Metal Oxide Nanoparticles: A Critical Review. Journal of the Chinese Chemical Society 2016;63:385–93.

[12] Miller, K.P. 2015. Bacterial Communication and its Role as a Target for Nanoparticle-Based Antimicrobial Therapy.

[13] Popov A, Priezzhev A, Lademann J, Myllylä R. TiO2 nanoparticles as an effective UV-B radiation skin-protective compound in sunscreens. Journal of Physics D: Applied Physics 2005;38:2564.

[14] Scott B, Shah SI. Photocatalytic Properties of TiO2 Nanoparticles Dekker Encyclopedia of Nanoscience and Nanotechnology. Taylor & Francis; 2007.

[15] Chava RK, Raj S, Yu Y-T. Synthesis and electrophoretic deposition of hollow-TiO2 nanoparticles for dye sensitized solar cell applications. Journal of Alloys and Compounds 2016;672:212–22.

[16] Zhang C, Hu Z, Deng B. Silver nanoparticles in aquatic environments: Physiochemical behavior and antimicrobial mechanisms. Water Research 2016;88:403–27.

[17] Sagadevan S, Murugasen P. Electrical Properties of Copper Oxide Nanoparticles. Journal of Nano Research 2015;30.

[18] Sharmila G, Thirumarimurugan M, Sivakumar VM. Optical, catalytic and antibacterial properties of phytofabricated CuO nanoparticles using Tecoma castanifolia leaf extract. Optik-International Journal for Light and Electron Optics 2016;127:7822–8.

[19] Gupta VK, Chandra R, Tyagi I, Verma M. Removal of hexavalent chromium ions using CuO nanoparticles for water purification applications. Journal of Colloid and Interface Science 2016;478:54–62.

[20] Sarwar S, Chakraborti S, Bera S, Sheikh IA, Hoque KM, Chakrabarti P. The antimicrobial activity of ZnO nanoparticles against Vibrio cholerae: Variation in response depends on biotype. Nanomedicine: Nanotechnology, Biology and Medicine 2016;12:1499–509.

[21] Mandal S, Natarajan S, Tamilselvi A, Mayadevi S. Photocatalytic and antimicrobial activities of zinc ferrite nanoparticles synthesized through soft chemical route: A magnetically recyclable catalyst for water/wastewater treatment. Journal of Environmental Chemical Engineering 2016;4:2706–12.

[22] Bindhu MR, Umadevi M, Kavin Micheal M, Arasu MV, Abdullah Al-Dhabi N. Structural, morphological and optical properties of MgO nanoparticles for antibacterial applications. Materials Letters 2016;166:19–22.

[23] Mageshwari K, Mali SS, Sathyamoorthy R, Patil PS. Template-free synthesis of MgO nanoparticles for effective photocatalytic applications. Powder Technology 2013;249:456–62.

[24] Marquis G, Ramasamy B, Banwarilal S, Munusamy AP. Evaluation of antibacterial activity of plant mediated CaO nanoparticles using Cissus quadrangularis extract. Journal of Photochemistry and Photobiology B: Biology 2016;155:28–33.

[25] Lu Z, Mao C, Meng M, Liu S, Tian Y, Yu L, et al. Fabrication of CeO2 nanoparticle-modified silk for UV protection and antibacterial applications. Journal of Colloid and Interface Science 2014;435:8–14.

[26] Ahmed A, Nadeem S. The study of (Cu, TiO2, Al2O3) nanoparticles as antimicrobials of blood flow through diseased arteries. Journal of Molecular Liquids 2016;216:615–23.

[27] Prasannakumar JB, Vidya YS, Anantharaju KS, Ramgopal G, Nagabhushana H, Sharma SC, et al. Bio-mediated route for the synthesis of shape tunable Y2O3: Tb3+ nanoparticles: Photoluminescence and antibacterial properties. Spectrochimica Acta Part A: Molecular and Biomolecular Spectroscopy 2015;151:131–40.
[28] Gupta SM, Tripathi M. A review of TiO2 nanoparticles. Chinese Science Bulletin 2011;56:1639–57.
[29] Visai L, De Nardo L, Punta C, Melone L, Cigada A, Imbriani M, et al. Titanium oxide antibacterial surfaces in biomedical devices. International Journal of Artificial Organs 2011;34:929–46.
[30] Sunada K, Watanabe T, Hashimoto K. Studies on photokilling of bacteria on TiO 2 thin film. Journal of Photochemistry and Photobiology A: Chemistry 2003;156:227–33.
[31] Dizaj SM, Lotfipour F, Barzegar-Jalali M, Zarrintan MH, Adibkia K. Antimicrobial activity of the metals and metal oxide nanoparticles. Materials Science and Engineering: C 2014;44:278–84.
[32] Thomas A, Venkataramana J. Antimicrobial activity of tio2 nanoparticles against microbial isolates causing dental plaques. International Journal of Bioassays 2014;3: 3106–10.
[33] Ahmad R, Sardar M. TiO 2 nanoparticles as an antibacterial agents against E. coli. Int J Innovative Res Sci Eng Technol 2013;2:3569–74.
[34] Soenen SJ, Parak WJ, Rejman J, Manshian B. Intra) Cellular stability of inorganic nanoparticles: effects on cytotoxicity, particle functionality, and biomedical applications. Chemical Reviews 2015;115:2109–35.
[35] Salari Z, Danafar F, Dabaghi S, Ataei SA. Sustainable synthesis of silver nanoparticles using macroalgae Spirogyra varians and analysis of their antibacterial activity. Journal of Saudi Chemical Society 2014.
[36] Zafar N, Shamaila S, Nazir J, Sharif R, Rafique MS, Ul-Hasan J, et al. Antibacterial Action of Chemically Synthesized and Laser Generated Silver Nanoparticles Against Human Pathogenic Bacteria. Journal of Materials Science & Technology 2016.
[37] Abd-Elnaby HM, Abo-Elala GM, Abdel-Raouf UM, Hamed MM. Antibacterial and anticancer activity of extracellular synthesized silver nanoparticles from marine Streptomyces rochei MHM13. The Egyptian Journal of Aquatic Research 2016.
[38] De Aragão AP, De Oliveira TM, Quelemes PV, Perfeito MLG, Araújo MC, Santiago JDAS, et al. Green synthesis of silver nanoparticles using the seaweed Gracilaria birdiae and their antibacterial activity. Arabian Journal of Chemistry 2016.
[39] Thuc DT, Huy TQ, Hoang LH, Tien BC, Van Chung P, Thuy NT, et al. Green synthesis of colloidal silver nanoparticles through electrochemical method and their antibacterial activity. Materials Letters 2016.
[40] Naika HR, Lingaraju K, Manjunath K, Kumar D, Nagaraju G, Suresh D, et al. Green synthesis of CuO nanoparticles using Gloriosa superba L. extract and their antibacterial activity. Journal of Taibah University for Science 2015;9:7–12.
[41] Ahamed M, Alhadlaq HA, Khan M, Karuppiah P, Al-Dhabi NA. Synthesis, characterization, and antimicrobial activity of copper oxide nanoparticles. Journal of Nanomaterials 2014:17. 2014.
[42] Das D, Nath BC, Phukon P, Dolui SK. Synthesis and evaluation of antioxidant and antibacterial behavior of CuO nanoparticles. Colloids and Surfaces B: Biointerfaces 2013;101:430–3.
[43] Khashan KS, Sulaiman GM, Abdulameer FA. Synthesis and Antibacterial Activity of CuO Nanoparticles Suspension Induced by Laser Ablation in Liquid. Arabian Journal for Science and Engineering 2016;41:301–10.

[44] Pandey P, Packiyaraj MS, Nigam H, Agarwal GS, Singh B, Patra MK. Antimicrobial properties of CuO nanorods and multi-armed nanoparticles against B. anthracis vegetative cells and endospores. Beilstein Journal of Nanotechnology 2014;5:789–800.
[45] Sirelkhatim A, Mahmud S, Seeni A, Kaus NHM, Ann LC, Bakhori SKM, et al. Review on zinc oxide nanoparticles: antibacterial activity and toxicity mechanism. Nano-Micro Letters 2015;7:219–42.
[46] Espitia PJP, Soares NDFF, Dos Reis Coimbra JS, De Andrade NJ, Cruz RS, Medeiros EAA. Zinc oxide nanoparticles: synthesis, antimicrobial activity and food packaging applications. Food and Bioprocess Technology 2012;5:1447–64.
[47] Xie Y, He Y, Irwin PL, Jin T, Shi X. Antibacterial activity and mechanism of action of zinc oxide nanoparticles against Campylobacter jejuni. Applied and Environmental Microbiology 2011;77:2325–31.
[48] Liu Y, He L, Mustapha A, Li H, Hu Z, Lin M. Antibacterial activities of zinc oxide nanoparticles against Escherichia coli O157: H7. Journal of Applied Microbiology 2009;107:1193–201.
[49] Gunalan S, Sivaraj R, Rajendran V. Green synthesized ZnO nanoparticles against bacterial and fungal pathogens. Progress in Natural Science: Materials International 2012;22:693–700.
[50] Tang Z-X, Lv B-F. MgO nanoparticles as antibacterial agent: preparation and activity. Brazilian Journal of Chemical Engineering 2014;31:591–601.
[51] Leung YH, Ng A, Xu X, Shen Z, Gethings LA, Wong MT, et al. Mechanisms of Antibacterial Activity of MgO: Non-ROS Mediated Toxicity of MgO Nanoparticles Towards Escherichia coli. Small 2014;10:1171–83.
[52] Sundrarajan M, Suresh J, Gandhi RR. A comparative study on antibacterial properties of MgO nanoparticles prepared under different calcination temperature. Digest J Nanomaterials Biostructures 2012;7:983–9.
[53] He Y, Ingudam S, Reed S, Gehring A, Strobaugh TP, Irwin P. Study on the mechanism of antibacterial action of magnesium oxide nanoparticles against foodborne pathogens. Journal of Nanobiotechnology 2016;14:1.
[54] Jin T, He Y. Antibacterial activities of magnesium oxide (MgO) nanoparticles against foodborne pathogens. Journal of Nanoparticle Research 2011;13:6877–85.
[55] Roy A, Gauri SS, Bhattacharya M, Bhattacharya J. Antimicrobial activity of CaO nanoparticles. Journal of Biomedical Nanotechnology 2013;9:1570–8.
[56] Das S, Dowding JM, Klump KE, Mcginnis JF, Self W, Seal S. Cerium oxide nanoparticles: applications and prospects in nanomedicine. Nanomedicine 2013;8:1483–508.
[57] Dos Santos, C.C.L., Farias, I.A.P., Dos Reis Albuquerque, A.D.J.E., Silva, P.M.D.F., Da Costa One, G.M. & Sampaio, F.C. Antimicrobial activity of nano cerium oxide (IV) (CeO2) against Streptococcus mutans. BMC Proceedings, 2014. BioMed Central, 1.
[58] Cuahtecontzi-Delint R, Mendez-Rojas MA, Bandala ER, Quiroz MA, Recillas S, Sanchez-Salas JL. Enhanced antibacterial activity of CeO2 nanoparticles by surfactants. International Journal of Chemical Reactor Engineering 2013;11:1–5.
[59] Ansari MA, Khan HM, Khan AA, Pal R, Cameotra SS. Antibacterial potential of Al2O3 nanoparticles against multidrug resistance strains of Staphylococcus aureus isolated from skin exudates. Journal of Nanoparticle Research 2013;15:1–12.
[60] Ansari MA, Khan HM, Alzohairy MA, Jalal M, Ali SG, Pal R, et al. Green synthesis of Al2O3 nanoparticles and their bactericidal potential against clinical isolates of multi-drug resistant Pseudomonas aeruginosa. World Journal of Microbiology and Biotechnology 2015;31:153–64.

[61] Yien L, Zin NM, Sarwar A, Katas H. Antifungal activity of chitosan nanoparticles and correlation with their physical properties. International Journal of Biomaterials, 2012.
[62] Alishahi A. Antibacterial effect of chitosan nanoparticle loaded with nisin for the prolonged effect. Journal of Food Safety 2014;34:111–8.
[63] De Paz LEC, Resin A, Howard KA, Sutherland DS, Wejse PL. Antimicrobial effect of chitosan nanoparticles on Streptococcus mutans biofilms. Applied and Environmental Microbiology 2011;77:3892–5.
[64] Ma Y, Liu P, Si C, Liu Z. Chitosan nanoparticles: preparation and application in antibacterial paper. Journal of Macromolecular Science, Part B 2010;49:994–1001.
[65] Mohammadi A, Hashemi M, Hosseini SM. Effect of chitosan molecular weight as micro and nanoparticles on antibacterial activity against some soft rot pathogenic bacteria. LWT-Food Science and Technology 2016;71:347–55.
[66] Piras AM, Maisetta G, Sandreschi S, Gazzarri M, Bartoli C, Grassi L, et al. Chitosan nanoparticles loaded with the antimicrobial peptide temporin B exert a long-term antibacterial activity in vitro against clinical isolates of Staphylococcus epidermidis. Frontiers in Microbiology 2015;6:372.
[67] Chheda, A. & Vernekar, M. 2014. A natural preservative ε-poly-L-lysine: fermentative production and applications in food industry.
[68] El-Sersy NA, Abdelwahab AE, Abouelkhiir SS, Abou-Zeid DM, Sabry SA. Antibacterial and Anticancer activity of ε-poly-L-lysine (ε-PL) produced by a marine Bacillus subtilis sp. Journal of Basic Microbiology 2012;52:513–22.
[69] Shi C, Zhao X, Liu Z, Meng R, Chen X, Guo N. Antimicrobial, antioxidant, and antitumor activity of epsilon-poly-L-lysine and citral, alone or in combination. Food & Nutrition Research 2016:60.
[70] Shima S, Matsuoka H, Iwamoto T, Sakai H. Antimicrobial action of. EPSILON-Poly-L-lysine. The Journal of Antibiotics 1984;37:1449–55.
[71] Majumdar P, He J, Lee E, Kallam A, Gubbins N, Stafslien SJ, et al. Antimicrobial activity of polysiloxane coatings containing quaternary ammonium-functionalized polyhedral oligomeric silsesquioxane. Journal of Coatings Technology and Research 2010;7:455–67.
[72] Cui X, Qiao C, Wang S, Ding Y, Hao C, Li J. Synthesis, surface properties, and antibacterial activity of polysiloxane quaternary ammonium salts containing epoxy group. Colloid and Polymer Science 2015;293:1971–81.
[73] Lin Y, Liu Q, Cheng L, Lei Y, Zhang A. Synthesis and antimicrobial activities of polysiloxane-containing quaternary ammonium salts on bacteria and phytopathogenic fungi. Reactive and Functional Polymers 2014;85:36–44.
[74] Yazdankhah SP, Scheie AA, Høiby EA, Lunestad B-T, Heir E, Fotland TØ, et al. Triclosan and antimicrobial resistance in bacteria: an overview. Microbial Drug Resistance 2006;12:83–90.
[75] Suller M, Russell A. Triclosan and antibiotic resistance in Staphylococcus aureus. Journal of Antimicrobial Chemotherapy 2000;46:11–18.
[76] Braid JJ, Wale MC. The antibacterial activity of triclosan-impregnated storage boxes against Staphylococcus aureus, Escherichia coli, Pseudomonas aeruginosa, Bacillus cereus and Shewanella putrefaciens in conditions simulating domestic use. Journal of Antimicrobial Chemotherapy 2002;49:87–94.
[77] Fan F, Yan K, Wallis NG, Reed S, Moore TD, Rittenhouse SF, et al. Defining and combating the mechanisms of triclosan resistance in clinical isolates of Staphylococcus aureus. Antimicrobial Agents and Chemotherapy 2002;46:3343–7.
[78] Bahar AA, Ren D. Antimicrobial peptides. Pharmaceuticals 2013;6:1543–75.

[79] Izadpanah A, Gallo RL. Antimicrobial peptides. Journal of the American Academy of Dermatology 2005;52:381–90.
[80] Ganz T. The role of antimicrobial peptides in innate immunity. Integrative and Comparative Biology 2003;43:300–4.
[81] Guilhelmelli F, Vilela N, Albuquerque P, Derengowski LDS, Silva-Pereira I, Kyaw CM. Antibiotic development challenges: the various mechanisms of action of antimicrobial peptides and of bacterial resistance. New edge of antibiotic development: antimicrobial peptides and corresponding resistance 2014;63.
[82] Giuliani A, Pirri G, Nicoletto S. Antimicrobial peptides: an overview of a promising class of therapeutics. Open Life Sciences 2007;2:1–33.
[83] Brigger I, Dubernet C, Couvreur P. Nanoparticles in cancer therapy and diagnosis. Advanced Drug Delivery Reviews 2002;54:631–51.
[84] Ahn S, Seo E, Kim K, Lee SJ. Controlled cellular uptake and drug efficacy of nanotherapeutics. Scientific Reports 2013:3.
[85] Krishnan, S.R. & George, S.K. 2014. Nanotherapeutics in cancer prevention, diagnosis and treatment. Pharmacology and Therapeutics, (Ed. Thatha SJ). Gowder, ISBN, 978–953.
[86] Lytton-Jean AK, Kauffman KJ, Kaczmarek JC, Langer R. Cancer nanotherapeutics in clinical trials Nanotechnology-Based Precision Tools for the Detection and Treatment of Cancer. Springer; 2015.
[87] Bhattacharyya S, Kudgus RA, Bhattacharya R, Mukherjee P. Inorganic nanoparticles in cancer therapy. Pharmaceutical Research 2011;28:237–59.
[88] Tang M, Russell PJ, Khatri A. Magnetic nanoparticles: prospects in cancer imaging and therapy. Discovery Medicine 2009;7:68–74.
[89] El-Deeb NM, El-Sherbiny IM, El-Aassara MR, Hafez EE. Novel trend in colon cancer therapy using silver nanoparticles synthesized by honey bee. Journal of Nanomedicine & Nanotechnology 2015:2015.
[90] Jeyaraj M, Sathishkumar G, Sivanandhan G, Mubarakali D, Rajesh M, Arun R, et al. Biogenic silver nanoparticles for cancer treatment: an experimental report. Colloids and Surfaces B: Biointerfaces 2013;106:86–92.
[91] Lalitha P. Apoptotic efficacy of biogenic silver nanoparticles on human breast cancer MCF-7 cell lines. Progress in Biomaterials 2015;4:113–21.
[92] Gurunathan S, Han JW, Eppakayala V, Jeyaraj M, Kim J-H. Cytotoxicity of biologically synthesized silver nanoparticles in MDA-MB-231 human breast cancer cells. BioMed Research International 2013 2013.
[93] Jain S, Hirst D, O'sullivan J. Gold nanoparticles as novel agents for cancer therapy. The British Journal of Radiology 2014.
[94] Kodiha M, Wang YM, Hutter E, Maysinger D, Stochaj U. Off to the organelles—killing cancer cells with targeted gold nano-particles. Theranostics 2015;5:357–70.
[95] Kumar A, Ma H, Zhang X, Huang K, Jin S, Liu J, et al. Gold nanoparticles functionalized with therapeutic and targeted peptides for cancer treatment. Biomaterials 2012;33:1180–9.
[96] Kennedy LC, Bickford LR, Lewinski NA, Coughlin AJ, Hu Y, Day ES, et al. A New Era for Cancer Treatment: Gold-Nanoparticle-Mediated Thermal Therapies. Small 2011;7:169–83.
[97] Hainfeld JF, Slatkin DN, Smilowitz HM. The use of gold nanoparticles to enhance radiotherapy in mice. Physics in Medicine and Biology 2004;49:N309.
[98] Laurent S, Mahmoudi M. Superparamagnetic iron oxide nanoparticles: promises for diagnosis and treatment of cancer. Int J Mol Epidemiol Genet 2011;2:367–90.

[99] Santhosh PB, Ulrih NP. Multifunctional superparamagnetic iron oxide nanoparticles: promising tools in cancer theranostics. Cancer Letters 2013;336:8–17.

[100] Bakhtiary Z, Saei AA, Hajipour MJ, Raoufi M, Vermesh O, Mahmoudi M. Targeted superparamagnetic iron oxide nanoparticles for early detection of cancer: Possibilities and challenges. Nanomedicine: Nanotechnology, Biology and Medicine 2016;12: 287–307.

[101] Peng X-H, Qian X, Mao H, Wang AY, Chen Z, Nie S, et al. Targeted magnetic iron oxide nanoparticles for tumor imaging and therapy. Int J Nanomedicine 2008;3:311–21.

[102] Quinto CA, Mohindra P, Tong S, Bao G. Multifunctional superparamagnetic iron oxide nanoparticles for combined chemotherapy and hyperthermia cancer treatment. Nanoscale 2015;7:12728–36.

[103] Liu H, Chen D, Li L, Liu T, Tan L, Wu X, et al. Multifunctional gold nanoshells on silica nanorattles: a platform for the combination of photothermal therapy and chemotherapy with low systemic toxicity. Angewandte Chemie 2011;123:921–5.

[104] Zhao J, Wallace M, Melancon MP. Cancer theranostics with gold nanoshells. Nanomedicine 2014;9:2041–57.

[105] Morton JG, Day ES, Halas NJ, West JL. Nanoshells for photothermal cancer therapy. Cancer Nanotechnology: Methods and Protocols 2010:101–17.

[106] Bardhan R, Lal S, Joshi A, Halas NJ. Theranostic nanoshells: from probe design to imaging and treatment of cancer. Accounts of Chemical Research 2011;44:936–46.

[107] Trouiller B, Reliene R, Westbrook A, Solaimani P, Schiestl RH. Titanium dioxide nanoparticles induce DNA damage and genetic instability in vivo in mice. Cancer Research 2009;69:8784–9.

[108] Fujiwara R, Luo Y, Sasaki T, Fujii K, Ohmori H, Kuniyasu H. Cancer therapeutic effects of titanium dioxide nanoparticles are associated with oxidative stress and cytokine induction. Pathobiology 2015;82:243–51.

[109] You DG, Deepagan V, Um W, Jeon S, Son S, Chang H, et al. ROS-generating TiO2 nanoparticles for non-invasive sonodynamic therapy of cancer. Scientific Reports 2016;6.

[110] Sungkaworn T, Triampo W, Nalakarn P, Triampo D, Tang I, Lenbury Y, et al. The effects of TiO2 nanoparticles on tumor cell colonies: fractal dimension and morphological properties. World Academy of Science, Engineering and Technology, International Journal of Medical, Health, Biomedical, Bioengineering and Pharmaceutical Engineering 2008;2:20–7.

[111] Lin W, Stayton I, Huang Y-W, Zhou X-D, Ma Y. Cytotoxicity and cell membrane depolarization induced by aluminum oxide nanoparticles in human lung epithelial cells A549. Toxicological and Environmental Chemistry 2008;90:983–96.

[112] Arul Prakash F, Babu GD, Lavanya M, Vidhya KS, Devasena T. Toxicity studies of aluminium oxide nanoparticles in cell lines. Int J Nanotechnol Appl 2011;5:99–107.

[113] Di Virgilio A, Reigosa M, Arnal P, De Mele MFL. Comparative study of the cytotoxic and genotoxic effects of titanium oxide and aluminium oxide nanoparticles in Chinese hamster ovary (CHO-K1) cells. Journal of Hazardous Materials 2010;177:711–8.

[114] Sun Z, Wang W, Wang R, Duan J, Hu Y, Ma J, et al. Aluminum nanoparticles enhance anticancer immune response induced by tumor cell vaccine. Cancer Nanotechnology 2010;1:63–9.

[115] Fang M, Peng C-W, Pang D-W, Li Y. Quantum dots for cancer research: current status, remaining issues, and future perspectives. Cancer Biology & Medicine 2012;9:151.

[116] Zhang H, Yee D, Wang C. Quantum dots for cancer diagnosis and therapy: biological and clinical perspectives. Nanomedicine 2008;3:83–91.

[117] Malik P, Gulia S, Kakkar R. Quantum dots for diagnosis of cancers, 2013.
[118] Xing Y, Rao J. Quantum dot bioconjugates for in vitro diagnostics & in vivo imaging. Cancer Biomarkers 2008;4:307–19.
[119] Chen C, Peng J, Xia H-S, Yang G-F, Wu Q-S, Chen L-D, et al. Quantum dots-based immunofluorescence technology for the quantitative determination of HER2 expression in breast cancer. Biomaterials 2009;30:2912–8.
[120] Parveen S, Sahoo SK. Polymeric nanoparticles for cancer therapy. Journal of Drug Targeting 2008;16:108–23.
[121] Masood F. Polymeric nanoparticles for targeted drug delivery system for cancer therapy. Materials Science and Engineering: C 2016;60:569–78.
[122] Arya G, Vandana M, Acharya S, Sahoo SK. Enhanced antiproliferative activity of Herceptin (HER2)-conjugated gemcitabine-loaded chitosan nanoparticle in pancreatic cancer therapy. Nanomedicine: Nanotechnology, Biology and Medicine 2011;7:859–70.
[123] Park K, Kim J-H, Nam YS, Lee S, Nam HY, Kim K, et al. Effect of polymer molecular weight on the tumor targeting characteristics of self-assembled glycol chitosan nanoparticles. Journal of Controlled Release 2007;122:305–14.
[124] Zhang J, Chen XG, Liu CS, Park HJ. Investigation of polymeric amphiphilic nanoparticles as antitumor drug carriers. Journal of Materials Science: Materials in Medicine 2009;20:991–9.
[125] Kumar A, Glaum M, El-Badri N, Mohapatra S, Haller E, Park S, et al. Initial observations of cell-mediated drug delivery to the deep lung. Cell Transplantation 2011;20:609–18.
[126] Ekinci M, Ilem-Ozdemir D, Gundogdu E, Asikoglu M. Methotrexate loaded chitosan nanoparticles: Preparation, radiolabeling and in vitro evaluation for breast cancer diagnosis. Journal of Drug Delivery Science and Technology 2015;30:107–13.
[127] Ortiz R, Prados J, Melguizo C, Arias JL, Ruiz MA, Alvarez PJ, et al. 5-Fluorouracil-loaded poly (ε-caprolactone) nanoparticles combined with phage E gene therapy as a new strategy against colon cancer. International Journal of Nanomedicine 2012.
[128] Chawla JS, Amiji MM. Biodegradable poly (ε-caprolactone) nanoparticles for tumor-targeted delivery of tamoxifen. International Journal of Pharmaceutics 2002;249:127–38.
[129] Mei L, Zhang Y, Zheng Y, Tian G, Song C, Yang D, et al. A novel docetaxel-loaded poly (ε-caprolactone)/pluronic F68 nanoparticle overcoming multidrug resistance for breast cancer treatment. Nanoscale Research Letters 2009;4:1530.
[130] Rai R. Biosynthesis of polyhydroxyalkanoates and its medical applications. University of Westminster; 2010.
[131] Rai R, Keshavarz T, Roether J, Boccaccini AR, Roy I. Medium chain length polyhydroxyalkanoates, promising new biomedical materials for the future. Materials Science and Engineering: R: Reports 2011;72:29–47.
[132] Choiniere, P. 2015. Development of Polyhydroxyalkanoate Nanoparticles for Cancer Therapy.
[133] Zhang W, Zhang Z, Zhang Y. The application of carbon nanotubes in target drug delivery systems for cancer therapies. Nanoscale Research Letters 2011;6:1.
[134] Liu Z, Chen K, Davis C, Sherlock S, Cao Q, Chen X, et al. Drug delivery with carbon nanotubes for in vivo cancer treatment. Cancer Research 2008;68:6652–60.
[135] Elhissi A, Ahmed W, Hassan IU, Dhanak VR, D'emanuele A. Carbon nanotubes in cancer therapy and drug delivery. Journal of Drug Delivery, 2012.
[136] Madani SY, Naderi N, Dissanayake O, Tan A, Seifalian AM. A new era of cancer treatment: carbon nanotubes as drug delivery tools. Int J Nanomedicine 2011;6:2963–79.
[137] Mahmood M, Karmakar A, Fejleh A, Mocan T, Iancu C, Mocan L, et al. Synergistic enhancement of cancer therapy using a combination of carbon nanotubes and anti-tumor drug. Nanomedicine 2009;4:883–93.

[138] Wang L, Zhang M, Zhang N, Shi J, Zhang H, Li M, et al. Synergistic enhancement of cancer therapy using a combination of docetaxel and photothermal ablation induced by single-walled carbon nanotubes. Int J Nanomedicine 2011;6:e52.

[139] Bharali, D.J., Khalil, M., Gurbuz, M., Simone, T.M. & Mousa, S.A. 2009. Nanoparticles and cancer therapy: a concise review with emphasis on dendrimers.

[140] Padilla De Jesús OL, Ihre HR, Gagne L, Fréchet JM, Szoka FC. Polyester dendritic systems for drug delivery applications: in vitro and in vivo evaluation. Bioconjugate Chemistry 2002;13:453–61.

[141] Bhadra D, Bhadra S, Jain S, Jain N. A PEGylated dendritic nanoparticulate carrier of fluorouracil. International Journal of Pharmaceutics 2003;257:111–24.

[142] Shi X, Wang S, Meshinchi S, Van Antwerp ME, Bi X, Lee I, et al. Dendrimer-entrapped gold nanoparticles as a platform for cancer-cell targeting and imaging. Small 2007;3:1245–52.

[143] Brown S, Khan DR. The treatment of breast cancer using liposome technology. Journal of Drug Delivery, 2012.

[144] Pandey H, Rani R, Agarwal V. Liposome and their applications in cancer therapy. Brazilian Archives of Biology and Technology 2016;59.

[145] Cortes JE, Goldberg SL, Feldman EJ, Rizzeri DA, Hogge DE, Larson M, et al. Phase II, multicenter, randomized trial of CPX-351 (cytarabine: daunorubicin) liposome injection versus intensive salvage therapy in adults with first relapse AML. Cancer 2015;121:234–42.

[146] Sriraman SK, Salzano G, Sarisozen C, Torchilin V. Anti-cancer activity of doxorubicin-loaded liposomes co-modified with transferrin and folic acid. Eur J Pharmaceut Biopharmaceut 2016.

Nanostructured coatings for biomaterials

10

Farideh Ordikhani, Fatemeh Mohandes and Abdolreza Simchi
Sharif University of Technology, Tehran, Iran

10.1 Introduction

To improve human health, the use of various natural, synthetic, and semisynthetic materials to fabricate implantable devices such as drug-eluting stents, artificial organs, biosensors, catheters, tissue engineering scaffolds, and heart valves is rapidly growing [1]. Although many kinds of implants, particularly orthopedic and dental implants, have been developed to repair defects, implant-mediated inflammation, and bacterial infections are critical issues that determine the implantation success [2,3]. Among different strategies adopted to control these critical aspects, surface modifications of biomedical materials by organic, inorganic, and composite coatings have attracted much interest in recent years. This is a flexible and versatile approach to modify biomaterial surfaces with regard to surface energy, adhesion, bioactivity, biocompatibility, hydrophilicity, corrosion, and degradation as well as providing special functionality such as drug delivery and cellular differentiation by loading growth factors [4].

Smart design and functionalization of biomaterial surfaces with coatings highly depend on interactions between the surface and the surrounding tissues [5]. Generally, biomaterials are divided into three classes based on their interactions with the living tissues and organs including bioinert, bioactive, and bioresorbable materials [6]. Bioinert materials do not form chemical or biological bond at the interface between the implant and the host tissue and the consequent relative movements are likely to cause inflammatory reactions. Several polymers (high molecular weight polyethylene and poly(etheretherketone)), ceramics (Al_2O_3, ZrO_2), and metals (Ti and Cr-Co alloys) appertain to this class [6]. In order to improve the adhesion between bioinert materials and living tissues and organs, some strategies including cementation [7] as well as morphological and biological fixation are introduced [8]. The cementation is achieved when the prosthesis is fixed by an inorganic or a polymeric cementing paste. Morphological and biological fixation may occur with porous implants due to bone ingrowth. Although mechanical attachment of bone to the bioinert devices takes place using fixation methods, the adhesion problems cannot completely be solved. Bioactive coatings are commonly used on bioinert metallic implants (stainless steel, cobalt chrome alloys, titanium alloys, etc.), where no cement for fixation is applied. The second generation of biomaterials, called "bioactive materials," have been evolved after L.L. Hench [9] who developed bioactive glasses that were able to bond to hard and soft tissues without any rejection. Surface modifications of bioinert materials with bioactive coatings have then become a golden approach to enhance

Nanobiomaterials Science, Development and Evaluation. DOI: http://dx.doi.org/10.1016/B978-0-08-100963-5.00010-0

their biofunctionality and to resolve the fixation shortcomings. The coatings must include several important criteria [10]:

- Biocompatibility without immune response with the human body.
- Sufficient mechanical strength when under physiological stresses associated with locomotion to not detach from the implant surface.
- Osteoconductivity to stimulate the osteoblast cells for making new bone surrounding the implant.
- Osteoinductivity and be able to recruit various stem cells from surrounding tissue and induce differentiation into osteogenic cells.
- Antibacterial property and antiinfective surface to minimize prosthetic infection.

Bioresorbable materials with a potential of gradual degrading in body environment and replacing by the living host tissue are promising candidates for the surface modifications of biomedical articles [11,12]. Although apatite formation might not be observed on the surface of some bioresorbable materials such as β-tricalcium phosphate [13] and natural calcite [14] after soaking in simulated body fluid (SBF) or in vivo condition, these materials enable to bond to living bone due to their high resorbability. Bioresorbable inorganic materials and some bioresorbable polymers including polylactic acid and polycaprolactone have been developed and utilized for coating of drug-eluting stents [15].

To boost the performance of bioactive coatings, nanotechnology has opened up new opportunities for surface modifications of biomedical implants by mechanical (blasting, attrition for obtaining nanosized grains), chemical (acid etching, chemical vapor deposition (CVD), electrochemical processes) and physical (thermal and plasma spray, sputtering, physical vapor deposition (PVD)) methods or by their combination [16]. Such evidences affect surface area, surface energy, roughness, and hydrophilic properties of the biomedical implants, and can thus enhance adhesion and epitenon cells [17], proliferation [18], endocytotic activity [19], and gene regulation [20] of fibroblasts [21], osteoblasts and osteoclasts [22], endothelial [23], and epithelial [24]. In this chapter, a brief introduction to surface modifications of biomaterials based on nanostructured coatings and their potential applications are presented.

10.2 Biocompatible nanostructured coatings

Biocompatibility refers to the interaction of a living system with medical devices or component materials. The common definition of biocompatibility is "the quality of being compatible with living system by not being toxic or injurious and not causing immunological rejection" [25]. A tetrazolium-based colorimetric assay (3-(4,5-dimethylthiazol-2-yl)-2,5-diphenyltetrazolium bromide (MTT)), blood compatibility, and numerous other strategies such as mimicking cell membranes, enhancing the surface affinity for serum proteins, promoting cell adhesion, inclusion, or immobilization of anticoagulants are commonly utilized to evaluate biocompatibility [26,27]. Most of these approaches are based on an underlying hydrophilic surface. Hydrophilic coatings on medical devices may also be used as the basis for active coatings, the elution of drugs or other species, and for imaging purposes [28]. For instance, contrast agents for magnetic resonance imaging (MRI) are often coated with polymers to increase their solubility and biocompatibility [29]; the coating of Ti surface with poly(amino acid) diblock copolymer nanoparticles (NPs) as a novel surface modification approach is introduced to load and controllably release bone morphogenetic protein-2 (BMP-2) for 40 days due to the decreased hydrophilicity of Ti substrate [30].

10.2.1 Nanocomposites based on synthetic and natural polymeric coatings

Poly(ethyleneglycol) (PEG), poly(lactic-co-glycolic acid) (PLGA), dendrimers molecules, polyvinylpyrrolidone (PVP), and polyvinyl alcohol (PVA) are the most successfully developed synthetic polymers to prepare nanocomposite coating for biomedical applications [31,32]. Under physiological conditions, the polymers hydrolyze in the body and produce original monomers. Since the produced monomers are by-products of various metabolic pathways in the body, there is minimal toxicity with the use of the polymer for drug delivery, vaccine adjuvant, or other biomedical applications [31]. Among the natural polymers, polysaccharides including chitosan, sodium alginate, and dextran are frequently used to cover NPs. Excellent properties of these polymers including rapid blood clotting, biodegradability, nontoxicity, high charge density, gelling, and mucoadhesivity led to their wide pharmaceutical applications. It has further been suggested that polysaccharides may structurally mimic extracellular glycoprotein carbohydrate and they may play a role in reorganizing collagen fibers in reconstructed tissues to provide efficient physiological functioning [31]. Electrospun nanofibrous polymers coated by biocompatible NPs have been introduced as an interesting and controllable architecture to fabricate three-dimensional (3D) scaffolds [33] for wound dressings and skin repair [34], tooth regeneration [35], and drug delivery [36]. PVA nanofibers coated by Ag NPs through dip-coating methods can be utilized as an antibacterial wound healing mat with high porosity and excellent pore-interconnectivity, which is particularly important for exuding fluid from the wound [34]. This polymeric nanocomposite inhibits the invasion of exogenous microorganisms and assists the control of fluid drainage due to its small pores and very high specific surface area of PVP nanofibers.

10.2.2 Coatings based on nanostructured calcium phosphates

So far, many studies have been performed to determine the behavior of different calcium phosphate phases under in vitro and in vivo conditions with respect to bioactivity, osteoinductivity, and osteoconductivity [37,38]. Their long-term stability as well as their suitability as a corrosion-protective coating for biodegradable metallic implants have also been examined [39,40]. For example, in vitro studies have determined that dicalcium phosphate dehydrate (DCPD) is a promising biodegradable and bioresorbable coating for metallic substrates because of its high release rate of calcium and phosphate ions [41]. Recently, biodegradable Mg alloys were coated with plate-like DCPD/MgF_2 nanostructures via fluoride conversion processes followed by an electrochemical deposition method [42]. It was shown that the DCPD/MgF_2 coatings improved the nucleation sites of apatite more than those of the uncoated implants.

Additionally, clinical studies involving the implantation of dicalcium phosphate anhydrous (DCPA) granules in the alveolar sockets of humans showed an increased bone regeneration, indicating its osteoconductivity [43]. Xu et al. [44] studied the effect of particle size of DCPA on the Ca and PO_4 release in dental composites including nanosilica-fused whiskers and DCPA particles at DCPA:whisker mass ratio of 1:1. They showed that dental resin (bisphenol A-glycidyl methacrylate (Bis-GMA)) composites containing DCPA with an average particle size of 112 nm released Ca to a concentration of 0.85 mmol/L and PO_4 of 3.48 mmol/L, which were more than the composites containing 12 μm DCPA (Ca of 0.67 mmol/L and PO_4 of 1.11 mmol/L).

Several studies have demonstrated the stability of octacalcium phosphate (OCP) at a physiological pH and temperature, and its ability to convert to a bone-like apatite when exposed to slightly more acidic conditions. Wang and coworker [45] electrochemically fabricated a novel micro/nanostructured OCP/protein composite coating on titanium substrate by using an induced deposition technique. Enhanced in vitro adhesion of osteoblast cells to the nanosized OCP/protein coating compared with the microsized OCP/protein coating was observed [45]. In another study, Jiang et al. [39] investigated the effect of micro- and nanosponge-like OCP coatings on titanium surface on in vitro biological response to osteoblast cells. Enhanced *MC3T3-E1* cell proliferation, alkaline phosphatase activity, and extracellular matrix mineralization on the nanocoating was shown. They suggested that the OCP nanocoating could be considered as a favorable implant for osseointegration in vivo.

Tricalcium phosphate (TCP) is often investigated as a biphasic coating in combination with hydroxyapatite (HA). Several studies have indicated that better biocompatibility is attained when a mixture of HA and TCP ratios are utilized due to the greater solubility of TCP compared to HA [46–48]. Tanzer et al. [47] showed that TCP/HA coatings applied to titanium hip implants exhibited an increased biocompatibility and decreased bone loss compared to untreated implants without the coatings. Other researchers have successfully used antibiotic-loaded TCP to prevent bone infections in bovine cancellous bone defects during healing [49]. Fibroblast cell attachment on collagen scaffolds modified with nano-TCP and fibroblast growth factor 2 (FGF2) confirmed improved cytocompatibility compared with micro-TCP [50].

HA is the most attractive member of calcium phosphates with a chemical composition similar to the inorganic phase of natural bone (Ca/P = 1.67) [51]. In vitro and in vivo bioactivity, biocompatibility, and osteoconductive properties of HA have been shown in many studies [52,53]. The brittle nature of HA renders it unsuitable for use in load-bearing orthopedic applications [54]; however, as a coating material of metallic implants, a combination of high mechanical strength of metals with superior biological compatibility of HA can be attained. Nanosized HA coatings with high surface area show a significant improvement in bioactivity as extracellular matrix proteins, growth factors, and numerous osteogenic potential cells interact with nanostructured surfaces [18,20,23]. Zhao et al. [55] reported the effect of zinc-substituted nano-HA coatings on bone integration with implant surfaces. They showed that rod-like Zn–HA coatings significantly improved the bone area within all threads after 4 and 8 weeks. Jafari et al. [56] employed a sol–gel dip-coating method following sintering process to prepare nano-HA coatings on Ti-14Zr13Nb alloy for orthopedic applications. It was found that sintering at elevated temperatures led to a higher surface integrity and crystallinity of nano-HA (to ~89%) with improved mechanical strength. A better corrosion resistance to biological environment was also attained [56]. Surmeneva et al. studied in vitro biocompatibility of nanostructured Si–HA coatings on Ti substrates with the aid of MTT assay, and reported good attachment and growth of MG63 osteoblast-like cells after 7 days of incubation [57].

Recently, composites of HA with carbon nanostructures including graphene [58,59] and carbon nanotubes (CNTs) [60] have been prepared and utilized. Uniform bioactive coatings with improved mechanical strength and favorable corrosion stability were prepared from HA/graphene nanocomposite by electrophoretic deposition (EDP) on titanium [61]. EDP of nanostructured HA and HA/CNT coatings on Ti6Al4V alloy followed by sintering at 800°C was also examined, and increased surface hardness, adhesion strength, and bone-bioactivity were shown [60].

10.2.3 Nanostructured bioactive glass coatings

Bioactive glasses (BG) consist of oxides from the SiO_2–CaO–MgO–NaO–K_2O–P_2O system, and are commonly used in cranial repair and dental implants [62]; however, their usage in load-bearing applications is limited due to their poor mechanical properties and intrinsic brittleness. The release of silicate and calcium ions are thought to promote the growth and osteogenic differentiation of primary osteoblast cells and activation of some families of genes in osteoprogenitor cells [63]. As a result, the chemical composition of BG and their dissolution rate in physiological environment (which depends on their surface area and morphology) determine bioactivity depending on its morphology [62,64]. BG NPs with a high surface-to-volume ratio are very interesting not only because they present a larger specific surface area, but also a higher surface energy compared to micrometric-sized particles. Therefore, BG NPs are potentially very attractive for surface modifications of metallic implants and ceramic scaffolds due to the enhancement of bioactivity and mechanical properties. Many studies have focused on the development of coatings made of BG NPs and their composites. For instance, Roohani-Esfahani et al. [65] prepared a polycaprolactone/BG (40 nm; 30 wt%) nanocomposite coating on HA/β-tricalcium phosphate scaffolds with improved compressive strength and modulus; Esfahani et al. [66] showed enhancement in the compressive strength of cancellous bone extracted from an adult bovine femur surface modified with polyvinyl alcohol/BG nanocomposites; Rego et al. [67] prepared nanocomposite coatings with an architecture similar to nacre from BG NPs/chitosan/hyaluronic acid through layer-by-layer deposition techniques. They showed good adhesive properties and bioactivity of the coatings for dentistry and orthopedics.

10.2.4 Other inorganic nanoparticulate coatings

Dense or porous SiO_2 with low toxicity in vitro is commonly used to shell different NPs for gene and drug delivery applications. Increased cell damage has been shown for silica microsized particles compared with NPs [68]. Napierska et al. [69] studied the effect of particle size of amorphous SiO_2 on human endothelial cells function, and they found that the exposure of human endothelial cells to nanosized SiO_2 (18–54 nm) enhanced their adhesive properties. Besides SiO_2, Au-shelled NPs have been architected for biomedicine, especially for drug delivery [70] and cancer applied hyperthermia treatments [71]. Hashimoto et al. [71] compared the exposure of cultured macrophages RAW264.7 to Au and Ag NPs. Although an inflammatory response was observed for both materials, the harmful cytotoxic effects of gold were smaller than that of silver. As described for other kinds of nanomaterials, the interaction between cells and Au NPs could be mediated by unspecific adsorption of serum proteins onto the gold surface.

Diamond-like carbon (DLC) coatings have been emerged in orthopedic, cardiovascular, and dental applications due to their superior tribological and mechanical properties with corrosion resistance, biocompatibility, hemocompatibility, and cells growth without any cytotoxity and inflammation [72]. In vitro and in vivo studies on stents with DLC films has confirmed that the release of metal ions (Ni, Cr, Mo, and Mn) from the stents in contact with human plasma for 4 days was suppressed by the DLC coating [73,74]. In spite of several successful applications of DLC, there are some reports of failure of DLC coating in orthopedic implants [75,76]. A clinical test reported that the failure rate of the DLC-coated Ti-6Al-4V femoral head is much higher than the alumina femoral head because of the instability of DLC in aqueous environments caused by delamination or spallation [75].

10.3 Antibacterial coatings

Biomaterials-associated infections are one of the most common postoperative complications in health care environments. These infections may lead to a variety of complications such as chronic inflammation and implant failure, to delay in wound healing and proper tissue union, or even death [77]. Annually, about 750,000 surgical site infections arise in the United States that cost more than $1.6 billion in extra hospital charge and more than 3.7 million extra hospital days [78]. Cure of these infections is usually achieved by removal of the implant, debridement of all infected tissue, and long-term antibiotic drug therapy [79]. Several strategies have been developed to lower the risk of the infections after implant surgery including progressing in operating standards, minimizing the possibility of contamination during surgery, routine antimicrobial prophylaxis, and use of antimicrobial coatings [80]. The biomaterials-associated infections are very recalcitrant to treatment with antibiotics. Once the biomaterials are implanted in the body there will be a race between the bacteria and the host cells. If the bacteria win the race, they adhere to the surface of biomaterials and produce extracellular polysaccharide, resulting in the formation of a biofilm [81].

Bacteria cells in biofilms are up to 1000-fold more resistant to antimicrobial agents as compared with planktonic bacteria [82]. Biofilms may form on a wide variety of surfaces from water pipes and natural aquatic systems to medical devices and implants. Various kind of implants such as venous catheters, heart valves, stents, neurosurgical ventricular shunts, implantable neurologic stimulators, arthroprostheses, fracture fixation devices, breast implants, intraocular lenses, bone and dental implants are prone to be infected [83].

Current research studies are centered on strategies to prevent infections at the site of the implants by disrupting the ability of microorganisms to colonize on the surface of the biomaterials, as well as to prevent their propagation in the space surrounding the implant. Physiochemical modifications of implant surfaces, decorating the implant surfaces with antimicrobial agents such as Ag NPs or antibiotic drugs are some ways to inhibit the bacterial adhesion [84,85]. The following sections highlight some of the most recent progress at antibacterial nanostructured coatings to decrease and prevent the bacterial infection of biomaterials.

10.3.1 Antibiotic-releasing coatings

Local and controlled release of antimicrobial agents directly at the implant site may represent an effective approach to treat biomaterials-associated infections. The local release of antimicrobial agents provides a high concentration of the therapeutics at or near the desired target tissue, which reduces systemic side effects [86]. Recent studies have shown the effectiveness of local drug delivery to prevent bone infections and/or promote osteointegration [87,88]. The antibiotic-releasing coatings can act as reservoir for the antibiotic drugs and allow drug release during the implantation time or for a special period of time inside the body. In order to achieve an optimal effect of the drugs, many parameters such as physicochemical nature of the used coating material and the drug, porosity, thickness, and preparation method should be taken into consideration. Moreover, molecular weight and drug solubility in water as well as drug/coating affinity and interaction can influence the drug release behavior from the coatings. In a recent study, Ordikhani et al. [89] have utilized chitosan as a biodegradable carrier and vancomycin as an antibiotic drug model to modify the surface of bone implants. In vitro antibacterial assay against Gram-positive *Staphylococcus aureus* bacteria determined the effect of vancomycin release on preventing bacterial adhesion and reduction of infection risk. To enhance the bone-bioactivity and drug-release capacity of the coatings, BG NPs were incorporated into the chitosan–vancomycin coatings. The nanocomposite coatings exhibited high bone-bioactivity in terms of apatite-forming ability in simulated body fluid and showed better cellular affinity as compared to the chitosan coatings [90]. However, the elution kinetics of vancomycin from chitosan-bioactive glass nanocomposite coatings revealed a high initial burst release of the drug within the first elution step [90]. The burst release can be undesirable because it causes a high drug loss and adverse side effects or tissue irritation in vivo [91]. To overcome these limitations, Ordikhani et al. [92] introduced a multilayer chitosan-bioactive glass nanocomposite coating with a prolonged sustained vancomycin release for up to 6 weeks with a zero-order release kinetics (Fig. 10.1a).

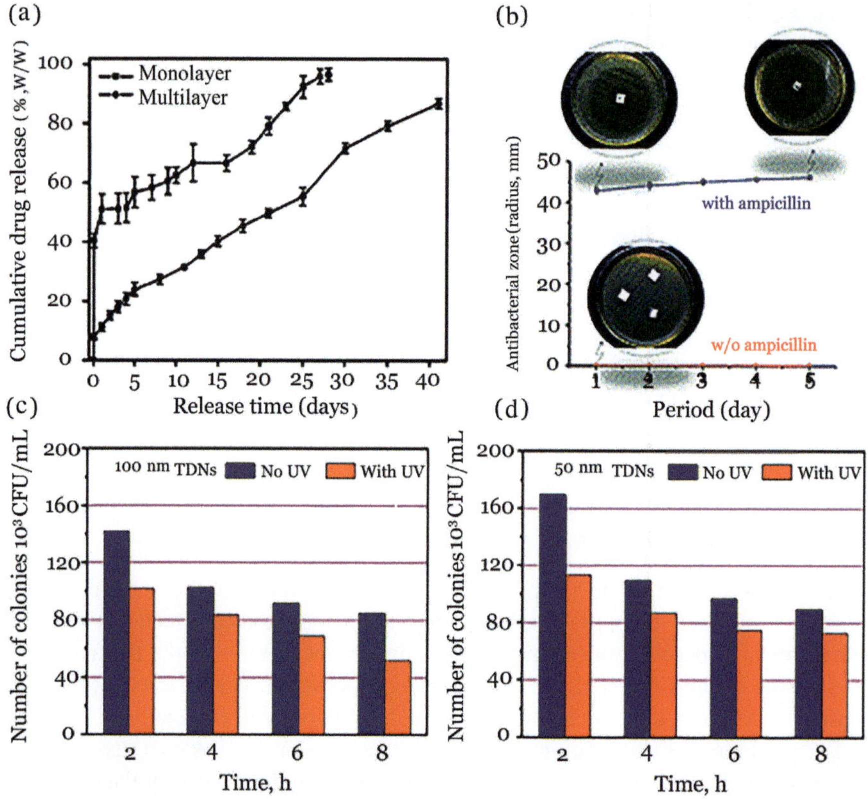

Figure 10.1 (a) Cumulative drug release in PBS solution at 37°C for multilayer nanocomposite coating as compared to monolayer nanocomposite coatings prepared from chitosan/BG suspension containing 2 mg/mL vancomycin [92]; (b) Antibacterial tests of the ampicillin-loaded BG nanoparticles coating against Streptococcus mutants using an agar diffusion plate. Antibacterial effective zone was formed around the ampicillin-loaded coating at 24 h and was maintained and even increased for up to 5 days, which was not observed in the coating without ampicillin loading, confirming the efficacy of the drug delivery through the composite coating layer [93]; Bactericidal activity of TiO_2 nanostructures with two diameters of (c) 100 nm and (d) 50 nm with and without UV irradiation [120].

Similarly, Patel et al. [93] developed chitosan-bioactive glass nanocomposite coatings containing ampicillin with a long-term drug delivery capacity over 10–11 weeks, and appropriate antibacterial effect against Streptococcus mutants (Fig. 10.1b) [93]. Chitosan matrix coatings containing graphene oxide (GO) nanosheets [94], Laponite nanolayers [95], and gelatin nanospheres [96] have also been used to locally deliver antibiotic drugs to combat implant-associated infections. Ciprofloxacin-loaded chitosan nanoparticle-based coatings on titanium implants exhibit a strong antibacterial efficacy against nosocomial strains of *S. aureus* bacteria, approximately 20 times more reduction than controls [80]. No interfering with MG63 osteoblast-like cells proliferation, adhesion, and gene expression up to 2 weeks is also noticeable [97].

Besides chitosan coatings, poly(D,L-lactide-co-glycolide acid) PLGA coatings have been utilized to temporarily and locally deliver antibiotics after implantation in the treatment of periodontal and bone infections [98]. In vitro drug release studies illustrated that the drug-loaded PLGA films were capable of effectively delivering metronidazole in a controlled way, that is 80% drug released within 2 weeks of incubation [98]. Resorbable and biocompatible thin silica hydrogels films containing vancomycin showed bactericidal properties against *S. aureus* and a great promise to prevent and treat bone infections [99].

Besides polymeric materials, nanoporous inorganic coatings on implants such as aluminum oxide [100], titanium oxide [101], and porous silica [102] can also provide sustained release of therapeutics. For example, titania nanotubes–loaded gentamicin exhibited effective results in minimizing initial bacterial adhesion with no adverse effects on adhesion, proliferation, and differentiation of osteoblast precursor cells [101]. Titania nanotubes capped with HA coating exhibited better drug-loading capacity of gentamicin (800 $\mu g/cm^2$) compared to the bare anodized substrate (660 $\mu g/cm^2$) [103]. Besides orthopedic implants, middle-ear prostheses are prone to infections, which may result in healing disorders after surgery and the extrusion of the implants. To this end, Hesse et al. [102] introduced nanoporous silica coatings as a drug delivery system for ciprofloxacin and they studied the impact of either a "slow release" or a "burst release" of ciprofloxacin in the infected middle-ear of white New Zealand rabbits. Their results showed a better outcome for animals of the burst release group [102]. The kinetics of drug release is an important issue, which influences the outcome of drug-releasing coatings. Fast release provides high doses of drugs in limited time with short-term actions, while slow release of drugs may not reach the required therapeutic level, and can cause bacterial resistance at the release site [104]. However, the high dosage of burst release may cause severe side effects inside the body.

10.3.2 Silver-release coatings

Although considerable research studies have been conducted on the efficacy of nanostructured drug-releasing coatings, clinical effectiveness of these implants is mainly dependent on the infections caused by bacteria that are sensitive to the used antibiotics in their surface modifications [105,106]. On the other hand, with the emergence of antibiotic-resistant strains of bacteria, the need for new classes of disinfection materials has increased [107]. Silver NPs are one of the most promising antimicrobial agents, which have been widely used in the formulation of many biomedical applications such as drinking water filter [108], textile fabrics [109], wound dressing [110], and implant coatings [111].

Recent studies have shown that Ag NPs can provide efficient antimicrobial properties mainly because of their high surface-to-volume area, which results in better contact with microorganisms and penetration inside them. Silver NPs interact with sulfur-containing proteins on the bacterial membrane and the phosphorus-containing compounds like DNA inside the bacteria [112]. The antibacterial properties of Ag NPs larger than 10 nm is mainly attributed to the release of silver ions (Ag^+) [113].

The mechanism of inhibitory action of Ag^+ on microorganisms is based on the loss of DNA replication ability and inactivation of cellular proteins [114].

One promising approach to provide antimicrobial coatings on the surface of biomaterials is incorporating Ag NPs into the biocompatible coatings. There are several methods to introduce silver NPs into the coatings, such as sol–gel [115], layer-by-layer assembly [116], electrophoretic deposition [117], and arc plasma deposition [118]. Tian et al. [111] showed that silver nanoparticle–doped HA coatings had excellent antimicrobial activity toward both Gram-negative *Escherichia coli* and Gram-positive *S. aureus* bacteria, without impeding the human bone marrow stromal cells proliferation, attachment, and osteoinductivity [111]. Polyelectrolyte-silver nanocomposite coatings containing polyethyleneimine as polycations, poly(sodium 4-styrenesulfonate) as polyanions and negatively charged Ag NPs exhibited strong antimicrobial effects against three Gram-negative bacterial strains with strong adhesive properties including *E. coli, Aeromonas hydrophila, and Asaia lannenesis* [116]. The antibacterial activity and cytotoxicity of silver-containing coatings are directly proportional to the silver content embedded in the matrix. For example, by increasing the amount of silver ions the bioactivity and biocompatibility of the calcium silicate glasses–based coatings decreased, while the antibacterial activity of the films against the *S. aureus* increased [119].

The antibacterial potency of Ag NPs can be enhanced in combination with titanium dioxide nanotube arrays, owing to electrical coupling between Ag NPs and TiO_2 nanotubes and improved hydrophobicity of the coating [120]. In a recent study, Jia et al. [121] developed hierarchical TiO_2/Ag coating with a sustained release of Ag^+ up to 4 weeks. The resultant coatings showed "trap-killing" antimicrobial potency without negatively affecting cell functions of osteoblast-like MG-63 in vitro or causing serious inflammatory response in a rabbit model in vivo [121]. Ultraviolet (UV) irradiation also enhances the antibacterial efficacy of TiO_2 coatings, as Esfandiari et al. [120] have shown; a decrease in the number of bacteria colonies upon UV radiation for two different sizes of TiO_2 nanotubes (100 nm and 50 nm) have been demonstrated (Figs. 10.1c and 10.1d).

PEEK coating containing BG and Ag NPs show antibacterial properties as well as better cell attachment and spreading behavior in in vitro experiments using *E. coli* bacteria and MG-63 osteoblast-like cells, respectively [117]. Composite orthopedic coatings containing chitosan/BG/Ag NPs deposited on the surface of stainless steel support proliferation of MG-63 osteoblast-like cells up to 7 days of culture [122]. The low released concentration of Ag^+ ions (<2.5 ppm) is efficiently inhibit activity of *Staphyloccocus aureus* up to 10 days [122].

Silver NPs are mostly made by physical and chemical methods that can be accompanied with toxic substances to be absorbed onto their surfaces [123]. Green synthesis of Ag NPs, as a safe, cost-effective, and ecofriendly method [124], does not require elaborate processes such as multiple purification steps and microbial culture maintenance [125]. Ciobanu et al. [126] deposited HA-Ag NP layers on porous polyurethane scaffold through HA biomimetic deposition combined with silver ions reduction from $AgNO_3$ solution [126]. Their results showed that by deposition of Ag NPs on the surface of HA/polyurethane scaffold, the antimicrobial activity against either *E. coli* or *S. aureus* bacteria has attained high values, up to 94.3% and 92.5% respectively [126]. Mishra et al.

[127] synthesized monodispersed and crystalline PVA-capped Ag NPs through a green facile microwave irradiating approach. They incorporated the PVA-capped Ag NPs in chitosan matrix and deposited on the surface of titanium substrates by "spread casting" followed by solvent evaporation. In vitro bactericidal activity against *E. coli* and *S. aureus* showed that the resultant coatings kept their antimicrobial activity for 8h due to the slow sustained release of silver ions [127]. Starch-capped Ag NPs incorporated into nanoporous silica coatings on titanium surface also exhibited strong antibacterial properties. The resultant coatings not only killed the adherent bacteria but also decreased the extent of biofilm formation by more than 70% compared to the control [128].

Animal studies have determined promising achievements by the incorporation of Ag NPs into the coatings. Secinti et al. [129] demonstrated the effect of Ag NPs coated on screws in bacteria-infected rabbits. They observed that biofilm formation was inhibited on all silver-coated screws, but all uncoated screws developed a biofilm on their surfaces [129]. Although the use of Ag NPs in biomaterials' coatings has shown a great promise in lowering the risk of infections in vitro and in animal models, this area needs more research, especially to reveal the potential adverse effects of circulating the NPs in human body.

In addition to Ag NPs, other nanoparticles such as zinc oxide, tungsten oxide, titanium dioxide, copper oxide, and magnesium oxide have shown reasonable antibacterial and antibiofilm properties [130,131]. Memarzadeh et al. [130] studied the minimum inhibitory concentration (MIC) and minimum bactericidal concentration (MBC) values of zinc oxide and tungsten oxide nanoparticulate coating against *S. aureus*, *E. coli*, *Staphylococcus epidermidis*, and *Pseudomonas aeruginosa* bacteria. Their findings showed that 2500μg/mL or above of the oxides were required to kill the species of bacteria tested. They also observed that while tungsten oxide was more effective in suspension using growth inhibition tests, the coated samples with zinc oxide was more bactericidal. Abdulkareem et al. [131] studied bactericidal potential of nanoparticulate coatings based on zinc oxide, HA, and a combination of both deposited on the surface of titanium substrates. A better antibacterial activity of ZnO NPs and the zinc oxide/HA composite coatings compared with pristine HA and the uncoated titanium surface was shown [131].

10.3.3 Other antimicrobial coatings

Apart from antibacterial release coatings, bacterial antiadhesive nanostructured coatings have been gained considerable research interests in biomaterial applications and health care environment. The surface characteristics of biomaterials such as topography, roughness, chemistry, hydrophilicity, surface charge, and energy play important roles on protein absorption and subsequently bacterial adhesion and biofilm formation [132]. Thereby, by manipulating the surface properties of biomaterials such as coating with bactericidal materials, a new class of antibiofilm-formation coatings without the use of antibiotic drugs or Ag NPs have been introduced. For example, nanostructured noble metal coating consisting of palladium, gold, and silver showed appropriate antiadhesive properties against *S. aureus* bacteria in vitro, without impeding osseointegration in vivo [133].

Nanostructured silica–copper films also showed potential applications for the reduction of microbial environmental contaminations [134]. Chitosan polymeric coatings have exhibited strong antimicrobial properties [135]. The antimicrobial mechanism of chitosan is mostly attributed to the interactions between charged amino-groups of chitosan with anionic groups on the bacteria cell walls, which enhance the cell-wall permeability and consequently causing osmotic imbalances and intracellular protein leakage [136]. Another proposed mechanism is to subdue bacterial growth by inhibiting enzymes via chelating transition metal ions [136,137]. The incorporating of GO nanosheets [94] could increase bactericidal capacity of chitosan coatings due to both membrane and oxidative stress as well as the direct contact of the sharp edges of the GO sheets with bacterial cell membranes [138]. Santos et al. [139] observed that the antimicrobial activity of a nanocomposite film containing poly-N-vinyl carbazole polymer containing GO was 90% more effective in preventing bacterial colonization relative to the unmodified surface.

Recent researches have shown that while antiadhesive nanostructured coatings are more biocompatible, active release therapeutic agents are more effective in the prevention of bacteria adhesion and biofilm formation [140]. However, toxicity issues and the emergence of microbial resistance compromise their applications; hence, there is an urgent need for translational science of these strategies. Close collaboration should be between the materials scientists, biologists, and clinicians in the development of nanostructured antimicrobial coatings to successfully combat biomaterial-associated infections.

10.4 Conclusion and future directions

When biomedical devices and implants come in contact with physiological environment, bioactivity, biocompatibility, and degradation are strongly dependent on their interactions with the surrounding tissues. Therefore, surface modifications of implants and medical devices to make them as compatible as with the body are very important and crucial. Many studies have determined that cell responses to surfaces with nanostructured features are different to microtextured surfaces due to the specific surface area, surface energy, roughness, and hydrophilic properties of nanotextured surfaces. The contents of this chapter propose a good opportunity to researchers from academia and industry to discuss the achievements in this field and outline future directions in terms of technological developments and product commercialization in the fields of biomedical devices.

References

[1] Khan W, Muntimadugu E, Jaffe M, Domb AJ. Implantable medical devices. Focal Controlled Drug Delivery 2014;33–59.

[2] Tang L, Jennings TA, Eaton JW. Mast cells mediate acute inflammatory responses to implanted biomaterials. Proceedings of the National Academy of Sciences 1998;95(15):8841–6.

[3] Song Z, Borgwardt L, Høiby N, Wu H, Sørensen TS, Borgwardt A. Prosthesis infections after orthopedic joint replacement: the possible role of bacterial biofilms. Orthopedic reviews 2013;5(2).

[4] Zhang BG, Myers DE, Wallace GG, Brandt M, Choong PF. Bioactive coatings for orthopaedic implants—recent trends in development of implant coatings. International journal of molecular sciences 2014;15(7):11878–921.

[5] Ikada Y. Surface modification of polymers for medical applications. Biomaterials 1994;15(10):725–36.

[6] Park J, Lakes RS. Biomaterials: an introduction. : Springer Science & Business Media; 2007.

[7] Hoffmann A, Goldberg T, Tanner A. Surface cementation of stemmed tibial components in primary total knee arthroplasty. J Arthroplastv 2006;21:353–7.

[8] Hench LL. Biomaterials: a forecast for the future. Biomaterials 1998;19(16):1419–23.

[9] Hench LL. The story of Bioglass®. Journal of Materials Science: Materials in Medicine 2006;17(11):967–78.

[10] Adiga SP, Jin C, Curtiss LA, Monteiro-Riviere NA, Narayan RJ. Nanoporous membranes for medical and biological applications. Wiley Interdisciplinary Reviews: Nanomedicine and Nanobiotechnology 2009;1(5):568–81.

[11] Hench LL. Genetic design of bioactive glass. Journal of the European Ceramic Society 2009;29(7):1257–65.

[12] Goodfriend AC, Welch TR, Barker G, Ginther R, Riegel MS, Reddy SV, et al. Novel bioresorbable stent coating for drug release in congenital heart disease applications. J Biomed Mater Res A 2015;103(5):1761–70.

[13] Ohtsuki C, Kokubo T, Neo M, Kotani S, Yamamuro T, Nakamura T, et al. Bone-bonding mechanism of sintered β-3CaO. P 2 O 5. Phosphorus Res Bull 1991;1:191–6.

[14] Ohtsuki C., Aoki Y., Kokubo T., Fujita Y., Kotani S., Yamamuro T., editors. Bioactivity of limestone and abalone shell. Transactions of the 11th annual meeting of Japanese society for biomaterials; 1989.

[15] Mano JF, Sousa RA, Boesel LF, Neves NM, Reis RL. Bioinert, biodegradable and injectable polymeric matrix composites for hard tissue replacement: state of the art and recent developments. Composites Science and Technology 2004;64(6):789–817.

[16] Kulkarni M, Mazare A, Schmuki P, Iglic A, Seifalian A. Biomaterial surface modification of titanium and titanium alloys for medical applications. Nanomedicine 2014;111:111.

[17] Gallagher J, McGhee K, Wilkinson C, Riehle M. Interaction of animal cells with ordered nanotopography. IEEE Trans Nanobioscience 2002;1(1):24–8.

[18] Dalby M, Riehle M, Johnstone H, Affrossman S, Curtis A. Polymer-demixed nanotopography: control of fibroblast spreading and proliferation. Tiss Eng 2002;8(6):1099–108.

[19] Dalby MJ, Berry CC, Riehle MO, Sutherland DS, Agheli H, Curtis AS. Attempted endocytosis of nano-environment produced by colloidal lithography by human fibroblasts. Exp Cell Res 2004;295(2):387–94.

[20] Dalby MJ, Yarwood SJ, Johnstone HJ, Affrossman S, Riehle MO. Fibroblast signaling events in response to nanotopography: a gene array study. IEEE Trans Nanobioscience 2002;1(1):12–17.

[21] Dalby MJ, Yarwood SJ, Riehle MO, Johnstone HJ, Affrossman S, Curtis AS. Increasing fibroblast response to materials using nanotopography: morphological and genetic measurements of cell response to 13-nm-high polymer demixed islands. Exp Cell Res 2002;276(1):1–9.

[22] Webster TJ, Ergun C, Doremus RH, Siegel RW, Bizios R. Enhanced osteoclast-like cell functions on nanophase ceramics. Biomaterials 2001;22(11):1327–33.

[23] Dalby M, Riehle M, Johnstone H, Affrossman S, Curtis A. In vitro reaction of endothelial cells to polymer demixed nanotopography. Biomaterials 2002;23(14):2945–54.
[24] Andersson A-S, Brink J, Lidberg U, Sutherland DS. Influence of systematically varied nanoscale topography on the morphology of epithelial cells. IEEE Trans Nanobioscience 2003;2(2):49–57.
[25] Oshida Y, Guven Y. 10 - Biocompatible coatings for metallic biomaterials A2 - Wen, Cuie Surface Coating and Modification of Metallic Biomaterials. : Woodhead Publishing; 2015; p. 287–343.
[26] Imai Y, Nose Y. A new method for evalution of antithrombogenicity of materials. J Biomed Mater Res 1972;6(3):165–72.
[27] Mosmann T. Rapid colorimetric assay for cellular growth and survival: application to proliferation and cytotoxicity assays. J Immunol Methods 1983;65(1–2):55–63.
[28] Wyman P. 1 - Hydrophilic coatings for biomedical applications in and ex vivo A2 - Driver, Mike Coatings for Biomedical Applications. : Woodhead Publishing; 2012; p. 3–42.
[29] Estelrich J, Sánchez-Martín MJ, Busquets MA. Nanoparticles in magnetic resonance imaging: from simple to dual contrast agents. Int J Nanomedicine 2015;10:1727.
[30] Lee HJ, Koo AN, Lee SW, Lee MH, Lee SC. Catechol-functionalized adhesive polymer nanoparticles for controlled local release of bone morphogenetic protein-2 from titanium surface. Journal of Controlled Release 2013;170(2):198–208.
[31] Gamucci O, Bertero A, Gagliardi M, Bardi G. Biomedical nanoparticles: overview of their surface immune-compatibility. Coatings 2014;4(1):139–59.
[32] Ma R. Nanocomposite Coatings for Biomedical Applications. 2010.
[33] Zafar M, Najeeb S, Khurshid Z, Vazirzadeh M, Zohaib S, Najeeb B, et al. Potential of electrospun nanofibers for biomedical and dental applications. Materials 2016;9(2):73.
[34] Liu X, Lin T, Fang J, Yao G, Zhao H, Dodson M, et al. In vivo wound healing and antibacterial performances of electrospun nanofibre membranes. J Biomed Mater Res A 2010;94(2):499–508.
[35] Kim J-J, Bae W-J, Kim J-M, Kim J-J, Lee E-J, Kim H-W, et al. Mineralized polycaprolactone nanofibrous matrix for odontogenesis of human dental pulp cells. J Biomater Appl 2013 0885328213495903.
[36] Hui Z, Feng L, Hong W, Jian-feng S, Guo-zhou R, Ang L, et al. Preliminary study of the dual release baicalin and rhBMP-2 system to improve periodontal tissue regeneration in minipigs. Shanghai Journal of Stomatology 2013;22(2).
[37] Johansson P, Jimbo R, Kozai Y, Sakurai T, Kjellin P, Currie F, et al. Nanosized hydroxyapatite coating on PEEK implants enhances early bone formation: A histological and three-dimensional investigation in rabbit bone. Materials 2015;8(7):3815–30.
[38] Mohandes F, Salavati-Niasari M. Influence of morphology on the in vitro bioactivity of hydroxyapatite nanostructures prepared by precipitation method. New Journal of Chemistry 2014;38(9):4501–9.
[39] Jiang P, Liang J, Song R, Zhang Y, Ren L, Zhang L, et al. Effect of Octacalcium-Phosphate-Modified Micro/Nanostructured Titania Surfaces on Osteoblast Response. ACS applied materials & interfaces 2015;7(26):14384–96.
[40] Shadanbaz S, Dias GJ. Calcium phosphate coatings on magnesium alloys for biomedical applications: a review. Acta Biomater 2012;8(1):20–30.
[41] Kumar M, Dasarathy H, Riley C. Electrodeposition of brushite coatings and their transformation to hydroxyapatite in aqueous solutions. J Biomed Mater Res 1999;45(4):302–10.
[42] Bakhsheshi-Rad HR, Idris MH, Abdul-Kadir MR. Synthesis and in vitro degradation evaluation of the nano-HA/MgF2 and DCPD/MgF2 composite coating on biodegradable Mg–Ca–Zn alloy. Surface and Coatings Technology 2013;222:79–89.

[43] Khairoun I, Magne D, Gauthier O, Bouler J-M, Aguado E, Daculsi G, et al. In vitro characterization and in vivo properties of a carbonated apatite bone cement. J Biomed Mater Res 2002;60(4):633–42.
[44] Xu HH, Weir MD, Sun L. Nanocomposites with Ca and PO 4 release: effects of reinforcement, dicalcium phosphate particle size and silanization. Dental materials 2007;23(12):1482–91.
[45] Wang H, Lin CJ, Hu R, Zhang F, Lin LW. A novel nano-micro structured octacalcium phosphate/protein composite coating on titanium by using an electrochemically induced deposition. J Biomed Mater Res A 2008;87(3):698–705.
[46] Yamada S, Heymann D, Bouler J-M, Daculsi G. Osteoclastic resorption of calcium phosphate ceramics with different hydroxyapatite/β-tricalcium phosphate ratios. Biomaterials 1997;18(15):1037–41.
[47] Tanzer M, Kantor S, Rosenthall L, Bobyn JD. Femoral remodeling after porous-coated total hip arthroplasty with and without hydroxyapatite-tricalcium phosphate coating: a prospective randomized trial. J Arthroplasty 2001;16(5):552–8.
[48] Roy M, Krishna BV, Bandyopadhyay A, Bose S. Laser processing of bioactive tricalcium phosphate coating on titanium for load-bearing implants. Acta Biomater 2008;4(2): 324–33.
[49] Luginbuehl V, Ruffieux K, Hess C, Reichardt D, Von Rechenberg B, Nuss K. Controlled release of tetracycline from biodegradable β-tricalcium phosphate composites. J Biomed Mater Res Part B Appl Biomater 2010;92(2):341–52.
[50] Ibara A, Miyaji H, Fugetsu B, Nishida E, Takita H, Tanaka S, et al. Osteoconductivity and biodegradability of collagen scaffold coated with nano-β-TCP and fibroblast growth factor 2. Journal of Nanomaterials 2013;2013:46.
[51] Boskey AL. Mineralization of Bones and Teeth. Elements 2007;3(6):385–91.
[52] Mohandes F, Salavati-Niasari M, Fereshteh Z, Fathi M. Novel preparation of hydroxyapatite nanoparticles and nanorods with the aid of complexing agents. Ceramics International 2014;40(8, Part A):12227–33.
[53] Johansson LA, Isaksson S, Adolfsson E, Lindh C, Sennerby L. Bone regeneration using a hollow hydroxyapatite space-maintaining device for maxillary sinus floor augmentation--a clinical pilot study. Clin Implant Dent Relat Res 2012;14(4):575–84.
[54] Oonishi H, Hench LL, Wilson J, Sugihara F, Tsuji E, Kushitani S, et al. Comparative bone growth behavior in granules of bioceramic materials of various sizes. J Biomed Mater Res 1999;44(1):31–43.
[55] Zhao S-F, Dong W-J, Jiang Q-H, He F-M, Wang X-X, Yang G-L. Effects of zinc-substituted nano-hydroxyapatite coatings on bone integration with implant surfaces. J Zhejiang Univ Sci B 2013;14(6):518–25.
[56] Jafari H, Hessam H, Shahri SMG, Assadian M, Shairazifard SHP, Idris MH. Characterizing Sintered Nano-Hydroxyapatite Sol-Gel Coating Deposited on a Biomedical Ti-Zr-Nb Alloy. Journal of Materials Engineering and Performance 2016;25(3):901–9.
[57] Surmeneva M., Surmenev R., Pichugin V., Ivanova A., Grubova I., Chaikina M., et al., editors. Biocompatible nanostructured coatings based on calcium phosphates prepared by means of rf-magnetron sputtering deposition. Strategic Technology (IFOST), 2012 7th International Forum on; 2012: IEEE.
[58] Mohandes F, Salavati-Niasari M. Freeze-drying synthesis, characterization and in vitro bioactivity of chitosan/graphene oxide/hydroxyapatite nanocomposite. RSC Advances 2014;4(49):25993–6001.
[59] Mohandes F, Salavati-Niasari M. In vitro comparative study of pure hydroxyapatite nanorods and novel polyethylene glycol/graphene oxide/hydroxyapatite nanocomposite. Journal of Nanoparticle Research 2014;16(9):1–12.

[60] Zhang B, Kwok CT, Cheng FT, Man HC. Fabrication of nano-structured HA/CNT coatings on Ti6Al4V by electrophoretic deposition for biomedical applications. J Nanosci Nanotechnol 2011;11(12):10740–5.
[61] Janković A, Eraković S, Mitrić M, Matić IZ, Juranić ZD, Tsui GCP, et al. Bioactive hydroxyapatite/graphene composite coating and its corrosion stability in simulated body fluid. Journal of Alloys and Compounds 2015;624:148–57.
[62] Sola A, Bellucci D, Cannillo V, Cattini A. Bioactive glass coatings: a review. Surface Engineering 2011;27(8):560–72.
[63] Kokubo T. Bioactive glass ceramics: properties and applications. Biomaterials 1991;12(2):155–63.
[64] Gerhardt L-C, Boccaccini AR. Bioactive glass and glass-ceramic scaffolds for bone tissue engineering. Materials 2010;3(7):3867–910.
[65] Roohani-Esfahani S, Nouri-Khorasani S, Lu Z, Appleyard R, Zreiqat H. Effects of bioactive glass nanoparticles on the mechanical and biological behavior of composite coated scaffolds. Acta Biomater 2011;7(3):1307–18.
[66] Esfahani SIR, Tavangarian F, Emadi R. Nanostructured bioactive glass coating on porous hydroxyapatite scaffold for strength enhancement. Materials Letters 2008;62(19):3428–30.
[67] Rego SJ, Vale AC, Luz GM, Mano JF, Alves NM. Adhesive Bioactive Coatings Inspired by Sea Life. Langmuir 2016;32(2):560–8.
[68] Dobrovolskaia MA, McNeil SE. Handbook of immunological properties of engineered nanomaterials. : World Scientific; 2013.
[69] Napierska D, Quarck R, Thomassen LC, Lison D, Martens JA, Delcroix M, et al. Amorphous Silica Nanoparticles Promote Monocyte Adhesion to Human Endothelial Cells: Size-Dependent Effect. Small 2013;9(3):430–8.
[70] Gangopadhyay P, Gallet S, Franz E, Persoons A, Verbiest T. Novel superparamagnetic core (shell) nanoparticles for magnetic targeted drug delivery and hyperthermia treatment. IEEE Trans Magn 2005;41(10):4194–6.
[71] Hashimoto M, Toshima H, Yonezawa T, Kawai K, Narushima T, Kaga M, et al. Responses of RAW264. 7 macrophages to water-dispersible gold and silver nanoparticles stabilized by metal–carbon σ-bonds. J Biomed Mater Res A 2014;102(6):1838–49.
[72] Cui FZ, Li DJ. A review of investigations on biocompatibility of diamond-like carbon and carbon nitride films. Surface and Coatings Technology 2000;131(1–3):481–7.
[73] Laube N, Kleinen L, Bradenahl J, Meissner A. Diamond-like carbon coatings on ureteral stents—a new strategy for decreasing the formation of crystalline bacterial biofilms? J Urol 2007;177(5):1923–7.
[74] Gutensohn K, Beythien C, Bau J, Fenner T, Grewe P, Koester R, et al. In Vitro Analyses of Diamond-like Carbon Coated Stents: Reduction of Metal Ion Release, Platelet Activation, and Thrombogenicity. Thromb Res 2000;99(6):577–85.
[75] Affatato S, Frigo M, Toni A. An in vitro investigation of diamond-like carbon as a femoral head coating. J Biomed Mater Res 2000;53(3):221–6.
[76] Roy RK, Lee KR. Biomedical applications of diamond-like carbon coatings: A review. J Biomed Mater Res Part B Appl Biomater 2007;83(1):72–84.
[77] Vester H, Wildemann B, Schmidmaier G, Stöckle U, Lucke M. Gentamycin delivered from a PDLLA coating of metallic implants: In vivo and in vitro characterisation for local prophylaxis of implant-related osteomyelitis. Injury 2010;41(10):1053–9.
[78] Edmiston CE, Spencer M, Lewis BD, Brown KR, Rossi PJ, Henen CR, et al. Reducing the Risk of Surgical Site Infections: Did We Really Think SCIP Was Going to Lead Us to the Promised Land? Surg Infect (Larchmt) 2011;12(3):169–77.

[79] Widmer AF. New Developments in Diagnosis and Treatment of Infection in Orthopedic Implants. Clinical Infectious Diseases 2001;33(Supplement 2):S94–S106.
[80] Campoccia D, Montanaro L, Arciola CR. The significance of infection related to orthopedic devices and issues of antibiotic resistance. Biomaterials 2006;27(11):2331–9.
[81] Donlan RM. Biofilm Formation: A Clinically Relevant Microbiological Process. Clinical Infectious Diseases 2001;33(8):1387–92.
[82] Feng G, Cheng Y, Wang S-Y, Borca-Tasciuc DA, Worobo RW, Moraru CI. Bacterial attachment and biofilm formation on surfaces are reduced by small-diameter nanoscale pores: how small is small enough? Npj Biofilms And Microbiomes 2015;1:15022.
[83] Subramani K, Jung RE, Molenberg A, Hammerle CHF. Biofilm on dental implants: a review of the literature. Int J Oral Maxillofac Implants 2009;24(4):616–26.
[84] Liu X, Chu PK, Ding C. Surface modification of titanium, titanium alloys, and related materials for biomedical applications. Materials Science and Engineering: R: Reports 2004;47(3–4):49–121.
[85] Goodman SB, Yao Z, Keeney M, Yang F. The future of biologic coatings for orthopaedic implants. Biomaterials 2013;34(13):3174–83.
[86] Hirabayashi H, Fujisaki J. Bone-Specific Drug Delivery Systems. Clin Pharmacokinet 2003;42(15):1319–30.
[87] Raphel J., Holodniy M., Goodman S.B., Heilshorn S.C. Multifunctional coatings to simultaneously promote osseointegration and prevent infection of orthopaedic implants. Biomaterials. 84:301–314.
[88] Mazaheri M, Eslahi N, Ordikhani F, Tamjid E, Simchi A. Nanomedicine applications in orthopedic medicine: state of the art. Int J Nanomedicine 2015;10:6039–54.
[89] Ordikhani F, Tamjid E, Simchi A. Characterization and antibacterial performance of electrodeposited chitosan–vancomycin composite coatings for prevention of implant-associated infections. Materials Science and Engineering: C 2014;41:240–8.
[90] Ordikhani F, Simchi A. Long-term antibiotic delivery by chitosan-based composite coatings with bone regenerative potential. Appl Surf Sci 2014;317:56–66.
[91] Hezaveh H, Muhamad II. Controlled drug release via minimization of burst release in pH-response kappa-carrageenan/polyvinyl alcohol hydrogels. Chemical Engineering Research and Design 2013;91(3):508–19.
[92] Ordikhani F, Zustiak SP, Simchi A. Surface Modifications of Titanium Implants by Multilayer Bioactive Coatings with Drug Delivery Potential: Antimicrobial, Biological, and Drug Release Studies. JOM 2016;68(4):1100–8.
[93] Patel KD, El-Fiqi A, Lee H-Y, Singh RK, Kim D-A, Lee H-H, et al. Chitosan-nanobioactive glass electrophoretic coatings with bone regenerative and drug delivering potential. J Mater Chem 2012;22(47):24945–56.
[94] Ordikhani F, Ramezani Farani M, Dehghani M, Tamjid E, Simchi A. Physicochemical and biological properties of electrodeposited graphene oxide/chitosan films with drug-eluting capacity. Carbon N Y 2015;84:91–102.
[95] Ordikhani F, Dehghani M, Simchi A. Antibiotic-loaded chitosan–Laponite films for local drug delivery by titanium implants: cell proliferation and drug release studies. Journal of Materials Science: Materials in Medicine 2015;26(12):1–12.
[96] Song J, Chen Q, Zhang Y, Diba M, Kolwijck E, Shao J, et al. Electrophoretic Deposition of Chitosan Coatings Modified with Gelatin Nanospheres To Tune the Release of Antibiotics. ACS Applied Materials & Interfaces 2016.
[97] Mattioli-Belmonte M, Cometa S, Ferretti C, Iatta R, Trapani A, Ceci E, et al. Characterization and cytocompatibility of an antibiotic/chitosan/cyclodextrins nanocoating on titanium implants. Carbohydrate Polymers 2014;110:173–82.

[98] Gentile P, Frongia ME, Cardellach M, Miller CA, Stafford GP, Leggett GJ, et al. Functionalised nanoscale coatings using layer-by-layer assembly for imparting antibacterial properties to polylactide-co-glycolide surfaces. Acta Biomater 2015;21:35–43.

[99] Radin S, Ducheyne P. Controlled release of vancomycin from thin sol–gel films on titanium alloy fracture plate material. Biomaterials 2007;28(9):1721–9.

[100] Kang H-J, Kim DJ, Park S-J, Yoo J-B, Ryu YS. Controlled drug release using nanoporous anodic aluminum oxide on stent. Thin Solid Films 2007;515(12):5184–7.

[101] Popat KC, Eltgroth M, LaTempa TJ, Grimes CA, Desai TA. Decreased Staphylococcus epidermis adhesion and increased osteoblast functionality on antibiotic-loaded titania nanotubes. Biomaterials 2007;28(32):4880–8.

[102] Hesse D, Ehlert N, Lüenhop T, Smoczek A, Glage S, Behrens P, et al. Nanoporous Silica Coatings as a Drug Delivery System for Ciprofloxacin: Outcome of Variable Release Rates in the Infected Middle Ear of Rabbits. Otology & Neurotology 2013;34(6):1138–45.

[103] Rajesh P, Mohan N, Yokogawa Y, Varma H. Pulsed laser deposition of hydroxyapatite on nanostructured titanium towards drug eluting implants. Materials Science and Engineering: C 2013;33(5):2899–904.

[104] Vasilev K, Cook J, Griesser HJ. Antibacterial surfaces for biomedical devices. Expert Rev Med Devices 2009;6(5):553–67.

[105] Gallo J, Holinka M, Moucha CS. Antibacterial Surface Treatment for Orthopaedic Implants. International Journal of Molecular Sciences 2014;15(8):13849–80.

[106] Antoci V, King SB, Jose B, Parvizi J, Zeiger AR, Wickstrom E, et al. Vancomycin covalently bonded to titanium alloy prevents bacterial colonization. Journal of Orthopaedic Research 2007;25(7):858–66.

[107] Le Ouay B, Stellacci F. Antibacterial activity of silver nanoparticles: A surface science insight. Nano Today 2015;10(3):339–54.

[108] Jain P, Pradeep T. Potential of silver nanoparticle-coated polyurethane foam as an antibacterial water filter. Biotechnol Bioeng 2005;90(1):59–63.

[109] Durán N, Marcato PD, De Souza GIH, Alves OL, Esposito E. Antibacterial Effect of Silver Nanoparticles Produced by Fungal Process on Textile Fabrics and Their Effluent Treatment. Journal of Biomedical Nanotechnology 2007;3(2):203–8.

[110] Maneerung T, Tokura S, Rujiravanit R. Impregnation of silver nanoparticles into bacterial cellulose for antimicrobial wound dressing. Carbohydrate Polymers 2008;72(1):43–51.

[111] Tian B, Chen W, Yu D, Lei Y, Ke Q, Guo Y, et al. Fabrication of silver nanoparticle-doped hydroxyapatite coatings with oriented block arrays for enhancing bactericidal effect and osteoinductivity. J Mech Behav Biomed Mater 2016;61:345–59.

[112] Rai M, Yadav A, Gade A. Silver nanoparticles as a new generation of antimicrobials. Biotechnol Adv 2009;27(1):76–83.

[113] Durán N, Durán M, de Jesus MB, Seabra AB, Fávaro WJ, Nakazato G. Silver nanoparticles: A new view on mechanistic aspects on antimicrobial activity. Nanomedicine: Nanotechnology, Biology and Medicine 2016;12(3):789–99.

[114] Sondi I, Salopek-Sondi B. Silver nanoparticles as antimicrobial agent: a case study on E. coli as a model for Gram-negative bacteria. J Colloid Interface Sci 2004;275(1):177–82.

[115] Procaccini R, Bouchet A, Pastore JI, Studdert C, Ceré S, Pellice S. Silver-functionalized methyl-silica hybrid materials as antibacterial coatings on surgical-grade stainless steel. Prog Org Coat 2016;97:28–36.

[116] Kruk T, Szczepanowicz K, Kręgiel D, Szyk-Warszyńska L, Warszyński P. Nanostructured multilayer polyelectrolyte films with silver nanoparticles as antibacterial coatings. Colloids and Surfaces B: Biointerfaces 2016;137:158–66.

[117] Seuss S., Heinloth M., Boccaccini A.R. Development of bioactive composite coatings based on combination of PEEK, bioactive glass and Ag nanoparticles with antibacterial properties. Surface and Coatings Technology.

[118] Park S-H, Kim SH, Park S-J, Ryoo S, Woo K, Lee JS, et al. Direct incorporation of silver nanoparticles onto thin-film composite membranes via arc plasma deposition for enhanced antibacterial and permeation performance. J Memb Sci 2016;513:226–35.

[119] Catauro M, Bollino F, Papale F, Vecchio Ciprioti S. Investigation on bioactivity, biocompatibility, thermal behavior and antibacterial properties of calcium silicate glass coatings containing Ag. Journal of Non-Crystalline Solids 2015;422:16–22.

[120] Esfandiari N, Simchi A, Bagheri R. Size tuning of Ag-decorated TiO2 nanotube arrays for improved bactericidal capacity of orthopedic implants. J Biomed Mater Res A 2014;102(8):2625–35.

[121] Jia Z, Xiu P, Li M, Xu X, Shi Y, Cheng Y, et al. Bioinspired anchoring AgNPs onto micro-nanoporous TiO2 orthopedic coatings: Trap-killing of bacteria, surface-regulated osteoblast functions and host responses. Biomaterials 2016;75:203–22.

[122] Pishbin F, Mouriño V, Gilchrist JB, McComb DW, Kreppel S, Salih V, et al. Single-step electrochemical deposition of antimicrobial orthopaedic coatings based on a bioactive glass/chitosan/nano-silver composite system. Acta Biomater 2013;9(7):7469–79.

[123] Prabhu S, Poulose E. Silver nanoparticles: mechanism of antimicrobial action, synthesis, medical applications, and toxicity effects. International Nano Letters C7 - 32 2012;2(1):1–10.

[124] Jeyaraj M, Rajesh M, Arun R, MubarakAli D, Sathishkumar G, Sivanandhan G, et al. An investigation on the cytotoxicity and caspase-mediated apoptotic effect of biologically synthesized silver nanoparticles using Podophyllum hexandrum on human cervical carcinoma cells. Colloids and Surfaces B: Biointerfaces 2013;102:708–17.

[125] Jeyaraj M, Sathishkumar G, Sivanandhan G, MubarakAli D, Rajesh M, Arun R, et al. Biogenic silver nanoparticles for cancer treatment: An experimental report. Colloids and Surfaces B: Biointerfaces 2013;106:86–92.

[126] Ciobanu G, Ilisei S, Luca C. Hydroxyapatite-silver nanoparticles coatings on porous polyurethane scaffold. Materials Science and Engineering: C 2014;35:36–42.

[127] Mishra SK, Ferreira JMF, Kannan S. Mechanically stable antimicrobial chitosan–PVA–silver nanocomposite coatings deposited on titanium implants. Carbohydrate Polymers 2015;121:37–48.

[128] Massa MA, Covarrubias C, Bittner M, Fuentevilla IA, Capetillo P, Von Marttens A, et al. Synthesis of new antibacterial composite coating for titanium based on highly ordered nanoporous silica and silver nanoparticles. Materials Science and Engineering: C 2014;45:146–53.

[129] Secinti KD, Özalp H, Attar A, Sargon MF. Nanoparticle silver ion coatings inhibit biofilm formation on titanium implants. Journal of Clinical Neuroscience 2011;18(3):391–5.

[130] Memarzadeh K, Vargas M, Huang J, Fan J, Allaker RP. Nano Metallic-Oxides as Antimicrobials for Implant Coatings. Key Engineering Materials 2012;493–494:489–94.

[131] Abdulkareem EH, Memarzadeh K, Allaker RP, Huang J, Pratten J, Spratt D. Anti-biofilm activity of zinc oxide and hydroxyapatite nanoparticles as dental implant coating materials. J Dent 2015;43(12):1462–9.

[132] Zhao L, Chu PK, Zhang Y, Wu Z. Antibacterial coatings on titanium implants. J Biomed Mater Res Part B Appl Biomater 2009;91B(1):470–80.

[133] Svensson S., Suska F., Emanuelsson L., Palmquist A., Norlindh B., Trobos M., et al. Osseointegration of titanium with an antimicrobial nanostructured noble metal coating. Nanomedicine: Nanotechnology, Biology and Medicine. 9(7):1048–1056.

[134] Varghese S, ElFakhri SO, Sheel DW, Sheel P, Bolton FEJ, Foster HA. Antimicrobial activity of novel nanostructured Cu-SiO2 coatings prepared by chemical vapour deposition against hospital related pathogens. AMB Express 2013;3(1):1–8.
[135] Di Martino A, Sittinger M, Risbud MV. Chitosan: A versatile biopolymer for orthopaedic tissue-engineering. Biomaterials 2005;26(30):5983–90.
[136] Xie W, Xu P, Wang W, Liu Q. Preparation and antibacterial activity of a water-soluble chitosan derivative. Carbohydrate Polymers 2002;50(1):35–40.
[137] Sarasam A, Brown P, Khajotia S, Dmytryk J, Madihally S. Antibacterial activity of chitosan-based matrices on oral pathogens. Journal of Materials Science: Materials in Medicine 2008;19(3):1083–90.
[138] Akhavan O, Ghaderi E. Escherichia coli bacteria reduce graphene oxide to bactericidal graphene in a self-limiting manner. Carbon N Y 2012;50(5):1853–60.
[139] Santos CM, Tria MCR, Vergara RAMV, Ahmed F, Advincula RC, Rodrigues DF. Antimicrobial graphene polymer (PVK-GO) nanocomposite films. Chemical Communications 2011;47(31):8892–4.
[140] Serrano C, García-Fernández L, Fernández-Blázquez JP, Barbeck M, Ghanaati S, Unger R, et al. Nanostructured medical sutures with antibacterial properties. Biomaterials 2015;52:291–300.

Evaluation techniques

11

Serap Yesilkir-Baydar[1,*], *Olga N. Oztel*[2,*], *Rabia Cakir-Koc*[1,*] *and Ayse Candayan*[3]
[1]Yildiz Technical University, Istanbul, Turkey
[2]Liv Hospital Center for Regenerative Medicine and Stem Cell Manufacturing (LivMedCell), Istanbul, Turkey
[3]Bogazici University, Istanbul, Turkey

11.1 Introduction

Nanomaterials are small-scale (<100 nm) materials with distinct optical, magnetic, electrical, and mechanical properties generated by molecular engineering. They are thought to enhance the properties of virtually all types of materials (Royal Society, 2004), and the use of these products with distinct properties is becoming even more prominent [1]. Nanomaterials bearing these unique chemical and physical properties can be used in various application fields such as biotechnology, medicine, electronics, photonics, telecommunication, aerospace, and energy [2]. Optical, electrical, and mechanical characterization of nanomaterials is a challenging issue for researchers [3] and several different optical microscopy techniques can be used to study nanomaterials [4]. Additionally, for the use of nanomaterials in regenerative medicine studies with stem cells (SCs), phototherapy, drug/gene delivery, and imaging, the interaction of the materials with cells has to be determined [5]. Thus, this section describes physical and chemical properties of nanomaterials, techniques for characterization and in vivo and in vitro interactions of nanomaterials.

11.2 Structural characterizations using microscopy techniques

Several types of optical microscopy, scanning probe microscopy (SPM), and electron microscopy (EM) may be accounted as advanced microscopy since they can produce high-resolution images at micrometer to subnanometer scale. All of these techniques have different advantages and disadvantages in studying nanomaterials.

1. *Optical microscopy* can monitor various species with great temporal resolution, but has limited spatial resolution due to diffraction of light through the microscope and light scattering in thick samples.
2. *SPM techniques* can image samples in subnanometer resolution, but cannot track multiple materials at the same time and cannot effectively image large surfaces.

* These authors equally contributed to the chapter.

Nanobiomaterials Science, Development and Evaluation. DOI: http://dx.doi.org/10.1016/B978-0-08-100963-5.00011-2

3. *Electron microscopy techniques* can produce excellent detail at the subnanometer scale, but only conductive, dry samples are compatible with EM imaging [4].

Therefore, the choice for advanced-microscopy techniques to image a nanomaterial strictly depends on the information to be investigated and the desired resolution.

11.2.1 Optical microscopy techniques

In order to observe micron-level samples with a certain resolution, optical microscopes can be used. Advanced magnification is not possible in optical microscopes due to limitations in light wavelength. Therefore, to observe submicron size samples, more advanced imaging techniques such as SEM, TEM, and AFM have been developed.

11.2.2 Scanning probe microscopy techniques

SPM is a group of techniques used in the characterization of nanostructures with atomic or subatomic resolution spatially that includes atomic force microscopy (AFM) and scanning tunneling microscopy (STM) [6–10]. By bringing a small sample probe into close proximity with the sample, SPM measures the interaction between these and an image is then generated by scanning the tip of the probe and collecting data pixel by pixel, which can be constructed as a three-dimensional (3D) display. SPM techniques are very useful in direct characterization of the surface of materials with high spatial resolution without a laborious specimen preparation process. They allow nanoscale observation and thus are best for characterization of nanomaterial structure [11].

11.2.3 Atomic force microscopy

AFM is an SPM technique with high resolution that is used for real-time imaging and ability to monitor surface topography at nanoscale. It is possible to investigate electronic structure and chemical bonding of atoms and molecules using AFM. This technique utilizes a sharp tip located at the end of a microcantilever and recognizes the interaction between this tip and the sample surface [12]. The radius of the tip ranges between a few angstroms with carbon nanotube (CNT) tips to a few nanometers with silicon-based tips and recognizes a potential resulting from van der Waals, chemical, electrostatic, capillary, and magnetic force interactions with the surface that changes with distance from the surface [13]. When the tip is brought closer to the sample, the cantilever is deflected due to increase in intermolecular forces. This deflection can be tracked using the laser displacement that is reflected off the cantilever and can be imaged onto a photodiode array. The resolution is dependent on the size of the tip and reaches 0.1 nm in vertical and 0.5 nm in lateral directions under optimal conditions [12].

AFM scanning is performed either by contact or tapping. When imaging is performed when the tip is in contact with the sample, the overall force is repulsive and this type is called static or contact mode of AFM. Tapping mode is performed by oscillating the cantilever at its resonant frequency with limited interaction between the tip and the specimen. The surface properties are determined by the change in the amplitude, phase, and frequency of the oscillations according to the tip–sample interactions. Amplitude modulation is the most common use in the noncontact mode where changes in the amplitude and phase of the oscillations provide the information for imaging [14]. Changes in amplitude provide information about the surface topography, while changes in phase discriminate between different types of materials. Therefore, surface topography, adhesion forces, viscosity, and rigidity can be investigated using noncontact AFM [15]. Another application of AFM is scanning force microscopy that enables nanomechanical studies by measuring magnetic, frictional, molecular, and electrostatic interaction forces. AFM is a more useful method for nonconductive nanomaterials [16,17].

11.2.4 Scanning tunneling microscopy

Another influential SPM technique is STM [18], which is based on monitoring the tunneling current between a sharp metal tip and the sample. Unlike AFM, STM tip does not usually touch the surface of the specimen, but a voltage between a few millivolts and a few volts is applied between the tip and the specimen and the tunneling current is measured. When the tip touches the surface of the specimen, the voltage will end up in an electrical current, but when the tip is further away, the system is an open circuit and the current will be zero. In fact, the distances between the tip and the surface of the specimen is extremely small, about only 0.5 to 1.0 nm, or only a few atomic diameters long, and electrons can tunnel between the tip and the surface creating a tunneling current. This current strictly depends on the distance between the tip and the surface. The distance between the tip and the surface of the specimen is controlled with a piezoelectric element attached to the STM tip and an electrical voltage. This voltage is adjusted to hold the tunneling current constant in the z direction, thus keeping the distance between the surface of the specimen and the tip constant using feedback electronics [19]. STM is useful for detecting and characterizing conductive samples such as CNTs and graphine layer. The instrument can also be used to move single nanotubes, molecules, and metal ions on smooth surfaces with great precision [20].

11.2.5 Electron microscopy techniques

EM is highly capable of analyzing nanoparticles to investigate their size, shape, and aggregation state, and also can aid interpretation of information generated using other techniques; hence considered one of the most powerful techniques in investigating nanomaterials [21]. For high-resolution imaging, electromagnetic radiation with shorter wavelengths, such as electron beams, must be utilized. The development of electron microscopes has enabled researchers to achieve magnifications of the order of one million and resolution of up to 0.1 nm. When an electron beam encounters the sample, electrons can be transmitted, diffracted, or backscattered generating measurable signals. Electrons may also get diffracted by particles oriented toward the beam, generating crystallographic information. Additionally, the electrons in the beam may encounter atoms in the sample, causing the electrons in the beam to be scattered back or remove more electrons from the atoms of the specimen. Because these processes increase the atomic number of the atom, backscattering and secondary electron generation are more effective. There are two main types of electron microscope the transmission EM (TEM) and the scanning EM (SEM) [22].

11.2.5.1 Transmission electron microscopy (TEM)

TEM is applicable for investigating particle size, shape, surface layers, or absorbates with high spatial resolution [23,24]. Recently, the technique has been improved so that the structural changes in nanoparticles resulting from interactions with substrates at gas, liquid, or solid phases can be studied. A modern TEM can image atoms in crystalline specimens with a resolution about 0.1 nm, which is smaller than interatomic distance. Additionally, a single nanocrystal can be chemically analyzed quantitatively by focusing an electron beam to a diameter less than 0.3 nm. Such analyses are essential for the characterization of materials at a differing length ranging from atoms to a few hundred nanometers. TEM can also be used to investigate particle shape, size, crystallinity, and interparticle interaction of nanomaterials [25]. Using two condenser lenses, a monochromatic electron stream from an electron gun is focused to form a beam. High-angle electrons in the beam are eliminated by the condenser aperture before they reach the sample to be analyzed. It is also essential that the sample is thin enough to permit some electrons in the beam to transmit through the specimen. Some electrons are elastically and inelastically scattered in the forward direction, while others are unscattered due to interactions between the beam and the specimen. The detected signal contains information about the sample.

Although TEM imaging has many advantages, it still exhibits several challenges such as image overlapping. In image overlaps, the surrounding matrix usually masks the supported nanoparticles. However, occasionally an epitaxial relationship between the nanoparticles and their support can provide information about size and shape. Besides, the electron beam irradiation in the usual high-resolution imaging conditions may cause damage to the nanoparticles. High-resolution transmission electron microscopy (HRTEM) generates images of the crystalloid structure of a sample at an atomic scale making use of the interference of the electron wave with itself in the image plane. Each imaging electron interacts with the specimen in an independent manner, the electron wave undergoes further phase change and interference as it goes through the microscope's imaging system. In order to obtain structural and chemical information with a spatial resolution at atomic level, such as the oxidation state of an element, TEM can be complemented with electron energy-loss spectroscopy (EELS) [21].

11.2.5.2 Scanning electron microscopy (SEM)

SEM is capable of imaging almost any surface with a resolution of about 1 nm. The properties of the electron probe and the interaction of the probe with the specimen determines the image resolution of SEM. Unlike TEM, SEM is inadequate for characterizing nanoparticles, because in some cases SEM is unable to differentiate nanoparticles from the substrate. The situation is worse when the nanoparticles under investigation tend to adhere to each other to form agglomerates. Still, surface topology, morphology, and chemical composition can be studied using SEM. Its high-resolution capability enables researchers to probe nanomaterials with critical structural properties. Nonetheless, SEM can provide information on the purity of a nanoparticle and an insight on their degree of aggregation.

11.2.6 Energy-dispersive X-ray analysis (EDX)

Energy-dispersive X-ray spectroscopy (EDX) is a technique used in combination with SEM and enables the analysis of near-surface elements and their amount at different positions providing a map of the sample. The material being examined determines the energy of the emitted X-rays. The X-rays are produced in a region about 2 microns deep, making EDX not a true surface science technique. Electron beam is moved across the material and an image of the elements in the specimen can be formed; however, due to low X-ray intensity, image generation usually takes a couple of hours. If the nanoparticles near or at the surface of a specimen are heavy metal ions, such as Au, Pd and Ag nanoparticles, the composition and the amount can be estimated with EDX; however, elements with low atomic numbers are difficult to detect because the Si–Li detector protected by beryllium window is unable to detect elements with atomic number below 11 (Na). Various X-ray techniques are utilized for the characterization of nanomaterials such as X-ray absorption fine structure (XAFS), X-ray photoelectron spectroscopy (XPS), small-angle X-ray scattering (SAXS), and X-ray diffraction (XRD) nowadays. For analyzing chemical composition, spectroscopies based on X-rays are useful, which include X-ray absorption spectroscopy (XAS) such as extended X-ray absorption fine structure (EXAFS), XPS, X-ray absorption near-edge structure (XANES), EDX, and X-ray fluorescence spectroscopy (XRF). These techniques mostly make use of the radiation absorbed or emitted by the sample after X-ray excitation (except for electrons in XPS). The spectroscopic techniques can be used for elemental analysis since spectroscopy properties are characteristic to specific elements [21,26].

11.3 Biomechanical properties

Molecules that have strong conjugation with the neighboring molecules end up with high mobility scores. Therefore, characterizing optical, mechanical, and electrical properties of newly developed molecules has always been an issue for researchers. On the other hand, mechanical properties of the materials are fundamentally related to stress and strain. By introducing structural changes in nanomaterials, mechanical property and structure correlation can be established. Thus, characterizing mechanical properties of nanomaterials is essential both for scientific purposes and device application. Quantifying mechanical properties of the nanomaterials will enable researchers to determine the operating limit of these materials in applicable devices [3].

The mechanical properties of nanomaterials would be enhanced than bulk materials, if their chemical stability could be enhanced. It is known that CNTs have excellent mechanical properties. Bulk ceramic and metallic materials, effect of porosity, grain size, and particle-filled polymers and polymer composites, superplasticity, and CNT-based composites are studied under "Mechanical Properties of Nanoparticles". The study of mechanical properties of nanomaterials is a basic interest, because it is very challenging to produce macroscopic materials of such great density with grain size less than 100 nm. Two materials, polymers that contain nanoparticles or nanotubes and severely plastic-deformed metals attract great interest for their potential industrial importance as they exhibit outstanding properties. However, the latter are not accounted as nanomaterials because of their large grain size. Procedures for studying mechanical properties of bulk nanomaterials are usually very limiting, because producing samples with defined porosities and grain sizes are strictly required [27].

Biomechanics is the study of movement and structure of living things using mechanical laws. Mechanics is a branch of physics that deals with motion and the forces that create motion. Motion can be created in living things as a consequent of forces such as a stimulus for growth and development. With the help of mathematical and conceptual tools, biomechanics help us understand how living things move and how we can improve movement to make it safer when needed [28].

11.4 Cell/biomaterials interactions

Cells of an organism obtained from any tissue require surface attachment to be able to proliferate, execute cellular activity, and maintain vitality. Therefore, it is very important that the cells utilized in tissue engineering applications to attach to the surface of the tissue scaffold. Furthermore, the molecular and topographical structure of the biomaterial forming the tissue scaffold is essential for the development of a microenvironment that mimics the extracellular matrix. Biological activities of the cells used in tissue engineering applications such as cellular growth, differentiation, and proliferation are regulated with stimuli from extracellular matrix (neurotransmitters, hormones, etc.). These signals are received by the cells using specific receptors on the cell surface [29]. In order to convert these signals into cellular responses, a complex cellular mechanism including molecules made of up carbohydrate, protein, and generally glycoconjugate plays a role. Carbohydrates found on the cell surface regulate the communication between the cell and its environment. The carbohydrate subunits of the glycoconjugates on the surface of animal cells regulate the adhesion of cells onto surfaces, act as receptors (integrins) or function as ligands (fibronectin, laminin, etc.) [30].

Nonspecific chemical interactions (electrostatical forces, van der Waals interactions, etc.) as well as receptor–ligand interactions are important in the attachment of a cell to the surface. Although there is constant nonspecific chemical interaction between interacting cells and the surface, specific receptor–ligand interactions are only achieved through the expression of the receptor molecules on the cell surface that recognize ligand molecules by their functional groups [30]. Once the cells adhere to the tissue scaffold, a series of physical and chemical reactions begin between the cells and the scaffold surface. After the placement of the tissue scaffold in the body or in cell culture, adsorption is initiated by cell surface molecules. These focal adhesions make up the primary cellular domains of complex assemblies that consist of cytoplasmic and transmembrane proteins and the integrin receptors [31].

11.5 Stem cells

Long-term cell division, proliferation potential and self-renewal capabilities of stem cells (SCs) earned them a central place in the field of regenerative medicine, particularly in tissue engineering. SCs can be isolated from various sources such as bone marrow, cord blood, cord matrix, peripheral blood, and adipose tissue [32]. Although therapeutic cloning seems to be a possibility in tissue engineering, the technology to precisely control stem cell behavior under culture conditions is still under development. For instance, a recent study reporting successful osteogenic differentiation of SCs for tissue engineering when gold nanoparticles were used in culture suggests the importance of including nanoparticles in culture [33]. Advances in nanomaterial research will definitely facilitate the advances in stem cell research. Scaffolds utilizing nanomaterials may assume specific roles in tissue engineering applications using SCs. Although research is ongoing on this topic, various limitations are encountered routinely. Several studies have reported different influences of nanoparticles on different cell lines based on the type and size of the particles; however, studies investigating interactions between nanoparticles and SCs are inconclusive [34–39]. Cytotoxic effects, genetic analysis, and histological evaluation of SCs in nanomaterial-based tissue engineering applications urgently need to be studied in order to approve biosafety of use of nanoparticles in stem cell cultures [40–42].

11.6 Biocorrosion

Nanomaterial research is leading to novel and exciting applications, because of unique properties of nanomaterials such as high grain boundary volume fraction and extremely fine grain size [43]. Nanomaterials lie in the high-energy local-minima region and are thermodynamically metastable; however their kinetics is rapid, thus retaining active metal nanoparticles is very challenging. They are prone to attack and transformation, which may cause poor corrosion resistance, phase change, high solubility, deterioration, and difficulty in retaining structure [27].

In most laboratory investigations, the cause of corrosion is primarily attributed to microbes, instead of CO_2 or other factors that cause corrosion [44].

Corrosion was associated with microbes as early as 1910 [45,46]. It is known that the presence of microorganisms on surfaces affect the performance of the material; and such microbial growth on surfaces, namely biofilms, promote biofouling. Biofilms may also promote undesired physicochemical reactions that do not occur under abiotic conditions. For metallic materials, formation of a biofilm or a biofouling layer that cause changes in the material's properties are called biocorrosion or microbially influenced corrosion (MIC) [47]. Biocorrosion or MIC refers to the rapid deformation of metals due to biofilms on their surfaces. Although biocorrosion and microbial corrosion suggest microbes as the main cause of corrosion, the term *MIC* does not specify whether the microbe association is direct or indirect. Recent investigations on biocorrosion mostly focused on the effect of mineralization on the surface of metallic materials and the effect of extracellular enzymes of the biofilm on electrochemical reactions such as redox reactions at biofilm–metal interface [45–47].

Anaerobic iron corrosion results from electron loss from elemental iron (Fe^0) that releases soluble ferrous iron (Fe^{+2}). Under anaerobic conditions, the electrons must be accepted by an oxidant other than oxygen [44] and it is important to identify the terminal acceptor in corrosion research. Several biocorrosion studies have focused on biocorrosion of aluminum and its alloys in jet fuels by fungal contaminants, corrosion of steel due to sulfate-reducing bacteria (SRB), strategies to monitor biocorrosion in industrial water systems, and electrochemical techniques for evaluating the effects of biocorrosion [48].

It has been shown that Cu-containing stainless steel has high antibacterial activity (99.9%) against *Escherichia coli* and *Staphylococcus aureus*, but for this efficiency, Cu concentration must be at least 5 wt.%. Such high Cu content creates a Ti_2Cu intermetallic phase that rapidly deteriorates mechanical properties of the steel. In addition to that, Ag has even higher antibacterial ability than Cu and has been used in antibacterial coatings and alloys [49].

The research is now more focused on the manufacture of materials or coatings that have greater abrasion and corrosion resistance [43].

Nanomaterials have distinct physical, chemical, and physicochemical properties; therefore nanocoating is becoming a hot topic in nanotechnology applications for prevention and management of corrosion. Nanocoating is the integration of nanoparticles in the coating material forming denser products and provide enhanced properties regarding thermal and electrical conductivity, corrosion resistance, chemical resistance, and better surface appearance [50,51]. Examples of these are antimicrobial coatings with enhanced corrosion resistance, zeolite coatings, and epoxy coatings, as well as titanium coatings with hydroxyapatite nanoparticles that are used in biomedical implants [43,51].

Despite their wide use in medical devices for their ability to resist corrosion, their biocompatibility and mechanical properties, titanium and its alloys may cause loosening or even the failure of implants due to bacterial infections, because they do not have antibacterial activity [49]. Additionally, magnesium and its alloys have been shown to have outstanding biocompatibility in several studies; however, their tendency to undergo swift degradation and corrosion usually damages the surrounding tissue and limits their clinical applications [52].

Early implant failure has been shown to be caused by local corrosion of the surface of metals and alloys that affect their bioactivity [53]. Titanium alloys in medical implants spontaneously form a protective oxide coating on their surface; still, surface modifications are employed to enhance the antibacterial function of these implants like the addition of antibacterial materials such as Ag, Cu, and Zn into surface coatings [49]. Unfortunately, these antibacterial implants that have undergone surface modification usually present solid coating shedding and the sustainability periods are short.

Physical and dielectric properties of the oxide film have been proposed to be vital for implant biocompatibility. Titanium alloys have unique corrosion resistance ability; however, the release of metal ions into the physiological environment such as vanadium still raises questions due to studies reporting potential adverse effects. In order to reduce ion release from surgical implants, passivation strategies such as nitric acid or heat treatment and aging in 100°C water are employed. However, some of these procedures have been reported to cause significant increase in Ti, Al, and V trace levels in passivated Ti alloys; thus are controversial. Such high ion and protein concentration in the body creates an aggressive environment, which may cause compositional change in the implant, eventually causing early failure. The corruption process can occur across multiple layers. It is also important that the surface coating is able to promote tissue engineering of the implant. Coatings modified with hydroxyapatite, calcium, or phosphate have been shown to promote bone formation and cellular growth on implants [53].

Future prospects in this field are very much related to the studies on the development of innovative microscopy techniques, novel spectroscopic techniques, and electrochemistry [48].

11.7 Biodegradation

Nanocomposites with ultralarge surface area to volume ratio, so-called clay nanocomposites or nanoclays, are formed by nanoparticles. Using nanoparticles for filling up spaces, enhance mechanical properties of the material as well as their degradation resistance. Nanoparticles can also help achieve activation energy faster.

Various nanoparticles also enhance thermal, mechanical, physicochemical stability, as well as biodegradability [54]. Biodegradation is defined as the microbial decomposition of an organic substance, suggesting that this process does not account for inorganic nanomaterials. Therefore, biotic degradation is usually out of question for most nanomaterials including silver, titanium oxide, cerium oxide, nano-zero-valent iron, zinc oxide, copper oxide, and quantum dots [55].

Biodegradation of particles is an essential issue to be questioned because of the knowledge gap in biodegradation mechanisms [54]. When particles are not biodegraded or excreted from the body, adverse effects may occur and to study particle accumulation in various organs and tissues, long-term in vivo studies of model organisms are required [56].

Biodegradation of carbon-based nanomaterials, especially certain CNTs, has been a major concern, because it is thought that they may display asbestos-like pathogenicity due to their fiber-like morphology and/or biopersistency. Several studies have suggested that carbon-based nanomaterials may be liable to biodegradation. According to our knowledge, limited mineralization occurs under very specific test conditions. Carbon-based nanomaterials, such as CNTs, graphene oxide, and nanodiamonds are also resistant to biodegradation due to their inorganic nature and they are potential candidates for medical applications such as imaging and drug delivery [54,57]. Thus, biodegradation is an insignificant issue for the fate of carbon-based nanomaterials such as CNT and carbon black (CB), and their behavior in the environment. Nevertheless, biological degradation of organic surface coatings may occur and should not be overlooked [55].

It has been shown that particle shape plays an important role in the degradation properties of nanoparticles. Surface area and diameter are also important for cellular uptake of nanoparticles. Although hemispherical particles are used as sustained release devices to achieve zero-order; spherical particles have shapes that are susceptible to degradation and can present different degradation profiles. In addition to that, deterioration rate of spherical nanoparticles is especially important for spleen filtration, because the filtering units of the spleen are asymmetrical. Biocompatible nanoparticle polymers are also used to extend the drug release period because they have biodegradation periods that range from days to months. Molecular weight of polymers is especially an important parameter for biodegradation rate [58].

Low-density polyethylene (LDPE) accumulates daily, thus its degradation is a solemn problem. Many different degradation procedures have been studied, but the efficiency is strictly dependent on certain conditions. LDPE was successfully degraded by nanobarium titanate (NBT), Fullerene 60, and super magnetic iron oxide (SPION) with the enhancement of microbial activity [59].

Many carbon-based nanomaterials have been produced for investigation in the use of diagnostics and therapeutics. Nonetheless, the biological interactions of these materials are still largely unknown [57].

Nanoparticle bioreactivity is based on interactions between proteins and nanoparticles and provides the formation of a nanoparticle-protein corona, which is quite dynamic. This protein corona may affect various cellular and molecular processes such as cellular uptake, degradation, and clearance of nanoparticles and inflammation [60]. Undeniably, the so-called "bio-corona" of biomolecules on nanomaterials in the body has a potential significance. A special example of biocorona interactions, which is enzymatic degradation of carbon-based nanomaterials by immune cells, serve as an important example for medical use of these nanomaterials [57].

11.8 In vitro assessments

Scientists generally use in vitro tests to evaluate biomaterial toxicity, dose–response relationship of chemicals and the risk when a patient is potentially exposed to toxic chemicals [61]. In vitro tests have lower cost and test time than in vivo tests [62], but the properties of the material to be tested, the fitness of the test, and the biocompatibility analysis affects the choice of test and physiological and inflammatory responses against the materials to be tested cannot be assessed by in vitro tests [63]. Replacing in vivo tests with in vitro methods enables us to screen multiple compounds at a time, can be used to produce preliminary data for further screening newly developed materials and has ethical importance regarding animal welfare. In vitro tests generally focus on evaluating the toxicity of a material [64]. Although the methods available for assessing toxicity of nanomaterials are the same as the techniques for macromolecules, nanomaterial toxicity is more diverse than other materials [65].

The technique to be used depends on the properties of the material, biocompatibility data analysis, and the fitness of the test [63].

Compared to in vivo tests, more specific and sophisticated in vitro tests are being developed to overcome the high cost of experiments, to reduce the use of experimental animals and to avoid time and energy consumption for ethical committee approvals [66]. These tests must consistently predict and evaluate possible influences of the nanomaterial in a spectrum of benefits to risks, including potential health threats upon exposure to the material as they begin to be commonly used in medicine and manufacturing [67].

11.8.1 Cell cultures for cytotoxicity

Cell responses against the tested materials are assessed using in vitro biocompatibility tests [68]. When nanomaterials are exposed to in vivo conditions, they immediately encounter an enormous amount of biological and physiological stimuli such as surface-active molecules, inflammatory or pathological conditions, and many different cell types. In order to evaluate nanomaterial compatibility or toxicity, it is essential to understand the interactions of nanomaterials with different proteins and cells. Interactions between cells and nanomaterials include cellular uptake of nanomaterials for further processing, effects on membrane perturbations and cell signaling, effects on electron transfer machinery, cytokine, chemokine, and reactive oxygen species (ROS) production, gene regulation, programmed and unprogrammed cell death, and toxic reactivity [67]. Additionally, the physicochemical properties of nanomaterials such as particle size, composition, shape, surface area, and chemistry, crystallinity, redox potential, and solubility, are also very important as they are associated with potential toxicity [69].

Using numerous cell lines in in vitro systems provide many advantages including the observation of primary effects on target cells without inflammation, efficiency, and cost-effectiveness, ability to assess multiple parameters at the same time and information made available for the design of further whole animal studies [70]. Other advantages being discussed are the potential use of transgenic cell lines, reduced variability between experiments, and reduced amount of test materials. On the other hand, the conditions of many commercially available cell lines, such as being overpassaged, lacking validity for phenotype, and contamination with other cells cause significant disadvantages. Moreover, in vitro models cannot completely mimic the physiological and biological organization and complexity of cell, tissue, or organs in vivo [71].

For the last 40 years, cell culture in two dimensions has been used as a routine application in thousands of laboratories worldwide [72]. The most common evaluation method is cell reactivity assay using in vitro cell culture either with commercial, usually genetically modified cells or primary cells freshly harvested from tissue on plastic plates, with or without serum, exposed to nanomaterials [67]. Different models of in vitro studies provide information about different levels information associated with in vivo organization. Moreover, two-dimensional cell culture is suggested to be primitive and cannot reproduce the anatomy of a tissue in its physiological state in the body [72]. In organ culture, whole or a part of an organ (explant) is cultured to preserve histological architecture and it is possible to study in vivo processes *ex vivo*. Organotypic culture is another in vitro assay method that uses several different cell types to reconstitute cell heterogeneity as in vivo conditions. Using multiple cell types in these models is essential to generate complex cellular organization and function [71]. With multidisciplinary approach and expertise, it would be possible to create a third dimension in cell culture, which will be more relevant to study. For the third dimension, scaffolds need to be designed for supporting cells and bioreactors for nutrient and waste exchange. Since 3D culture systems are becoming more mature and they reflect animal physiology more every day, soon we will be able to develop co-cultures with possible stem cell integration [72].

In vitro cell viability tests generally assess cell morphology, proliferation, membrane permeability, and cell function [73].

11.8.2 Cell proliferation and membrane permeability

The effect of biomaterials on cell proliferation can easily be assessed by making a cell count. Cell counting can be performed either under microscope by different types of counting chambers such as Petroff-Hausser and Hemocytometer or by using automatized devices such as flow cytometer [16].

Cell count can also be performed by directly evaluating the increase in cell amount in culture or by using dyes that differentiate between living and dead cells. Staining living/dead cells enables us to calculate percent viability [69]. This assay is generally based on changes in cell permeability of living and dead cells, because living cells maintain a functional membrane transport, whereas dead cells do not. Although some dyes stain only dead or membrane-damaged cells, some others will only stain living cells because they are taken into cells by active transport [74]. For instance, release of cytosolic lactate dehydrogenase enzyme (LDH) can be used as an indicator of membrane damage, because it is found in the soluble fraction of the cell and a damage to the cell membrane will cause leakage of this enzyme to the extracellular fluid [75]. Additionally, DNA synthesis and proliferation can be evaluated using fluorescence dyes.

11.8.3 Morphological analysis

Cells are exposed to some materials to be tested, and differences in the morphology can be detected by a light microscope or an electron microscope with great detail [76]. Changes in morphology of any cells usually correlate with the cytotoxicity results of the cells [69]. Observations that help us to evaluate the morphology of a cell include lysosome formation in dying cells, condensation and fragmentation of cells, lysosomal disintegration of cell fragments in neighboring cells through phagocytosis, detachment of cells from the surface, and breakdown of cells into fragments [77].

11.8.4 Metabolic tests of cell

Viable cells have different abilities to convert certain chemicals into measurable forms and these differences can be utilized to measure metabolic activity of the cells [78]. Cellular functions and metabolic activity is assessed with these tests. Mossman described one of the most common metabolic tests that uses (3-(4,5-dimethylthiazol-2-yl)-2,5-diphenyltetrazolium bromide) (MTT). MTT is an indirect test and measures the activity of mitochondrial dehydrogenase enzyme when MTT is applied to cells in culture. Metabolically active living cells convert MTT reactant into purple formazan crystals using mitochondrial dehydrogenase enzyme and the quantification of the purple color determines the activity of dehydrogenase, thus indirectly cell viability [79]. Resazurin, a redox-sensitive dye, is another example that can be used as a metabolic test. On the other hand, ATP detection is accounted to be the gold standard, because cell death causes loss of ability to synthesize ATP and a swift loss of cytoplasmic ATP by means of endogenous ATPases, both of which influence ATP levels of the cell, thus indicating cell viability, which closely regulates ATP levels [78].

11.8.5 Other tests

Some other in vitro tests are available to serve different purposes. The cytotoxicity of the materials that are directly in contact with the cells can be measured by the morphological changes in the cells, which is the basis of ***direct contact test*** [66]. This test can be used to determine the toxicity of biomaterials, since it tests the toxicity of solid materials directly [80]. On the other hand, ***agar overlay method*** was developed as a standard for the assessment of cytotoxicity of biomaterials by Guess *et al.* In this method, briefly, L929 cells are grown as a monolayer on the bottom of a petri dish for 24 hours, then overlayed by a 1.5% agar nutrient layer. Subsequently, the cells are stained with neutral red, the material to be tested is applied to the top of the agar and according to the size of the decolored zone and the degree of cell lysis, the toxicity of the material is determined after 24 hours [81].

In vivo rabbit test was replaced by the in vitro skin irritating test in order to reduce animal experiments. Artificial skin samples such as EPISKIN [82] and EpiDerm [83] can be utilized to predict skin irritancy. Embryonic cultures for in vitro teratogenicity tests are also suitable for reducing animal use. Sister chromatid exchange tests, chromosomal abnormality tests, micronuclei test, and comet test are genotoxicity tests that can be used on cell cultures. Hemocompatibility assays, including hemolytic test, clotting time test, platelet adhesion and activation test, and anticoagulant assays, also provide another parameter [84].

11.9 In vivo assessments

Animal models make up an essential step for testing biomaterials before clinical use of those in humans. When a material is tested with in vivo tests, it comes into contact with various cell types and responses and interacts with proteins, enzymes, and hormones. Although there are numerous animal models available to test implants, it is always critical to decide on which model to use. Short-term in vivo studies usually take up to 12 weeks and use small animals such as mice, rats, rabbits, or guinea pigs. Long-term studies generally use animals with longer life expectancy such as rabbits, guinea pigs, dogs, goat, sheep, and pigs [85].

According to the ISO 10993-1 and FDA Biological Response Test, in vivo tests to evaluate tissue compatibility include assays for cytotoxicity, irritation, sensitization, systemic/acute toxicity, subchronic toxicity, chronic toxicity, intracutaneous reactivity, genotoxicity, hemocompatibility, carcinogenicity, and biodegradation [86]. Several of these tests are briefly explained below.

11.9.1 Systemic toxicity

Preclinical toxicology testing is important in determining the adverse effects profile of the tested compound according to Principles of Safety Pharmacology [87]. Although many effects can be predicted using the information from animal testing, there are still some toxic effects observed in humans that were not predicted from animal studies, which cause a major limitation to the tests [107].

According to WHO report (Principles for preclinical testing of drug safety) procedures are categorized into two classes: studies that use single administration and studies that use repeated administration that may use short-term (subacute) or long-term studies (chronic).

11.9.2 Skin sensitization

Skin sensitization testing is important in determining potential sensitization of chemicals prior to human exposure [88]. Skin sensitization risk is a crucial issue for especially cosmetic products [89].

Local lymph node assay (LLNA) has been authenticated as an alternative to skin sensitization test using comparisons between guinea pigs and humans. LLNA evaluates the effect of contact allergens on the function of lymphocyte proliferation in draining lymph nodes. This method is objective, time- and cost-effective, and provides important animal welfare benefits.

Nonanimal skin sensitization tests increasingly gain importance due to cost, animal welfare issues, and technological limitations. It is believed that nonanimal skin sensitization tests will be developed based on cell culture [90].

11.9.3 Irritation

During manufacturing, use, and disposal of nanomaterials, risk of exposure through surficial organs such as eyes and skin is very high. Information of surficial organ irritation and sensitization is an essential part of research on potentially hazardous chemicals [91]. Both in vivo and in vitro toxicity tests aim to assess irritation or sensitization risk of these materials when in contact with human skin or eye [92,93]. Rabbit skin irritation test described by Draize *et al.* is the most common of these tests [94].

11.9.4 Intracutaneous reactivity

The skin contains numerous highly potent immune-related cells, thus is one the most immunostimulatory tissues [95].

The rabbit intracutaneous reactivity test is a commonly used method for evaluating irritant chemicals. Test solutions that contain specific amounts of test compounds are prepared, the fur of the animal at the upper back is clipped, and a small gauge needle is used to inject the solution into the skin. The injection site forms a swelling resembling a mosquito bite and these sites can be scored by the investigators [96].

11.9.5 Genotoxicity

Genotoxicity is the ability of a physical or chemical agent to damage genetic material. This damage on DNA can be single- or double-strand breaks, DNA adducts, or alkali labile sites. In vivo and in vitro genotoxicity tests have been used since 1970s [97]. It would be essential to collect information from whole animal carcinogenicity assays with nanomaterials, in order to prepare a basis for genotoxicity assays [98].

Chromosomal abnormalities occur when normal chromosome structure or chromosome number are altered due to chemical mutagens or induced radiation [99]. Colchicine, which is a tubulin polymerization inhibitor, is injected to the experimental animals to inhibit cell division at metaphase stage, and animals are scarred 2–4 hours after injection. Abnormalities in bone marrow cells of the animals are then detected [100].

Micronuclei (MN) form during mitosis and can be derived from acentric chromosome fragments or whole chromosomes. An increase in the number of MN indirectly refers to structural or numerical aberrations in chromosomes that may be caused by various agents [101].

11.9.6 Carcinogenicity

Carcinogenicity is aberrant growth or cell division caused by damage to DNA. The mutagenic capacity of a substance defines its carcinogenic potential [102]. It has been suggested that the increased surface area of a given volume of biomaterial results in an increased foreign body reaction and a decrease in carcinogenicity or tumorigenesis potential. This may have crucial consequences for nanoparticles and tissue engineering scaffolds due to their high surface area in medical devices [103].

When nanoparticles are inhaled, the primary route of entry is the lungs, which raises a major issue of identifying nanoparticles that could potentially be lung carcinogens [104].

Long-term animal studies are crucial for reliable risk evaluation, especially for potential carcinogens. The standard procedure for carcinogenicity potential is testing a chemical in two rodent species of both sexes, usually mice and rats, at three doses (zero, low, and high) for up to 2 years [105].

11.9.7 Reproductive and developmental toxicity

Teratogenicity testing is used for determining materials that are toxic during the development of an organism. Four indicators of developmental toxicity are embryonic or fetal death, retardation, malformation, and functional impairment [106]. Teratogenicity tests are generally performed on mice, rats, and rabbits [107], as well as zebrafish and chick embryos [108].

11.10 Conclusion

Owing to their unique properties and novel application areas, it is obvious that nanoparticles have come into prominence recently [2]. Nanoparticles are considered to find various other application fields as well. However, the characterization of nanoparticles and determination of their interactions with living/nonliving materials is essential because nanoparticles have different physical and chemical properties at nanoscale in bulk form or as a result of different engineering processes.

Advanced imaging systems including optical and scanning microscopies can be used for imaging of the engineered nanoparticles. Nevertheless, these imaging systems are expensive, laborious, and sometimes inadequate for characterization of nanoparticles, thus there is a need for the improvement of available techniques, finding complements for them, and also development of novel systems.

Determination of the interactions between nanoparticles and other materials/equipment/biological products that will be used in medical, cosmetic, electronic, and so on areas together with nanoparticles is one of the most essential studies required for the improvement of nanotechnology. For instance, the interactions between nanoparticles and cellular structures, biological materials and polymers must be studied for tissue engineering studies. Studying cell/stem cell responses, biodegradability, and corrosive properties of the nanomaterials using in vitro and in vivo techniques is among the most common research techniques. However, these techniques are considerably complicated, costly, and laborious.

Nanotechnology studies will make progress especially in multidisciplinary fields such as tissue engineering with imaging and characterization of nanoparticles and determining their interactions with biological products or materials related to the area of use. Since the techniques used for this purpose are laborious and expensive, the staff working in these areas need to be specialized in nanomaterials. Thus, considering all these techniques and their needs, improvement and optimization of the available techniques and development of novel ones are required.

11.11 Future aspects

The physicochemical characteristics of nanomaterials at nanoscale are novel and still require investigation; thus the effect of nanomaterials in physiological interactions both at a molecular and systemic level is an interesting research topic, especially in the case of in vivo administration of nanomedicines [109].

The evaluation techniques for nanomaterials that are developed for use in biological systems often emphasize on safety and risk assessment.

In order to develop reliable protocols and techniques for characterization of nanomaterials and their interactions within biological systems, investigations using multidisciplinary collaborations including physical scientists, engineers, and toxicologists are essential [110].

Most of the safety tests regarding nanomaterials are based on in vivo animal models; however, only a few reports present assays utilizing in vitro techniques. Studies in assay biology, computation, and screening will continue an innovative course to open up new possibilities for mechanistic, efficient, and predictive chemical toxicology [111].

Nevertheless, full replacement of animal studies with in vitro techniques in reproductive hazard assessment does not appear to be prominent in near future [112].

References

[1] Tsuji JS, et al. Research strategies for safety evaluation of nanomaterials, part IV: risk assessment of nanoparticles. Toxicol Sci 2006;89(1):42–50.

[2] Dahotre NB, Seal S. Nanomaterials and surfaces: processing, characterization, and applications. JOM 2004;56(10):35.

[3] Ghorai S. Chemical, physical and mechanical properties of nanomaterials and its applications; 2013.

[4] Joshi M, Bhattacharyya A, Wazed Ali S. Characterization techniques for nanotechnology applications in textile. Indian J Fibre Text Res 2008;33:304–17.

[5] Verma A, Stellacci F. Effect of surface properties on nanoparticle–cell interactions. Small 2010;6(1):12–21.

[6] Liu GY, Xu S, Qian Y. Nanofabrication of self-assembled monolayers using scanning probe lithography. Acc Chem Res 2000;33(7):457–66.

[7] Giessibl FJ, et al. Subatomic features on the silicon (111)-(7x7) surface observed by atomic force microscopy. Science 2000;289(5478):422–6.

[8] Bonnell DA. Scanning tunneling microscopy A2 Buschow KHJ, editor. Encyclopedia of materials: science and technology (3rd ed.). Oxford: Elsevier; 2001. p. 8269–81.

[9] Meyer E. Atomic force microscopy: fundamentals to most advanced applications, Vol. 1. New York: Springer-Verlag Telos. 2007.

[10] Bonnel D. Scanning probe microscopy and spectroscopy: theory, techniques, and applications. New York: Wiley-VCH; 2000.

[11] Yarbrough JM, Himmel ME, Ding SY. Plant cell wall characterization using scanning probe microscopy techniques. Biotechnol Biofuels 2009;2:17.

[12] Fotiadis D, et al. Imaging and manipulation of biological structures with the AFM. Micron 2002;33(4):385–97.

[13] Israelachvili JN. Intermolecular and surface forces. Burlington, MA: Academic Press; 2011.

[14] Deniz AA, Mukhopadhyay S, Lemke EA. Single-molecule biophysics: at the interface of biology, physics and chemistry. J R Soc Interface 2008;5(18):15–45.

[15] Ando T, et al. High-speed AFM and nano-visualization of biomolecular processes. Pflugers Arch 2008;456(1):211–25.

[16] Guntherodt HJ, Anselmetti D, Meyer E. *Applied sciences*. NATO ASI series, Vol. 286. Dordrecht: Kluwer Academic; 1995.

[17] Binnig G, Quate CF, Gerber C. Atomic force microscope. Phys Rev Lett 1986;56(9):930–3.
[18] Bai C. Scanning tunneling microscopy and its applications. New York: Springer-Verlag Telos; 2007.
[19] Baro AM, Binnig G, Rohrer H, Gerber C, Stoll E, Baratoff A, et al. Real-space observation of the 2× 1 structure of chemisorbed oxygen on Ni(110) by scanning tunneling microscopy. Phys Rev Lett 1984;52:1304–7.
[20] Endo M, et al. Applications of carbon nanotubes in the twenty-first century. Philos Trans A Math Phys Eng Sci 2004;362(1823):2223–38.
[21] Laborda F, et al. Detection, characterization and quantification of inorganic engineered nanomaterials: a review of techniques and methodological approaches for the analysis of complex samples. Anal Chim Acta 2016;904:10–32.
[22] Blank H, et al. Application of low-energy scanning transmission electron microscopy for the study of Pt-nanoparticle uptake in human colon carcinoma cells. Nanotoxicology 2014;8(4):433–46.
[23] Henry CR. Morphology of supported nanoparticles. Prog Surf Sci 2005;80(3–4):92–116.
[24] Brydson R, Brown A. An investigation of the surface structure of nanoparticulate systems using analytical electron microscopes corrected for spherical aberration Turning Points in Solid-State, Material and Surface Science. London: RSC Publishing; 2008.778.91
[25] Wang ZL, Poncharal P, de Heer WA. Nanomeasurements in transmission electron microscopy. Microsc Microanal 2000;6(3):224–30.
[26] Barr TL, et al. X-ray photoelectron spectroscopic studies of kaolinite and montmorillonite. Vacuum 1995;46(12):1391–5.
[27] Alagarasi A. Introduction to nanomaterials. National Center for Environmental Research; 2011.
[28] Knudson D. Fundamentals of biomechanics. Springer Science & Business Media; 2007.
[29] Polak JM, Bishop AE. Stem cells and tissue engineering: past, present, and future. Ann N Y Acad Sci 2006;1068:352–66.
[30] Chen W, et al. Nanotopography influences adhesion, spreading, and self-renewal of human embryonic stem cells. ACS Nano 2012;6(5):4094–103.
[31] Chang H, Wang Y. Cell responses to surface and architecture of tissue engineering scaffolds. In: Regenerative medicine and tissue engineering—cells and biomaterials; 2011. p. 569–581.
[32] Allahverdiyev AM, et al. Microcapillary culture method: a novel tool for in vitro expansion of stem cells from scarce sources. Arch Med Res 2012;43(6):423–30.
[33] Li J, et al. Gold nanoparticle size and shape influence on osteogenesis of mesenchymal stem cells. Nanoscale 2016;8(15):7992–8007.
[34] Ahmad I. Nanotoxicity of natural minerals: an emerging area of nanotoxicology. J Biomed Nanotechnol 2011;7(1):32–3.
[35] Ai J, et al. Nanotoxicology and nanoparticle safety in biomedical designs. Int J Nanomedicine 2011;6:1117–27.
[36] Feliu N, Fadeel B. Nanotoxicology: no small matter. Nanoscale 2010;2(12):2514–20.
[37] Ferreira AJ, Cemlyn-Jones J, Cordeiro CR. Nanoparticles, nanotechnology and pulmonary nanotoxicology. Rev Port Pneumol 2013;19(1):28–37.
[38] Greish K, Thiagarajan G, Ghandehari H. In vivo methods of nanotoxicology. Methods Mol Biol 2012;926:235–53.
[39] Hubbs AF, et al. Nanotoxicology--a pathologist's perspective. Toxicol Pathol 2011;39(2):301–24.
[40] Bolt HM, Marchan R, Hengstler JG. Recent developments in nanotoxicology. Arch Toxicol 2013;87(6):927–8.

[41] Chou LY, Chan WC. Nanotoxicology. No signs of illness. Nat Nanotechnol 2012;7(7):416–7.
[42] Clark KA, White RH, Silbergeld EK. Predictive models for nanotoxicology: current challenges and future opportunities. Regul Toxicol Pharmacol 2011;59(3):361–3.
[43] Saji VS, Thomas J. Nanomaterials for corrosion control. Curr Sci 2007;92(1):51–5.
[44] Gu T. New understandings of biocorrosion mechanisms and their classifications. J Microb Biochem Technol 2012;2012.
[45] Morsi RE, Labena A, Khamis EA. Core/shell (ZnO/polyacrylamide) nanocomposite: In-situ emulsion polymerization, corrosion inhibition, anti-microbial and anti-biofilm characteristics. J Taiwan Inst Chem Eng 2016;63:512–22.
[46] Beech IB, Sunner J. Biocorrosion: towards understanding interactions between biofilms and metals. Curr Opin Biotechnol 2004;15(3):181–6.
[47] Beech IB, Sunner JA, Hiraoka K. Microbe-surface interactions in biofouling and biocorrosion processes. Int Microbiol 2010;8(3):157–68.
[48] Videla HA, Herrera LK. Microbiologically influenced corrosion: looking to the future. Int Microbiol 2005;8(3):169.
[49] Chen M, Zhang E, Zhang L. Microstructure, mechanical properties, bio-corrosion properties and antibacterial properties of Ti–Ag sintered alloys. Mater Sci Eng C 2016;62:350–60.
[50] Popoola A, Olorunniwo O, Ige O. Corrosion resistance through the application of anti-corrosion coatings. Pretoria, South Africa: Developments in Corrosion Protection, Intech; 2014.241.70
[51] Rathish RJ, et al. Corrosion resistance of nanoparticle-incorporated nano coatings. Eur Chem Bull 2013;2(12):965–70.
[52] Abdal-hay A, et al. Biocorrosion behavior of biodegradable nanocomposite fibers coated layer-by-layer on AM50 magnesium implant. Mater Sci Eng C 2016;58:1232–41.
[53] Advincula MC, et al. Surface analysis and biocorrosion properties of nanostructured surface sol–gel coatings on Ti6Al4V titanium alloy implants. J Biomed Mater Res Part B Appl Biomater 2007;80(1):107–20.
[54] Bhatia M, et al. Implicating nanoparticles as potential biodegradation enhancers: a review. J Nanomed Nanotechnol 2013;2013.
[55] Hartmann NIB, et al. Environmental fate and behaviour of nanomaterials: new knowledge on important transfomation processes. : Danish Environmental Protection Agency; 2014.
[56] Alkilany AM, Murphy CJ. Toxicity and cellular uptake of gold nanoparticles: what we have learned so far? J Nanopart Res 2010;12(7):2313–33.
[57] Bhattacharya K, et al. Biological interactions of carbon-based nanomaterials: from coronation to degradation. Nanomed Nanotechnol Biol Med 2016;12(2):333–51.
[58] Aslan B, et al. Nanotechnology in cancer therapy. J Drug Target 2013;21(10): 904–13.
[59] Pandey P, et al. Nanoparticles accelerated in vitro biodegradation of LDPE: a review. Adv Appl Sci Res 2015;6(4):17–22.
[60] Saptarshi SR, Duschl A, Lopata AL. Interaction of nanoparticles with proteins: relation to bio-reactivity of the nanoparticle. J Nanobiotechnol 2013;11(1):1.
[61] Ratner BD, et al. Biomaterials science: an introduction to materials in medicine. Elsevier Science; 2012.
[62] Peppas NA, Langer R. New challenges in biomaterials. Science 1994;263(5154):1715–9.
[63] Ratner BD, et al. Biomaterials science: an introduction to materials in medicine. Academic press; 2004.

[64] Ukelis U, et al. Replacement of in vivo acute oral toxicity studies by in vitro cytotoxicity methods: opportunities, limits and regulatory status. Regul Toxicol Pharmacol 2008;51(1):108–18.
[65] Lee J, et al. In vitro toxicity testing of nanoparticles in 3D cell culture. Small 2009;5(10):1213–21.
[66] Di Silvio L. Cellular response to biomaterials. Elsevier; 2008.
[67] Jones CF, Grainger DW. In vitro assessments of nanomaterial toxicity. Adv Drug Deliv Rev 2009;61(6):438–56.
[68] You ES, et al. In vitro biocompatibility of surface-modified poly (DL-lactide-co-glycolide) scaffolds with hydrophilic monomers. J Ind Eng Chem 2007;13(2):219.
[69] Farcal L, et al. Comprehensive in vitro toxicity testing of a panel of representative oxide nanomaterials: first steps towards an intelligent testing strategy. PLoS One 2015;10(5):e0127174.
[70] Huang Y-W, Wu C-H, Aronstam RS. Toxicity of transition metal oxide nanoparticles: recent insights from in vitro studies. Materials 2010;3(10):4842–59.
[71] Astashkina A, Mann B, Grainger DW. A critical evaluation of in vitro cell culture models for high-throughput drug screening and toxicity. Pharmacol Ther 2012;134(1):82–106.
[72] Haycock JW. 3D cell culture: a review of current approaches and techniques. 3D cell culture: methods and protocols; 2011. p. 1–15.
[73] Freshney RI. Culture of specific cell types. Wiley Online Library; 2005.
[74] Hudson L, Hay F. Isolation and structure of immunoglobulins. Pract Immunol 1980;3.
[75] Choksakulnimitr S, et al. In vitro cytotoxicity of macromolecules in different cell culture systems. J Controlled Release 1995;34(3):233–41.
[76] Dutta R. Fundamentals of biochemical engineering. Springer; 2010.
[77] Schweichel JU, Merker HJ. The morphology of various types of cell death in prenatal tissues. Teratology 1973;7(3):253–66.
[78] Riss TL, Moravec RA, Niles AL. Cytotoxicity testing: measuring viable cells, dead cells, and detecting mechanism of cell death. Mammalian cell viability: methods and protocols; 2011. p. 103–114.
[79] Mosmann T. Rapid colorimetric assay for cellular growth and survival: application to proliferation and cytotoxicity assays. J Immunol Methods 1983;65(1–2):55–63.
[80] Oleszczuk P. The toxicity of composts from sewage sludges evaluated by the direct contact tests phytotoxkit and ostracodtoxkit. Waste Manage 2008;28(9):1645–53.
[81] Schmalz G. Agar overlay method. Int Endod J 1988;21(2):59–66.
[82] Cotovio J, et al. The in vitro skin irritation of chemicals: optimisation of the EPISKIN prediction model within the framework of the ECVAM validation process. Altern Lab Anim 2005;33(4):329–49.
[83] Kandárová H, et al. The EpiDerm test protocol for the upcoming ECVAM validation study on in vitro skin irritation tests-an assessment of the performance of the optimised test. Altern Lab Anim 2005;33(4):351.
[84] Elahi MF, Guan G, Wang L. Hemocompatibility of surface modified silk fibroin materials: a review. Rev Adv Mater Sci 2014;38(2):148–59.
[85] Thrivikraman G, Madras G, Basu B. In vitro/in vivo assessment and mechanisms of toxicity of bioceramic materials and its wear particulates. RSC Adv 2014;4(25):12763–81.
[86] Morais JM, Papadimitrakopoulos F, Burgess DJ. Biomaterials/tissue interactions: possible solutions to overcome foreign body response. AAPS J 2010;12(2):188–96.
[87] Pugsley MK, Authier S, Curtis M. Principles of safety pharmacology. Br J Pharmacol 2008;154(7):1382–99.
[88] Robinson MK, et al. A review of the Buehler guinea pig skin sensitization test and its use in a risk assessment process for human skin sensitization. Toxicology 1990;61(2):91–107.

[89] Natsch A, Emter R. Skin sensitizers induce antioxidant response element dependent genes: application to the in vitro testing of the sensitization potential of chemicals. Toxicol Sci 2008;102(1):110–9.
[90] Sakaguchi H, et al. Development of an in vitro skin sensitization test using human cell lines; human Cell Line Activation Test (h-CLAT) II. An inter-laboratory study of the h-CLAT. Toxicol In Vitro 2006;20(5):774–84.
[91] Ema M, et al. Evaluation of dermal and eye irritation and skin sensitization due to carbon nanotubes. Regul Toxicol Pharmacol 2011;61(3):276–81.
[92] Tornier C, Rosdy M, Maibach HI. In vitro skin irritation testing on reconstituted human epidermis: reproducibility for 50 chemicals tested with two protocols. Toxicol In Vitro 2006;20(4):401–16.
[93] Kishore AS, Surekha P, Murthy PB. Assessment of the dermal and ocular irritation potential of multi-walled carbon nanotubes by using in vitro and in vivo methods. Toxicol Lett 2009;191(2):268–74.
[94] Draize JH, Woodard G, Calvery HO. Methods for the study of irritation and toxicity of substances applied topically to the skin and mucous membranes. J Pharmacol Exp Ther 1944;82(3):377–90.
[95] Alarcon JB, et al. Preclinical evaluation of microneedle technology for intradermal delivery of influenza vaccines. Clin Vaccine Immunol 2007;14(4):375–81.
[96] Bs LT. An analysis of ISO intracutaneous reactivity test results to justify a reduction in animal requirements. Lab Anim (NY) 2003;32(3):26.
[97] Bedir A, Bilgici B, Yurdakul Z. DNA Hasarı Analizinde µ-FADU ve COMET Yöntemlerinin Karşılaştırılması. Türk Klinik Biyokimya Derg 2004;2(3):97–103.
[98] Landsiedel R, et al. Genotoxicity investigations on nanomaterials: methods, preparation and characterization of test material, potential artifacts and limitations—many questions, some answers. Mutat Res 2009;681(2):241–58.
[99] Yüzbaşıoğlu D, Zengin N, Ünal F. Gıda Koruyucuları ve Genotoksisite Testleri. Gıda Dergisi 2014;39(3).
[100] Şekeroğlu ZA, Şekeroğlu V. Genetik toksisite testleri. TÜBAV Bilim Dergisi 2011;4(3):221–9.
[101] Demirel S, Zamani AG. Mikronükleus tekniği ve kullanım alanları. Genel Tıp Dergisi 2002;12(3):123–7.
[102] Güldaş E, Keçeci DA. Endodontik tedavidekullanılan kök kanal patlarınınsitotoksik özellikleri – Bölüm I. Türk Diş Hekimliği Dergisi 2011;81:72–5.
[103] Anderson JM. Future challenges in the in vitro and in vivo evaluation of biomaterial biocompatibility. Regener Biomater 2016:rbw001.
[104] Lindberg HK, et al. Genotoxicity of nanomaterials: DNA damage and micronuclei induced by carbon nanotubes and graphite nanofibres in human bronchial epithelial cells in vitro. Toxicol Lett 2009;186(3):166–73.
[105] Tsuda H, et al. Toxicology of engineered nanomaterials-a review of carcinogenic potential. Asian Pac J Cancer Prev 2009;10(6):975–80.
[106] Brown N. Teratogenicity testing in vitro May 27–29, 1986 Mechanisms and models in toxicology: proceedings of the European Society of Toxicology Meeting held in Harrogate. : Springer Science & Business Media; 2012.
[107] Baker J. Principles for the testing of drugs for teratogencity. Report of a WHO Scientific Group; 1967.
[108] Beedie SL, et al. In vivo screening and discovery of novel candidate thalidomide analogs in the zebrafish embryo and chicken embryo model systems. Oncotarget 2016;7(22):33237–45.

[109] Lin P-C, et al. Techniques for physicochemical characterization of nanomaterials. Biotechnol Adv 2014;32(4):711–26.
[110] Powers KW, et al. Research strategies for safety evaluation of nanomaterials. Part VI. Characterization of nanoscale particles for toxicological evaluation. Toxicol Sci 2006;90(2):296–303.
[111] Shukla SJ, et al. The future of toxicity testing: a focus on in vitro methods using a quantitative high-throughput screening platform. Drug Discov Today 2010;15(23):997–1007.
[112] Adler S, et al. Alternative (non-animal) methods for cosmetics testing: current status and future prospects—2010. Arch Toxicol 2011;85(5):367–485.

Nanotoxicity

12

Samad Ahadian and Milica Radisic
University of Toronto, Toronto, ON, Canada

12.1 Introduction

Nanomaterials have experienced a rapid growth in scientific, technological, and commercial applications leading to the spawn of nanoscience and nanotechnology fields. Several nanomaterial-based products have currently entered the market and new entries are coming on a daily base [1]. A large amount of nanomaterials are annually consumed to fulfill the market requirements [2]. Such manufacturing and utilization of nanomaterials open multiple routes of release and entry of these materials into the environment and human body [3]. Nanomaterials have also found wide applications in biomedicine, particularly in the context of bioimaging, biosensing, delivery of biomolecules, cancer therapy, and regenerative medicine [4]. Some nanotechnology products, such as imaging agents, diagnostic tools and materials, and drugs have already received (or expected to receive) regulatory approvals for human use [5]. Therefore, humans can be exposed to nanomaterials either inadvertently through an uncontrolled environment or deliberately through a known source (e.g., drugs or biomedical agents).

Increasing exposure of humans to nanomaterials and distinct characteristics of these materials need the development of reliable protocols and tools to characterize the nanomaterial properties and in particular their toxicity and hazard. These protocols and tools should be able to evaluate and predict health benefits and hazards associated with nanomaterials available in commercial products and medicine [6]. An ideal assessment regime considers both acute and chronic exposure of nanomaterials at different doses because they correspond to rigorous physicochemical characterization of materials. In addition, physiological reactivity of nanomaterials at molecular, cellular, tissue, and organ levels is considered in assessing the risk-benefit analyses of these materials [7,8]. To this end, many analytical approaches and devices have been developed to reveal the impact of nanomaterial properties on physiological responses and processes in vitro and in vivo. This assessment regime precedes any preclinical/clinical application of nanomaterials and their exposure to humans. A major challenge in the nanotoxicity assessment is that nanomaterials may have distinct properties from their micro- or macroscopic counterparts [9]. For example, a high fractional surface of nanoparticles (<20 nm in size) causes a significant change in physicochemical properties of particles compared with larger particles [10]. Therefore, the toxicological assessment of nanomaterials should be done for all developed nanomaterials regardless of their original nature.

Nanobiomaterials Science, Development and Evaluation. DOI: http://dx.doi.org/10.1016/B978-0-08-100963-5.00012-4

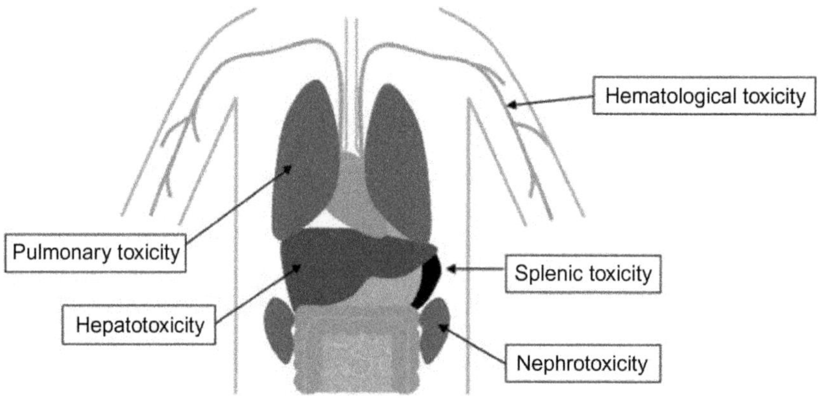

Figure 12.1 Major toxicity forms of nanomaterials in the body [49].

Major toxicity forms of nanomaterials in the body are shown in Fig. 12.1. Nanomaterials in the body can cause the toxicity via some molecular mechanisms. The major molecular mechanism is the formation of oxidative stress using free radicals [11]. The oxidative stress may enhance the inflammation response in the body via the upregulation of reduction-sensitive transcription factors (e.g., NF-κB), kinases, and activator protein-1 [12]. Such free radicals in large quantity can also oxidize and therefore damage biological components such as proteins, lipids, and DNA. Some organs, such as spleen and liver, are the main targets of oxidative stress due to slow removal and accumulation of free radicals along with the prevalence of large number of phagocytes. Other organs with high blood flow, such as lung and kidney, can also be affected by nanomaterials [13]. Nanomaterial interactions with cell nucleus and mitochondria may cause nanotoxicity. Some nanomaterials (e.g., fullerenes, gold nanoparticles, carbon nanotubes (CNTs), and block copolymer micelles) may be localized to the mitochondria and induce reactive oxygen species (ROS) formation and apoptosis [14]. Other toxicity mechanisms associated with nanomaterials may be due to their high interaction with the surrounding environment. Absorption of nanomaterials into the blood circulation may lead to thrombosis and hemolysis. Moreover, nanomaterial interactions with the immune system increase the risk of immunotoxicity [15].

This book chapter reviews commonly used approaches to identify nanomaterial toxicity in vitro and in vivo systems. These nanotoxicological assays are crucial in the characterization of nanomaterials prior to their applications in medicine, biotechnology, agriculture, and ecosystem. Toxicity of different nanomaterials is then discussed using some case studies. As the nanomaterials are quite complex in nature, there may be some inconsistent results showing the different views of nanomaterial safety. Finally, some concluding remarks are given on the nanomaterial toxicity, which may be useful in the design and development of nanomaterials and characterization tools.

12.2 In vitro cell-based toxicity assays

Nanomaterials encounter a wide and complex range of biological species and reactions in vivo, such as different cell types in different tissues and organs, soluble factors, and inflammatory or pathological reactions. Therefore, various in vitro cell-based toxicity assays were created to mimic physiological interactions of nanomaterials with cells and other physiological moieties. Nanomaterials affect cell behaviors and function in multiple ways, such as cell signaling, electron transfer cascades, membrane perturbations, production of chemokines, cytokines, and ROS, gene regulation, intercellular and transcytosis transport, and apoptosis or necrosis [16]. In vitro cell-based toxicity assays typically use primary cells harvested from tissues or cell lines cultured on plastic dishes. Nanomaterials are then applied to the cell culture plates and subsequent cell reactivity to nanomaterials is assessed [17]. A wide range of in vitro cell-based toxicity assays ideally reveal all possible physiological interactions with nanomaterials in vivo. However, there may not be a consistent correlation between the cell response in vitro and that observed in vivo because of complex and dynamic cellular environment in vivo. Therefore, further validation of in vitro cell-based toxicity results with in vivo conditions is crucial. Here, we review commonly used in vitro toxicity assays. In particular, the use of such assays to determine the toxicity of nanomaterials is highlighted.

12.2.1 Reactive oxygen species production assays

ROS can be directly measured in cell medium using fluorescein-based probes or electron paramagnetic resonance (EPR). Dichlorodihydrofluorescein diacetate [18] is a common material, which is oxidized using the ROS and produces the fluorescence light as a measure of nanoparticle concentration in cell media [19]. EPR is able to detect free radicals in the medium even in the presence of cells. For the EPR measurement, a radical-consuming spin probe (4-hydroxy-2,2,6,6-tetramethylpiperidine 1-oxyl) or a spin-trapping agent (5,5-dimethyl-1-pyrroline N-oxide) for superoxide or hydroxide radicals are added to the nanomaterial solution for a period of time. The supernatant is then analyzed on an EPR spectrometer [20,21].

Other ROS measurement assays can evaluate cells exposed to nanomaterials. Cells naturally use glutathione (an endogenous reducing agent derived from a ROS insult) to neutralize deleterious effects of ROS [22]. Therefore, glutathione assay was developed and used to detect the ROS [23]. Other ROS detection assays essentially analyze key oxidized species or aim to measure ROS effects on DNA or cell membrane. For example, immunocytochemistry is used to detect specific DNA lesions (e.g., 8-hydroxydeoxyguanosine) as a measure of ROS-affected DNA damage [20]. As an alternative, BODIPY-C_{11} (a fluorescent dye) is able to insert into lipid bilayers of cells exposed to ROS and distinguish between the unoxidized and oxidized lipids fluorescently as red and green colors, respectively [24].

12.2.2 Cell viability assays

Cell viability assays are mainly based on the cellular metabolism or membrane integrity [25]. Cell viability assays simply quantify the percentage of live cells versus dead cells in response to an external stimulus. Most assays involve the conversion of one or multiple dye precursors in live and/or dead cells, which can then distinguish the cells fluorescently or colorimetrically. Most commonly used cell viability assays to detect nanotoxicity are lactate dehydrogenase [26], trypan blue [20], formazan-based (e.g., 3-(4,5-dimethylthiazol-2-yl)-5-(3-carboxymethoxyphenyl)-2-(4-sulfophenyl)-2H-tetrazolium or MTS [27] and 3-(4,5-dimethylthiazol-2-yl)-2,5-diphenyltetrazolium bromide or MTT) [24] assays), Alamar blue (resazurin) [28], ATP-luciferin luminescence [29], and mitochondrial membrane potential [30] assays. However, there may be some side reactions or ambiguities associated with these assays. For example, cysteamine-coated quantum dots (QDs) catalytically reduced MTT to formazan without affecting the cellular metabolism [31]. The Alamar blue may reduce to a nonfluorescent material due to long incubation times or high density of cell cultures [32]. Therefore, careful calibration is required for all dye-based assays to assess potential interference of nanomaterials with the cell metabolism.

Cells can be sorted and quantified using fluorescence-activated cell sorting (FACS) in terms of live, dead, and apoptotic [33]. Moreover, FACS is able to reveal molecular mechanisms of nanotoxicity, such as measuring the upregulation of Fas receptor, an important signaling pathway in apoptosis [34]. FACS can be automated and simultaneously do the processing of several cells in one cell viability assay [35].

Other cell viability assays to evaluate nanotoxicity include specific enzyme-linked immunosorbent assay (ELISA) kits [36], Hoechst-DNA [37], Caspase [38], comet [39], and terminal deoxynucleotidyl transferase dUTP nick end labeling (TUNEL) assays [40]. The latter assays are sensitive to molecular pathways involving the apoptotic DNA fragmentation of cells. The ELISA uses antibodies (e.g., epidermal growth factor receptors) and fluorescence colorimeter to differentiate between live and dead cells [41]. The Hoechst-DNA, as a fluorescent probe, attaches to the double-stranded DNA with high amount of adenine-thymine extracted from the nucleus of cells under stress [42]. The Caspase measures the downstream regulators of the mitochondrial apoptotic pathway [43]. The comet assay uses gel electrophoresis to quantify the fragmented DNA [44]. The TUNEL quantifies the amount of fragmented DNA in cell nuclei as a measure of cell apoptosis [45]. These assays should be used with nanomaterials in cell-free medium as a control to detect any interference of nanomaterials with the assays.

12.2.3 Cell stress assays

Changes in cellular behavior or nonlethal injuries can be observed for cells exposed to nanomaterials. These injuries or changes can be revealed in gene or protein expression, inflammation reaction, and phagocytic ability of cells. Therefore, some characterization methods to determine the cell phenotype and its stability are used as cell stress assays to determine the nanotoxicity. These methods include polymerase chain reaction (PCR), Western blotting, and other protein assay analyses. In particular, the expression of GADD45β (DNA damage-dependent), CDKN1A (cell-cycle arrest gene), NFκBIA (inflammatory response), NF-κB (upregulator of cytokines, adhesion molecules, and fibrotic/inflammatory growth factors), EGFP (reporter gene), and IL-6 (inflammatory response) is assessed using quantitative, real-time PCR (qPCR) [46]. Major cellular proteins in the nanotoxicity pathways (e.g., chemokines and cytokines) are evaluated using the Western blotting [47].

12.3 Analysis of toxicity in vivo

Assessing nanotoxicity in vivo is a daunting task because the nanomaterial complexity has led to conflicting studies about the safe use of nanomaterials in vivo [48]. Unique properties of each nanomaterial make the generalization of nanotoxicity rather complicated. Therefore, it is necessary to evaluate all aspects of nanotoxicity for any underlying nanomaterial to predict its behaviors and fate in vivo. Examination of chronic exposure and long-term toxicity of nanomaterials are two important factors to understand the nanotoxicity in vivo [49]. In vivo toxicity assays are expensive, time-consuming, and involve ethical issues of using animals. However, they are more suitable to model the high complexity of human body than in vitro cell-based assays. There are some nanotoxicity studies reflecting contradictory results of toxicity analysis between in vitro and in vivo conditions [50]. For example, Sayes *et al.* employed in vitro cell-based assays to predict in vivo nanotoxicity of ZnO nanoparticles and showed that the in vitro assays did not demonstrate the toxicity associated with ZnO nanoparticles in vivo [51]. Therefore, it is crucial to do nanotoxicity analysis in vivo to precisely determine the safe use of a nanomaterial.

12.4 Nanomaterial toxicity

The nanotoxicity can result from composition, purity, size, and shape of nanomaterials [52]. Degradability of nanomaterial is also an important parameter affecting long-term and acute toxicity of nanomaterials. Accumulation of nondegradable nanomaterials in tissues and organs can cause detrimental problems for cells and tissues in the body [53]. On the other hand, biodegradation products of nanomaterials can cause unpredicted nanotoxicity [54]. Slow dissolution and shape of nanomaterials can affect the macrophage-mediated clearance of nanomaterials from the body. Champion and Mitragotri evaluated the interaction of alveolar macrophages with nanomaterials with different shapes [55]. They found that the macrophage spreading onto the nanomaterials is required for an effective clearance of nanomaterials. In this section, some research studies on the nanotoxicity of commonly used nanomaterials are summarized and discussed.

12.4.1 Gold nanoparticles

Facile synthesis, ease of surface functionalization, and stability have made gold nanomaterials an attractive option for protein and gene delivery, cancer treatment, implants (e.g., stents and pacemakers), and biological imaging [56]. Moreover, gold was reported to be an antirheumatic and antiinflammatory agent (e.g., Tauredon and Auranofin) to treat rheumatoid arthritis [57]. Some studies have assumed that gold nanomaterials are nontoxic most likely due to the well-known safety of bulk gold. However, gold behaves differently at the nanoscale dimensions compared with bulk gold. Some studies showed that gold nanomaterials may become toxic using cyanidation or oxidation in the body [58]. Gold nanomaterials can be heavily absorbed by the kidneys leading to eryptosis (erythrocyte suicidal death) or nephrotoxicity [59]. Shape, size, and surface charge are main design parameters to overwhelm the potential toxicity of gold nanomaterials [60].

12.4.2 Silver nanoparticles

Silver nanoparticles have widely been employed as antibacterial agents and thereby may exert toxic effects on the human health [61]. The toxicity of silver nanoparticles has been demonstrated for some cell types and animal models [62]. Silver nanoparticles can migrate to the olfactory bulb upon the inhalation or can enter into the kidneys, circulatory system, heart, and liver [63]. These nanoparticles were found in patients with colon cancer [64] and in patients with blood diseases [65]. In vivo toxicity of silver nanoparticles was evaluated using a mouse model [66]. The cytotoxic effects of nanoparticles on the sperm function and embryo development were studied (Fig. 12.2). The silver nanoparticles significantly decreased the rate of sperm fertilization and viability in a dose-dependent manner due to the internalization of nanoparticles into the sperms. In general, size, route of exposure, and concentration of silver nanoparticles are crucial parameters to determine the nanotoxicity of particles [67].

12.4.3 Metal oxides

Metal oxide nanoparticles (e.g., TiO_2 and magnetite) have been used in water treatment [68], groundwater remediation [69], pharmaceuticals [70], and removal of toxic elements from air [71]. Such wide applications of metal oxide nanoparticles increase their level of exposure to biological systems via dermal contact, inhalation, or ingestion. It was shown that CeO_2 nanoparticles can be introduced into human fibroblasts in vitro without affecting the cell viability [72]. Interestingly, Xu *et al.* showed that the nanotoxicity of metal oxide nanoparticles (CuO and ZnO) was associated with their electrical conductivity [73]. Karlsson *et al.* measured DNA damage and oxidative stress caused by different metal oxide nanoparticles (i.e., TiO_2, CuO, ZnO, Fe_2O_3, $CuZnFe_2O_4$, and Fe_3O_4) [74]. They showed that the nanotoxicity varied widely among the underlying nanoparticles. CuO nanoparticles caused the highest level of DNA damage and cytotoxicity. ZnO affected the cell viability and DNA damage, while the TiO_2 nanoparticles only led to the DNA damage. Iron oxide nanoparticles (Fe_2O_3 and Fe_3O_4) showed no or low cytotoxicity and $CuZnFe_2O_4$ particles had a moderate cytotoxicity effect.

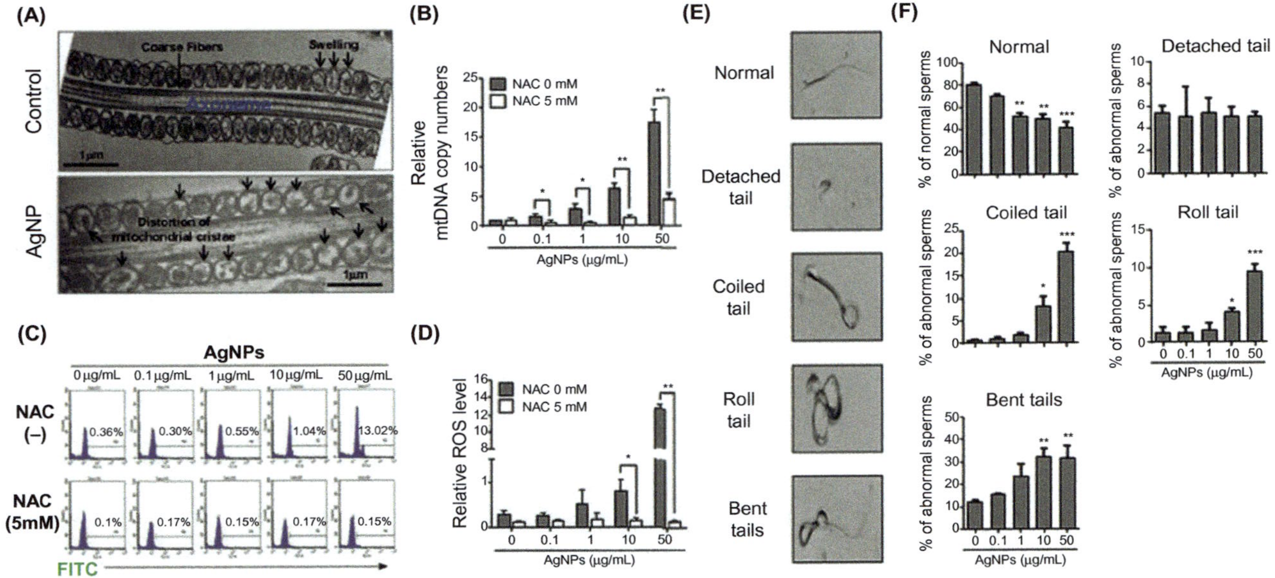

Figure 12.2 ROS analysis, mitochondrial damage, and sperm morphology after the treatment with different concentrations of silver nanoparticles. (A) The mitochondrial sheath in nanoparticle-treated and control sperm cells revealed by transmission electron microscopy. The arrows show the mitochondria swelling in the sheath. (B) Quantification of mitochondrial copy number in nanoparticle-treated sperms in the presence or absence of N-acetyl-L-cysteine (NAC) (a ROS inhibitor) pretreatment. The mitochondrial copy number was determined using qPCR. (C and D) Flow cytometry results showing the ROS in nanoparticle-treated sperms stained with 2′,7′-dichlorodihydrofluorescein diacetate-fluorescein isothiocyanate (DCFH-DA-FITC) in the presence or absence of NAC. (E) A morphological pattern picture of sperms taken by phase contrast microscopy. (F) The morphological analysis for five categories of normal morphology, coiled tail, detached head, bent tails, and roll tail (*$P < .05$, **$P < .01$, and ***$P < .001$) [66].

12.4.4 Carbon nanotubes

CNTs consist of one or multiple graphene sheets arranged into a cylindrical structure [75]. One single sheet of graphene forms single-walled CNTs, while multiwalled CNTs consist of more than one graphene sheets. CNTs have found wide biomedical applications ranging from tissue regeneration, bioimaging, biosensing, gene and drug delivery, and stem cell differentiation due to their unique structure, high mechanical strength, high electrical conductivity, and visibility in infrared region [76]. The safe use of CNTs is still under debate most likely due to the lack of complete and systematic toxicity analyses [77]. CNT characteristics, such as length, diameter, functionalization, and purity are potential factors to influence the nanotoxicity of CNTs in vitro and in vivo. We showed that highly pure and carboxyl-functionalized CNTs are not toxic to skeletal muscle cells and can be used to fabricate contractile skeletal muscle tissues [78,79]. Hydrophobic nature of CNTs can cause the CNT aggregation in aqueous media. The aggregate size is a primary concern for the nanotoxicity of CNTs in vivo. Therefore, pristine CNTs are usually dispersed in hydrogels [80] or biocompatible surfactants, such as Pluronic F108 or Tween 80 [81]. The accumulation of CNTs has been observed in the liver, lungs, and spleen [82]. However, no acute toxicity was reported for the tissues. It was discovered that single-walled CNTs were aggregated and wrapped by secreted proteins from cells [83]. Simultaneously, the upregulation of apoptosis-related genes occurred.

12.4.5 Graphene

Graphene consists of sp^2-hybridized carbons arranged in a single-layer and hexagonal structure [84]. Graphene was first fabricated from monocrystalline graphitic films [85]. Similar to CNTs, graphene-based nanomaterials have recently attracted much attention in tissue engineering, delivery of biomolecules, biosensing, and bioimaging due to extraordinary mechanical, electrical, and optical properties [86]. However, there have been less toxicity studies on graphene compared with CNTs. Chang *et al.* showed that graphene oxide has no obvious toxicity effect on A549 cells and the cells favorably proliferated on the graphene oxide films [87]. However, Zhang *et al.* demonstrated the stress-induced nanotoxicity of graphene oxide in vivo [88]. The formation of oxidizing cytochrome c and high production of hydroxyl radicals were responsible for the nanotoxicity of graphene oxide. Sadisharan *et al.* showed that pristine graphene was found on the Vero cell membrane causing high oxidative stress and apoptosis, while carboxyl-functionalized graphene showed no nanotoxicity despite internalizing the cell membrane (Fig. 12.3) [89]. Pristine graphene is hydrophobic and therefore has high potential of aggregation and toxicity in biological media. Therefore, some methods have been proposed to functionalize graphene and to make stable aqueous dispersions of graphene. In our recent work, bovine serum albumin (BSA) was used to make highly stable and aqueous dispersion of graphene in a facile and scalable manner [90]. The BSA physically interacted with the graphene sheets without compromising electrical and mechanical properties of pristine graphene. As recently reviewed by Kiew *et al.*, physicochemical properties of graphene (e.g., size,

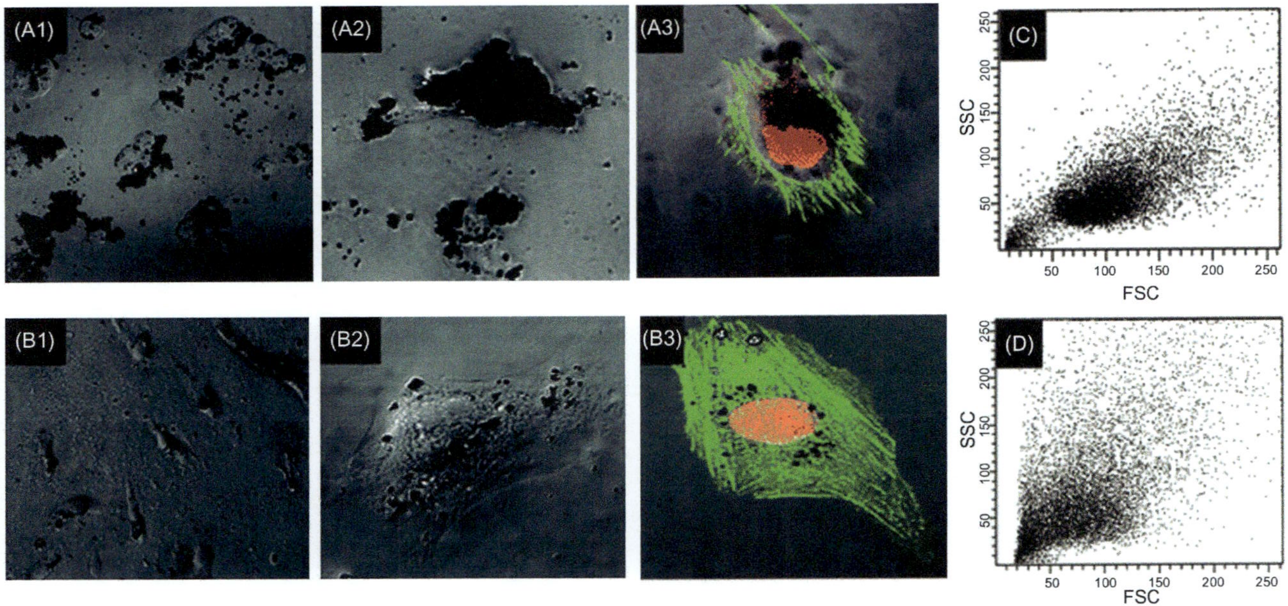

Figure 12.3 Confocal pictures and flow cytometry data showing the uptake of pristine graphene and carboxyl-functionalized graphene in Vero cells. (A1 and A2) Bright field images depicting the accumulation of carboxyl-functionalized graphene on the plasma membrane of cells. (B1 and B2) Intracellular uptake of carboxyl-functionalized graphene. Fluorescence confocal pictures of F-actin for the cells treated with the pristine graphene (A3) and carboxyl-functionalized graphene (B3). Flow cytometry data shows an enhanced forward scattering in (C) cells treated with the pristine graphene and an increase in side scattering in (D) cells treated with the carboxyl-functionalized graphene [89].

number of layers, functional groups, and reduction state) and exposure method are crucial parameters to evaluate the nanotoxicity of graphene-based nanomaterials [91].

12.4.6 Quantum dots

QDs are semiconductor nanocrystals having unique electrical and optical properties [92]. QDs have a broad absorption, high brightness, narrow line width in emission spectra, long fluorescence lifetime with little photobleaching over time, and tunable emission maxima [93]. These characteristics have made QDs popular in medicine and biotechnology as fluorescent probes in bioimaging for targeting DNA, peroxisomes, and cells [94]. The safe use of QDs in vivo is an ongoing research topic. The main problem of QD nanotoxicity in the body is nephrotoxicity due to their absorption and accumulation in the kidneys [95]. For instance, gadolinium-based contrast agents used in clinical magnetic resonance imaging were shown to cause acute renal failure [96]. While some researchers consider QDs as bioinert when their metallic core is completely passivated, other researchers still doubt the safety of QDs. Selenium and cadmium, as the most used metals in QD cores, may cause chronic and acute cytotoxicities in vertebrates and possess significant environmental and health concerns [97].

12.5 Future trends

Currently used nanotoxicology assays often lack high accuracy, sensitivity, and selectivity. Moreover, the complex nature of biological systems makes it difficult to obtain reliable information on the toxicity of nanomaterials [1]. There is no consensus among researchers regarding experimental designs and protocols of nanotoxicity studies. As a result, irreproducible and conflicting results can be found in the literature. Therefore, novel analytical tools and more importantly standardized methods are required to reliably and accurately determine the toxicology of nanomaterials. The latter requires a multidisciplinary team of molecular biologists, material scientists, and toxicologists to make sure that all aspects of nanotoxicology are considered. Such collaboration greatly helps us to fundamentally understand the biological interactions of nanomaterials with proteins, cells, tissues, and organs, which is important in the safe design and fabrication of nanomaterials. Prior to the use of nanomaterials in the clinic and industrial products, nanomaterials should show a high level of biocompatibility with minimal negative effects on cell viability and tissue function in vitro and in vivo [98].

Nanomaterials should not be considered biocompatible because of safety of their bulk materials. Physicochemical characteristics of nanomaterials (e.g., shape, size, surface charge, degree of aggregation, and surface chemistry) may affect the potential toxicity of nanomaterials. Long-term and chronic exposure of nanomaterials is important to understanding the nanotoxicity in vivo. Complex nature of nanomaterials may arise their unexpected interactions with biological moieties. Therefore, nanotoxicity experiments and assays should carefully be designed and performed to reveal all possible interactions of nanomaterials with biological components.

High-throughput analysis of advanced cell-based assays enables us to screen nanotoxicity of multiple nanomaterials at different concentrations on different cell types, simultaneously [99]. Such expanded experimental setup is useful to increase the level of accuracy and biomimicry of nanotoxicity assays. Moreover, high-throughput nanotoxicity assays may significantly reduce time and cost associated with commonly used nanotoxicity assays [100]. Numerous nanomaterial–cell interactions can be processed in high-throughput nanotoxicity assays in parallel to evaluating any potential cytotoxicity effect of nanomaterials in vivo [101]. As an example, Manshian *et al.* used a high-content imaging and PCR technique to reveal the nanotoxicity of silver nanoparticles coated with different polymers exposed to endothelial and neural cells [102]. They found that the particles coated with poly(ethylene glycol) had the highest level of toxicity.

Finally, nanotoxicity studies have significantly increased our understanding of environmental and health issues of nanomaterials. As a result, the human exposure to potentially toxic nanomaterials is substantially decreased. Nanotoxicity studies hold promise to further reveal molecular mechanisms associated with the nanomaterial toxicity and disease. In addition, these studies will be helpful in the development of safety policies regarding synthesis, commercial use, and recycling of nanomaterials.

12.6 Conclusions

Increasing exposure of humans to nanomaterials from synthetic and natural sources has motivated researchers to study nanotoxicity effects of nanomaterials. Herein, we described some commonly used assays to measure the toxicity of nanomaterials in vitro and in vivo. Some nanotoxicity studies were then discussed focusing on the toxicity of specific nanomaterials (i.e., metallic nanoparticles, metal oxides, CNTs, graphene, and QDs).

References

[1] Jones CF, Grainger DW. In vitro assessments of nanomaterial toxicity. Adv Drug Del Rev 2009;61:438–56.

[2] Park B. Chapter 1: Current and future applications of nanotechnology Hester RE, Harrison RM, editors. Nanotechnology: consequences for human health and the environment. The Royal Society of Chemistry; 2007. p. 1–18.

[3] Theodore L, Kunz RG. Chapter 1: Nanotechnology/environmental overview. Nanotechnology: environmental implications and solutions. Wiley; 2005. p. 1–60.

[4] Gurung S, Fei D, Ge Y. Chapter 16: Intersection of nanotechnology and healthcare Ge Y, Li S, Wang S, Moore R, editors. Nanomedicine. Springer; 2014. p. 341–54.

[5] Chakraborty M, Jain S, Rani V. Nanotechnology: emerging tool for diagnostics and therapeutics. Appl Biochem Biotechnol 2011;165:1178–87.

[6] Dhawan A, Sharma V. Toxicity assessment of nanomaterials: methods and challenges. Anal Bioanal Chem 2010;398:589–605.

[7] Nel A, Xia T, Mädler L, Li N. Toxic potential of materials at the nanolevel. Science 2006;311:622–7.
[8] Warheit DB. How meaningful are the results of nanotoxicity studies in the absence of adequate material characterization? Toxicol Sci 2008;101:183–5.
[9] Auffan M, Rose J, Bottero J-Y, Lowry GV, Jolivet J-P, Wiesner MR. Towards a definition of inorganic nanoparticles from an environmental, health and safety perspective. Nat Nano 2009;4:634–41.
[10] Campbell CT, Parker SC, Starr DE. The effect of size-dependent nanoparticle energetics on catalyst sintering. Science 2002;298:811–4.
[11] Lanone S, Boczkowski J. Biomedical applications and potential health risks of nanomaterials: molecular mechanisms. Curr Mol Med 2006;6:651–63.
[12] Rahman I, Biswas SK, Jimenez LA, Torres M, Forman HJ. Glutathione, stress responses, and redox signaling in lung inflammation. Antioxid Redox Signaling 2004;7:42–59.
[13] Arora S, Rajwade JM, Paknikar KM. Nanotoxicology and in vitro studies: the need of the hour. Toxicol Appl Pharmacol 2012;258:151–65.
[14] Unfried K, Albrecht C, Klotz L-O, Von Mikecz A, Grether-Beck S, Schins RPF. Cellular responses to nanoparticles: target structures and mechanisms. Nanotoxicology 2007;1:52–71.
[15] Dobrovolskaia MA, McNeil SE. Immunological properties of engineered nanomaterials. Nat Nanotechnol 2007;2:469–78.
[16] Veranth JM. Chapter 11: In vitro models for nanoparticle toxicology Grassian VH, editor. Nanoscience and nanotechnology: environmental and health impacts. Hoboken: Wiley; 2008. p. 261–86.
[17] Melo PS, Marcato PD, de Araújo DR, Durán N. Chapter 5: In vitro cytotoxicity assays of nanoparticles on different cell lines Durán N, Guterres SS, Alves OL, editors. Nanotoxicology. New York: Springer; 2014. p. 111–23.
[18] Hussain SM, Hess KL, Gearhart JM, Geiss KT, Schlager JJ. In vitro toxicity of nanoparticles in BRL 3A rat liver cells. Toxicol In Vitro 2005;19:975–83.
[19] Long TC, Tajuba J, Sama P, Saleh N, Swartz C, Parker J, et al. Nanosize titanium dioxide stimulates reactive oxygen species in brain microglia and damages neurons in vitro. Environ Health Perspect 2007;115:1631–7.
[20] Schins RPF, Duffin R, Höhr D, Knaapen AM, Shi T, Weishaupt C, et al. Surface modification of quartz inhibits toxicity, particle uptake, and oxidative DNA damage in human lung epithelial cells. Chem Res Toxicol 2002;15:1166–73.
[21] Singh S, Shi T, Duffin R, Albrecht C, van Berlo D, Höhr D, et al. Endocytosis, oxidative stress and IL-8 expression in human lung epithelial cells upon treatment with fine and ultrafine TiO_2: role of the specific surface area and of surface methylation of the particles. Toxicol Appl Pharmacol 2007;222:141–51.
[22] Chang H-H, Guo M-K, Kasten FH, Chang M-C, Huang G-F, Wang Y-L, et al. Stimulation of glutathione depletion, ROS production and cell cycle arrest of dental pulp cells and gingival epithelial cells by HEMA. Biomaterials 2005;26:745–53.
[23] Lewinski N, Colvin V, Drezek R. Cytotoxicity of nanoparticles. Small 2008;4:26–49.
[24] Choi AO, Cho SJ, Desbarats J, Lovrić J, Maysinger D. Quantum dot-induced cell death involves Fas upregulation and lipid peroxidation in human neuroblastoma cells. J Nanobiotechnol 2007;5:1–13.
[25] Astashkina A, Mann B, Grainger DW. A critical evaluation of in vitro cell culture models for high-throughput drug screening and toxicity. Pharmacol Ther 2012;134:82–106.
[26] Lin W, Huang Y-W, Zhou X-D, Ma Y. In vitro toxicity of silica nanoparticles in human lung cancer cells. Toxicol Appl Pharmacol 2006;217:252–9.

[27] Dong L, Joseph KL, Witkowski CM, Craig MM. Cytotoxicity of single-walled carbon nanotubes suspended in various surfactants. Nanotechnology 2008;19:255702.
[28] Srinivasan S, Jayasree R, Chennazhi KP, Nair SV, Jayakumar R. Biocompatible alginate/nano bioactive glass ceramic composite scaffolds for periodontal tissue regeneration. Carbohydr Polym 2012;87:274–83.
[29] Liu C, Zhang P, Zhai X, Tian F, Li W, Yang J, et al. Nano-carrier for gene delivery and bioimaging based on carbon dots with PEI-passivation enhanced fluorescence. Biomaterials 2012;33:3604–13.
[30] Xue C, Wu J, Lan F, Liu W, Yang X, Zeng F, et al. Nano titanium dioxide induces the generation of ROS and potential damage in HaCaT cells under UVA irradiation. J Nanosci Nanotechnol 2010;10:8500–7.
[31] Hoshino A, Fujioka K, Oku T, Suga M, Sasaki YF, Ohta T, et al. Physicochemical properties and cellular toxicity of nanocrystal quantum dots depend on their surface modification. Nano Lett 2004;4:2163–9.
[32] Rampersad SN. Multiple applications of Alamar Blue as an indicator of metabolic function and cellular health in cell viability bioassays. Sensors 2012;12:12347–60.
[33] Albrecht C, Borm PJA, Adolf B, Timblin CR, Mossman BT. In vitro and in vivo activation of extracellular signal-regulated kinases by coal dusts and quartz silica. Toxicol Appl Pharmacol 2002;184:37–45.
[34] Stel AJ, Cate B, Jacobs S, Kok JW, Spierings DCJ, Dondorff M, et al. Fas receptor clustering and involvement of the death receptor pathway in rituximab-mediated apoptosis with concomitant sensitization of Lymphoma B cells to Fas-induced apoptosis. J Immunol 2007;178:2287–95.
[35] Weissleder R, Kelly K, Sun EY, Shtatland T, Josephson L. Cell-specific targeting of nanoparticles by multivalent attachment of small molecules. Nat Biotechnol 2005;23:1418–23.
[36] Tian F, Cui D, Schwarz H, Estrada GG, Kobayashi H. Cytotoxicity of single-wall carbon nanotubes on human fibroblasts. Toxicol In Vitro 2006;20:1202–12.
[37] Griffin M, Nayyer L, Butler PE, Palgrave RG, Seifalian AM, Kalaskar DM. Development of mechano-responsive polymeric scaffolds using functionalised silica nano fillers for the control of cellular functions. Nanomed Nanotechnol Biol Med 2016.
[38] Kwon H-K, Lee J-H, Shin H-J, Kim J-H, Choi S. Structural and functional analysis of cell adhesion and nuclear envelope nano-topography in cell death. Sci Rep 2015;5:15623.
[39] Tice RR, Agurell E, Anderson D, Burlinson B, Hartmann A, Kobayashi H, et al. Single cell gel/comet assay: guidelines for in vitro and in vivo genetic toxicology testing. Environ Mol Mutag 2000;35:206–21.
[40] Yim EKF, Pang SW, Leong KW. Synthetic nanostructures inducing differentiation of human mesenchymal stem cells into neuronal lineage. Exp Cell Res 2007;313:1820–9.
[41] Fischer D, Li Y, Ahlemeyer B, Krieglstein J, Kissel T. In vitro cytotoxicity testing of polycations: influence of polymer structure on cell viability and hemolysis. Biomaterials 2003;24:1121–31.
[42] Crissman HA, Steinkamp JA. A new method for rapid and sensitive detection of bromodeoxyuridine in DNA-replicating cells. Exp Cell Res 1987;173:256–61.
[43] Chien W, Kumagai T, Miller CW, Desmond JC, Frank JM, Said JW, et al. Cyr61 suppresses growth of human endometrial cancer cells. J Biol Chem 2004;279:53087–96.
[44] McKelvey-Martin VJ, Green MHL, Schmezer P, Pool-Zobel BL, De Méo MP, Collins A. The single cell gel electrophoresis assay (comet assay): a European review. Mutat Res 1993;288:47–63.
[45] Kraupp BG, Ruttkay-Nedecky B, Koudelka H, Bukowska K, Bursch W, Schulte-Hermann R. In situ detection of fragmented DNA (TUNEL assay) fails to discriminate

among apoptosis, necrosis, and autolytic cell death: a cautionary note. Hepatology 1995;21:1465–8.
[46] Arenz A, Hellweg CE, Stojicic N, Baumstark-Khan C, Grotheer HH. Gene expression modulation in A549 human lung cells in response to combustion-generated nano-sized particles. Ann N Y Acad Sci 2006;1091:170–83.
[47] Karlsson M, Pålsgård E, Wilshaw PR, Di Silvio L. Initial in vitro interaction of osteoblasts with nano-porous alumina. Biomaterials 2003;24:3039–46.
[48] Powers KW, Brown SC, Krishna VB, Wasdo SC, Moudgil BM, Roberts SM. Research strategies for safety evaluation of nanomaterials. Part VI. Characterization of nanoscale particles for toxicological evaluation. Toxicol Sci 2006;90:296–303.
[49] Aillon KL, Xie Y, El-Gendy N, Berkland CJ, Forrest ML. Effects of nanomaterial physicochemical properties on in vivo toxicity. Adv Drug Del Rev 2009;61:457–66.
[50] Khlebtsov N, Dykman L. Biodistribution and toxicity of engineered gold nanoparticles: a review of in vitro and in vivo studies. Chem Soc Rev 2011;40:1647–71.
[51] Sayes CM, Reed KL, Subramoney S, Abrams L, Warheit DB. Can in vitro assays substitute for in vivo studies in assessing the pulmonary hazards of fine and nanoscale materials? J Nanopart Res 2009;11:421–31.
[52] Krug HF, Wick P. Nanotoxicology: an interdisciplinary challenge. Angew Chem Int Ed 2011;50:1260–78.
[53] Garnett MC, Kallinteri P. Nanomedicines and nanotoxicology: some physiological principles. Occup Med 2006;56:307–11.
[54] Baati T, Njim L, Neffati F, Kerkeni A, Bouttemi M, Gref R, et al. In depth analysis of the in vivo toxicity of nanoparticles of porous iron (III) metal–organic frameworks. Chem Sci 2013;4:1597–607.
[55] Champion JA, Mitragotri S. Role of target geometry in phagocytosis. Proc Natl Acad Sci USA 2006;103:4930–4.
[56] Chen PC, Mwakwari SC, Oyelere AK. Gold nanoparticles: from nanomedicine to nanosensing. Nanotechnol Sci Appl 2008;1:45–66.
[57] Murphy CJ, Gole AM, Stone JW, Sisco PN, Alkilany AM, Goldsmith EC, et al. Gold nanoparticles in biology: beyond toxicity to cellular imaging. Acc Chem Res 2008;41:1721–30.
[58] Williams ML. Core chemistry of gold and its complexes. Inflammopharmacology 2008;16:110–1.
[59] Sereemaspun A, Rojanathanes R, Wiwanitkit V. Effect of gold nanoparticle on renal cell: an implication for exposure risk. Ren Fail 2008;30:323–5.
[60] Tsoli M, Kuhn H, Brandau W, Esche H, Schmid G. Cellular uptake and toxicity of Au55 clusters. Small 2005;1:841–4.
[61] Antony JJ, Sivalingam P, Chen B. Toxicological effects of silver nanoparticles. Environ Toxicol Pharmacol 2015;40:729–32.
[62] Soto KF, Carrasco A, Powell TG, Garza KM, Murr LE. Comparative in vitro cytotoxicity assessment of some manufacturednanoparticulate materials characterized by transmissionelectron microscopy. J Nanopart Res 2005;7:145–69.
[63] Takenaka S, Karg E, Roth C, Schulz H, Ziesenis A, Heinzmann U, et al. Pulmonary and systemic distribution of inhaled ultrafine silver particles in rats. Environ Health Perspect 2001;109:547–51.
[64] Gatti AM. Biocompatibility of micro- and nano-particles in the colon. Part II. Biomaterials 2004;25:385–92.
[65] Gatti AM, Montanari S, Monari E, Gambarelli A, Capitani F, Parisini B. Detection of micro-and nano-sized biocompatible particles in the blood. J Mater Sci Mater Med 2004;15:469–72.

[66] Yoisungnern T, Choi Y-J, Han JW, Kang M-H, Das J, Gurunathan S, et al. Internalization of silver nanoparticles into mouse spermatozoa results in poor fertilization and compromised embryo development. Sci Rep 2015;5:11170.
[67] Gaillet S, Rouanet J-M. Silver nanoparticles: their potential toxic effects after oral exposure and underlying mechanisms-A review. Food Chem Toxicol 2015;77:58–63.
[68] Ferguson MA, Hoffmann MR, Hering JG. TiO_2-photocatalyzed As (III) oxidation in aqueous suspensions: reaction kinetics and effects of adsorption. Environ Sci Technol 2005;39:1880–6.
[69] Mattigod SV, Fryxell GE, Alford K, Gilmore T, Parker K, Serne J, et al. Functionalized TiO_2 nanoparticles for use for in situ anion immobilization. Environ Sci Technol 2005;39:7306–10.
[70] Ray PC, Yu H, Fu PP. Toxicity and environmental risks of nanomaterials: challenges and future needs. J Environ Sci Health C 2009;27:1–35.
[71] Esterkin CR, Negro AC, Alfano OM, Cassano AE. Air pollution remediation in a fixed bed photocatalytic reactor coated with TiO_2. AIChE J 2005;51:2298–310.
[72] Limbach LK, Li Y, Grass RN, Brunner TJ, Hintermann MA, Muller M, et al. Oxide nanoparticle uptake in human lung fibroblasts: effects of particle size, agglomeration, and diffusion at low concentrations. Environ Sci Technol 2005;39:9370–6.
[73] Xu M, Fujita D, Kajiwara S, Minowa T, Li X, Takemura T, et al. Contribution of physicochemical characteristics of nano-oxides to cytotoxicity. Biomaterials 2010;31:8022–31.
[74] Karlsson HL, Cronholm P, Gustafsson J, Möller L. Copper oxide nanoparticles are highly toxic: a comparison between metal oxide nanoparticles and carbon nanotubes. Chem Res Toxicol 2008;21:1726–32.
[75] Ahadian S, Kawazoe Y. An artificial intelligence approach for modeling and prediction of water diffusion inside a carbon nanotube. Nanoscale Res Lett 2009;4:1054–8.
[76] Ramón-Azcón J, Ahadian S, Obregón R, Shiku H, Ramalingam M, Matsue T. Applications of carbon nanotubes in stem cell research. J Biomed Nanotechnol 2014;10:2539–61.
[77] Fiorito S, Serafino A, Andreola F, Togna A, Togna G. Toxicity and biocompatibility of carbon nanoparticles. J Nanosci Nanotechnol 2006;6:591–9.
[78] Ahadian S, Ramón-Azcón J, Estili M, Liang X, Ostrovidov S, Shiku H, et al. Hybrid hydrogels containing vertically aligned carbon nanotubes with anisotropic electrical conductivity for muscle myofiber fabrication. Sci Rep 2014;4:4271.
[79] Ramón-Azcón J, Ahadian S, Estili M, Liang X, Ostrovidov S, Kaji H, et al. Dielectrophoretically aligned carbon nanotubes to control electrical and mechanical properties of hydrogels to fabricate contractile muscle myofibers. Adv Mater 2013;25:4028–34.
[80] Shin SR, Jung SM, Zalabany M, Kim K, Zorlutuna P, Kim Sb, et al. Carbon-nanotube-embedded hydrogel sheets for engineering cardiac constructs and bioactuators. ACS Nano 2013;7:2369–80.
[81] Cherukuri P, Gannon CJ, Leeuw TK, Schmidt HK, Smalley RE, Curley SA, et al. Mammalian pharmacokinetics of carbon nanotubes using intrinsic near-infrared fluorescence. Proc Natl Acad Sci USA 2006;103:18882–6.
[82] Yang S-T, Guo W, Lin Y, Deng X-Y, Wang H-F, Sun H-F, et al. Biodistribution of pristine single-walled carbon nanotubes in vivo. J Phys Chem C 2007;111:17761–4.
[83] Cherukuri P, Bachilo SM, Litovsky SH, Weisman RB. Near-infrared fluorescence microscopy of single-walled carbon nanotubes in phagocytic cells. J Am Chem Soc 2004;126:15638–9.
[84] Ahadian S, Zhou Y, Yamada S, Estili M, Liang X, Nakajima K, et al. Graphene induces spontaneous cardiac differentiation in embryoid bodies. Nanoscale 2016;8:7075–84.

[85] Novoselov KS, Geim AK, Morozov SV, Jiang D, Zhang Y, Dubonos SV, et al. Electric field effect in atomically thin carbon films. Science 2004;306:666–9.
[86] Zhang H, Grüner G, Zhao Y. Recent advancements of graphene in biomedicine. J Mater Chem B 2013;1:2542–67.
[87] Chang Y, Yang S-T, Liu J-H, Dong E, Wang Y, Cao A, et al. In vitro toxicity evaluation of graphene oxide on A549 cells. Toxicol Lett 2011;200:201–10.
[88] Zhang W, Wang C, Li Z, Lu Z, Li Y, Yin J-J, et al. Unraveling stress-induced toxicity properties of graphene oxide and the underlying mechanism. Adv Mater 2012;24:5391–7.
[89] Sasidharan A, Panchakarla LS, Chandran P, Menon D, Nair S, Rao CNR, et al. Differential nano-bio interactions and toxicity effects of pristine versus functionalized graphene. Nanoscale 2011;3:2461–4.
[90] Ahadian S, Estili M, Surya VJ, Ramón-Azcón J, Liang X, Shiku H, et al. Facile and green production of aqueous graphene dispersions for biomedical applications. Nanoscale 2015;7:6436–43.
[91] Kiew SF, Kiew LV, Lee HB, Imae T, Chung LY. Assessing biocompatibility of graphene oxide-based nanocarriers: A review. J Control Release 2016;226:217–28.
[92] Bruchez M, Moronne M, Gin P, Weiss S, Alivisatos AP. Semiconductor nanocrystals as fluorescent biological labels. Science 1998;281:2013–6.
[93] Riegler J, Nann T. Application of luminescent nanocrystals as labels for biological molecules. Anal Bioanal Chem 2004;379:913–9.
[94] Larson DR, Zipfel WR, Williams RM, Clark SW, Bruchez MP, Wise FW, et al. Water-soluble quantum dots for multiphoton fluorescence imaging in vivo. Science 2003;300:1434–6.
[95] Barbier O, Jacquillet G, Tauc M, Cougnon M, Poujeol P. Effect of heavy metals on, and handling by, the kidney. Nephron Physiol 2005;99:105–10.
[96] Akgun H, Gonlusen G, Cartwright JJ, Suki WN, Truong LD. Are gadolinium-based contrast media nephrotoxic: A renal biopsy study. Arch Pathol Lab Med 2006;130:1354–7.
[97] Zhang T, Stilwell JL, Gerion D, Ding L, Elboudwarej O, Cooke PA, et al. Cellular effect of high doses of silica-coated quantum dot profiled with high throughput gene expression analysis and high content cellomics measurements. Nano Lett 2006;6:800–8.
[98] Sharifi S, Behzadi S, Laurent S, Forrest ML, Stroeve P, Mahmoudi M. Toxicity of nanomaterials. Chem Soc Rev 2012;41:2323–43.
[99] Brayden DJ, Cryan S-A, Dawson KA, O'Brien PJ, Simpson JC. High-content analysis for drug delivery and nanoparticle applications. Drug Discov Today 2015;20:942–57.
[100] Nel A, Xia T, Meng H, Wang X, Lin S, Ji Z, et al. Nanomaterial toxicity testing in the 21st century: use of a predictive toxicological approach and high-throughput screening. Acc Chem Res 2013;46:607–21.
[101] Huo L, Chen R, Shi X, Bai R, Wang P, Chang Y, et al. High-content screening for assessing nanomaterial toxicity. J Nanosci Nanotechnol 2015;15:1143–9.
[102] Manshian BB, Pfeiffer C, Pelaz B, Heimerl T, Gallego M, Möller M, et al. High-content imaging and gene expression approaches to unravel the effect of surface functionality on cellular interactions of silver nanoparticles. ACS Nano 2015;9:10431–44.

Immune response to nanobiomaterials

13

Anzelika Schreiber and Frank Witte
Charité – Universitätsmedizin, Berlin, Germany

13.1 Introduction

The term "nanomaterial" has been defined by the Scientific Committee on Emerging and Newly Identified Health Risks of the European Commission on October 18, 2011 as followed: "nanomaterial" means a natural, incidental or manufactured material containing particles, in an unbound state or as an aggregate or as an agglomerate and where, for 50% or more of the particles in the number size distribution, one or more external dimensions is in the size range 1 nm–100 nm" [1].

The definition of "biomaterial" is mainly based on the interaction of the material with a biological environment and aimed to react with an appropriate host response in a specific application. A leading international journal defines "biomaterials" as those materials—which are natural or synthetic, alive or lifeless, and usually made of multiple components—that interact with biological systems. Biomaterials are often used in medical applications to augment or replace a natural function (http://www.nature.com/subjects/biomaterials). Thus, the material chemistry and properties are not defined solely by the term "biomaterial." The combination of both definition creates the term "nanobiomaterial" describing a material which is mainly characterized by its size and its biological host response. Thus, "nanobiomaterials" can be of natural and synthetic origin. In this chapter, we are mainly focusing on nanobiomaterials, their characteristics, possible application, and biological host response.

13.2 The effect of particle size

The reduced volume of nanoparticles produces an enhanced surface area with a rearrangement of atoms. The majority of atoms in a nanobiomaterial is on the surface of the particle [2] which is changing the catalytical, steric, magnetic, mechanical, biological, electrical, and optical properties of the nanobiomaterial particle [3]. The elemental composition in the nanoparticle determines the previously mentioned physical properties. Especially the size of a nanoparticle determines the property to cross natural and physiological barriers, which usually serve the organism to protect itself against foreign substances. The entry of nanoparticles is selected based on the physiological properties and transport mechanism of the host barriers [4]. The blood–brain barrier is crossed easily by particles with a size smaller than 100 nm [5]. In particular, the chemical and physical properties of the particles are important when crossing the

Nanobiomaterials Science, Development and Evaluation. DOI: http://dx.doi.org/10.1016/B978-0-08-100963-5.00013-6

blood–brain barrier. Investigations of Gao and Jiang showed that only particles with a coating based on colloidal molecules, in this case "polysorbate 80", passed the endothelial layer of the brain capillaries [5].

However, also cells have a protective outer layer, the cell membrane. The cytoplasma and all organelles are ensheeted by a double lipid layer and separated from the extracellular matrix. However, there are some mechanism, which allow particles to enter the internal part of a cell. Based on the particle size and the type of cell the entry mechanism of particles into the cell are different [6]. So-called "nonprofessional" phagocyting cells [7] seem to prefer the clathrin-endocytic and caveolin-endocytotic pathways when internalizing nanoparticles with a size of 40 nm. Particles with a size of more than 1 μm will not be internalized by these cells. In contrast, "professional phagozytes" [7] phagocyte or macro-pinocyte particles with a diameter of more than 1 μm. However, "professional phagocytes" can also internalize nanoparticles of 40 nm using the calthrin-mediated pathway as well as micropinocytosis or phagocytosis [6]. In general, studies show a huge variation in particle size for particles using non-phagocyting pathways in the range of 50 nm to 1 μm and particles of 250 nm to 3 μm preferring the phagocytosis pathway [8].

In total, five different particle internalization mechanisms have been identified. As mentioned before, cells are capable to take up particles depending on their size by phagocytosis, macro-pinocytosis, a clathrin (CME), or caveolae (CvME) cell mediated endocytosis or via a clathrin and caveolae independent endocytosis [9,10].

13.3 The immune system responds to nanobiomaterials

The size of the particles is one of the most important parameters in the biological internalization process. Particles with a diameter of 50 nm can enter cells directly using non-phagocyting pathways. However, nanoparticles of 20 nm can enter even the interstitium via gap junctions of endothelial cells [3]. As soon as the nanoparticles are leaving the isolated production conditions and get in contact with the natural or physiological environment, the "bare particles" are getting in contact with biological molecules [3,11–14]. The adsorption of proteins on the particles creates a shell called "corona." The surface properties and the particle material [15,16] as well as its location determine the composition of the "corona" and thus the response of the host organism against the particles [11,12,17]. The adhesion of proteins depends on the composition of the nanoparticles and the corresponding molecules [11,12]. Mainly non-covalent reversible forces, such as electrostatic, van der Waals, and hydrophobic forces so-called solvation forces [18], are determining the adhesion of proteins on the surface of the nanoparticle [19,20].

Body fluids provide a dynamic character, which results into high variations in potential "corona" proteins. Based on the adhesion of proteins to the nanoparticle surface, a "hard corona" is formed with strong interactions and a "soft corona" is formed with low binding strength [21]. The number of different adhered forms of serum proteins is even extended by the material-dependent change in protein conformation, which also constantly changes the contact area for immune cells [11,12,22,23]. These conformational changes are not only locally different depending on the application site but also dependent on the individual patient and therefore is never identical according to the high variation in protein concentrations and their changing protein relations in the serum or any other body liquid of a patient.

Depending on the health status of the patient the variation and number of proteins may rise. The shape and size of the particle have a direct effect on the composition of the protein "corona" [16]. The immune response to the particle is therefore also depending on the individual "corona" and thus hard to control. The most abundant proteins in the serum which are adsorbed on particles are immuno-globulins, lipoproteins, complement factors, acute phase proteins, and coagulation factors [11,12,16]. Immuno-globulins, complement factors, and acute phase proteins are part of the complement system. The most important physiological functions of the complement system is the defense of the organism against foreign particles by a process called "opsonization." But the complement system also acts via chemotactic recruitment of immune cells to the site of inflammation, vasodilatation, an anaphylactic effect, which intensifies the immune response via chemotactic effects, and activation of leukocytes by degranulation of the immune cells, and thus an activation of the adaptive immune system. Moreover, the complement system helps to eliminate cell detritus, denaturized proteins and promotes to eliminate particles via activation of phagocytes.

13.4 The effect of surface properties in biological systems

The surface of the nanoparticles seem to play an essential major role in the foreign body response. The nanoparticle's surface properties define the profile of the "corona". The proteins of the "corona" are the first parts of the nanoparticles to interact with the biological environment and thus determine the respective immune response. Thus, the surface properties of the nanoparticles are the key to control the kinetic of nanoparticles in the organism. The variance in charge, the structural properties, polarity, solubility, enzymatic, or immunologic properties of the nanoparticles have an influence on the resorption, distribution, metabolism, and excretion of the nanoparticles. In this respect, some research groups investigated some of the previously named parameters in depth. Bertholon et al. could demonstrate depending on the 3D orientation of the coated molecules on the nanoparticles a variation in the complement system activation. This effect is associated with the amplification of the steric-repulsive disability [15].

In nanoparticles, the outer surface can change, but also the inner surface of the nanoparticle can be varied to alter the functionality of the particle. Mesoporous silica nanoparticles have a hollow porous structure and provide further options to be used as a drug carrier or a diagnostic agent. The variable pore sizes of the nanoparticles [24] permit the loading and controlled as well as conditional release of various substances. The retention and release of the substances could be controlled by specific coatings and physical conditions (pH value and temperature). The important surface modifications of mesoporous silica nanoparticles and its role in drug delivery has been intensively reviewed elsewhere [25]. Several diseases are treated today by nanoparticles such as cancer, HIV, leukemia, neurological diseases, diabetes mellitus, and others [26]. The team of Li et al. from the Laboratory for Biological Effects of Nanomaterials and Nanosafety has investigated the increasing therapeutic challenge of multidrug resistant bacteria. The research team found an effective nanoparticle based treatment as an alternative for antibiotics. The combination of mesoporous silica nanoparticles and the antibacterial enzyme lysozyme has created a new and highly effective antibacterial medication. The enzyme lysozyme has been stabilized by the nanoparticles and promoted a multivalent binding of lysozyme to the bacterial wall and fast lysis, while it was completely biocompatible [27]. Aside the transport for pharmacolgical therapeutics, the nanoparticles can be used for diagnostic purposes. A coating of the nanoparticle surface with interleukin 10 enhances the detection of atherosclerotic plaques and thus helps for early discovery of the diseases. The integration of fluorescence molecules into the coating allows the detection of accumulated nanoparticles at the inflamed area of atherosclerotic plaques [28].

Further studies demonstrated that the charge of the nanoparticle [29] as well as its physiological polarity (lipophilic vs lipophobic) determines the effect on the immune status. The team of Ranit Kedmil et al. found that the positive charge of lipophilic nanoparticles has an increased immune response while negative and neutral particles have a less intense immune response, which is mainly linked to a temporarily enhancement of proinflammatory cytokines from TH1 and TH17 cells as well as an increased expression of interferon responsive genes in T cells, B cells, monocytes, and DCs [30–32]. Other research groups found that the increased immune response in the form of an acute hypersensitivity reaction to lipid-based nanoparticles was independent from the species [33]. Several studies prove that hydrophilic surfaces persist for longer periods in the body. This is an important observation for drug carriers. A specific solubility as well as other physical and chemical properties are determined by the material of the particle itself or can be created by a specific coating. One of the most popular nanoparticle coatings is polyethylene glycol (PEG) or *Macrogol* which provides an extended period inside the blood track. PEG is a water soluble, chemically inert, and nontoxic synthetic polymer. Until today, the mechanism for its long persistence in blood is addressed by its steric-repulsive disability and thus its reduced adsorption of blood proteins. The reduced adsorption results in a so-called "stealth effect," which means that the particle is not recognized as a foreign particle and thus its elimination via phagocytes is retarded until the carrier particle reaches the treatment location [34]. Latest studies demonstrated that with PEG coated particles not the quantity, but the quality of the adsorbed proteins are important. Specifically from the group of lipoproteins the apoliproteine J (clusterin) has a strong binding to PEG surfaces. This protein guarantees the so-called "stealth effect" of the coating [35]. This breakthrough discovery of the "stealth effect" has been combined with an absorbable particle alternative, which provides a non-toxic effect by using a temporary implant material (no material accumulation in the cells) [35]. In some cases synthetic polymer coatings have been also combined with naturally occurring glycoproteins such as

CD47 [36] and even whole membrane sections of leucozytes [37] and the red blood cells [38] to mimic the "self-status" of body own proteins and thus escape the immune response [39]. The glycoprotein CD47 induces after the contact with the suppressing partner CD172 a negative signal into the phagocytes and thus prevents by an activation [40]. The leucolike vectors as well as the erythrocyte-mimicking nanoparticles are fully covered by isolating membrane sections together with the characteristic surface marker and thus escape the immune system for some time [37,38]. The "stealth effect" can be combined with other functional structures and is thus used to optimize the property profile of the nanoparticles. Thus, Singh et al. have developed a gold-based nanoparticle, which was coated with PEG containing the cell-penetrating peptide trans-activator of a transcription peptide and a fluorescence marker. Both should enable the transport of a drug into the nucleus of HIV-infected cells. The fluorescence maker has been used to determine the location of the nanoparticles. The PEG coating guarantees the "immune-tolerated" stay of the nanoparticles in the blood stream until they reach their destination [41]. In general, nanoparticles can escape the contact with the immune system, but they can also intentionally be used to suppress the immune response.

13.5 How primary and secondary states of nanobiomaterials interfere with biological environments

The space occupied by a "primary" nanoparticle in a biological system is not always constant. Depending on the material properties, the chemical and physical properties of the particles as well as the environmental conditions, single "primary" nanoparticles can agglomerate and form complexes which increases the total diameter of their space in the biological environments. The bonding strength among the particle determines if they are called agglomerates or aggregates. In agglomerates, the nanoparticles are held together by weak forces such as van der Waals forces or electrostatic forces. Aggregates are formed by covalent or metallic bonds from primary nanoparticles. Both forms, aggregates and agglomerates, present the "secondary" status of nanoparticles. If the nanoparticles are in the "primary" state or change to the "secondary" determines the distribution of the nanoparticles in the biological organism (human) [42]. Another major parameter with a significant effect on the formation of the "secondary" status is the concentration of the nanoparticles. An increasing concentration of nanoparticles leads to an increasing particle agglomeration [43]. The nanoparticles tend to form "secondary" structures in fluids. The reversible agglomerates as well as the stable aggregate of nanoparticles sediment and accumulate in fluids [42,44]. If nanoparticles are linked to other complexes the volume and content of the "secondary" structure changes compared to the "primary" nanoparticles, but also the biological environment will be challenged differently. In this regard, cells in a cell culture will receive a higher concentration of nanoparticles, if they sediment, but receive less nanoparticles if they are staying dispersed in the solution. The status is influencing the uptake rate of the nanoparticles into cells [45]. Moreover, the increase in size of the "secondary" particle reduces the dissemination of the nanoparticle in the biological organism (human). Many external chemical and physical properties of the environment influence the formation of "secondary" structures [42]. The ionic strength is an environmental parameter which is influencing the agglomeration of the nanoparticles by changing the electrical double layer of the "primary" particles [46]. With increasing ionic strength of the solvent, the electrical double layer is reduced which enhances agglomeration. As an example, divalent cations have a promoting effect on the aggregation of 4–5 nm TiO_2 nanoparticles in $CaCl_2$ [47]. The calcium ions are adsorbed on the TiO_2 nanoparticle surface which neutralizes the negative charge and induces the particle agglomeration. A predominant effect in this process are van der Waals forces of the particles [48,49]. In contrast, a reduced ionic strength of the environment promotes a thicker electrical double layer which enhances electrostatic repulsion. In monovalent fluids (NaCl) as well as in deionized water, the pH value has a significant influence on the agglomeration of the nanoparticles via surface charge. In acid solutions the nanoparticles get a positive charge, while in alkaline solutions the nanoparticles get a negative charge. According to "Coulomb's law" particles of same charge push each other, while particles of opposite charge attract each other. Thus, nanoparticles of same charge in acid or alkaline milieu reduce the agglomeration, while the pH in the neutral range increases the effect of the van der Waals forces and thus increases the formation of clusters of nanoparticles [46]. The response of nanoparticles to various pH values in the environment depends if divalent or monovalent ions are present. In acidic milieu the nanoparticles have the same charge and push each other. In alkaline milieu the usually enhanced ionic strength reduces the electrical double layer of the negatively charged particles and thus reduces the repulsive force in favor of the van der Waals forces and the particles agglomerate. Not all divalent ions have the same strength to neutralize the particle's charge. As an example, it has been demonstrated that calcium ions have a stronger neutralization effect on agglomeration than magnesium ions [46] (Fig. 13.1).

The zeta-potential (ζ) is usually used to determine the stability of the dispersion. The zeta-potential represents the electrokinetic potential on the slipping plane of the double layer of the particles [50]. With increasing potential the electrokinetic repulsion increases and thus the agglomeration is less likely and the dispersion gets more stable [51,52] (Fig. 13.2).

The formation of agglomerates and aggregates are limiting the therapeutic use of nanoparticles. Intense research is focusing to control and reduce the formation of "secondary" states by specific coatings [49].

Figure 13.1 Environmental conditions influence the dispersion of the nanoparticle. (A) Strong surface charge, either positive or negative, increases the repulsive forces and thus continues a dispersion of nanoparticles in solutions. With weak surface charge, the repulsive forces are dominated by the van der Waals forces and particle clusters are formed. (B) Low ionic strength in the environmental milieu of the nanoparticles leads to an increased thickness of the electrical double layer and thus a continuation of the nanoparticles in the "primary," dispersed state. With an increased ionic strength, less ions are needed to neutralize the

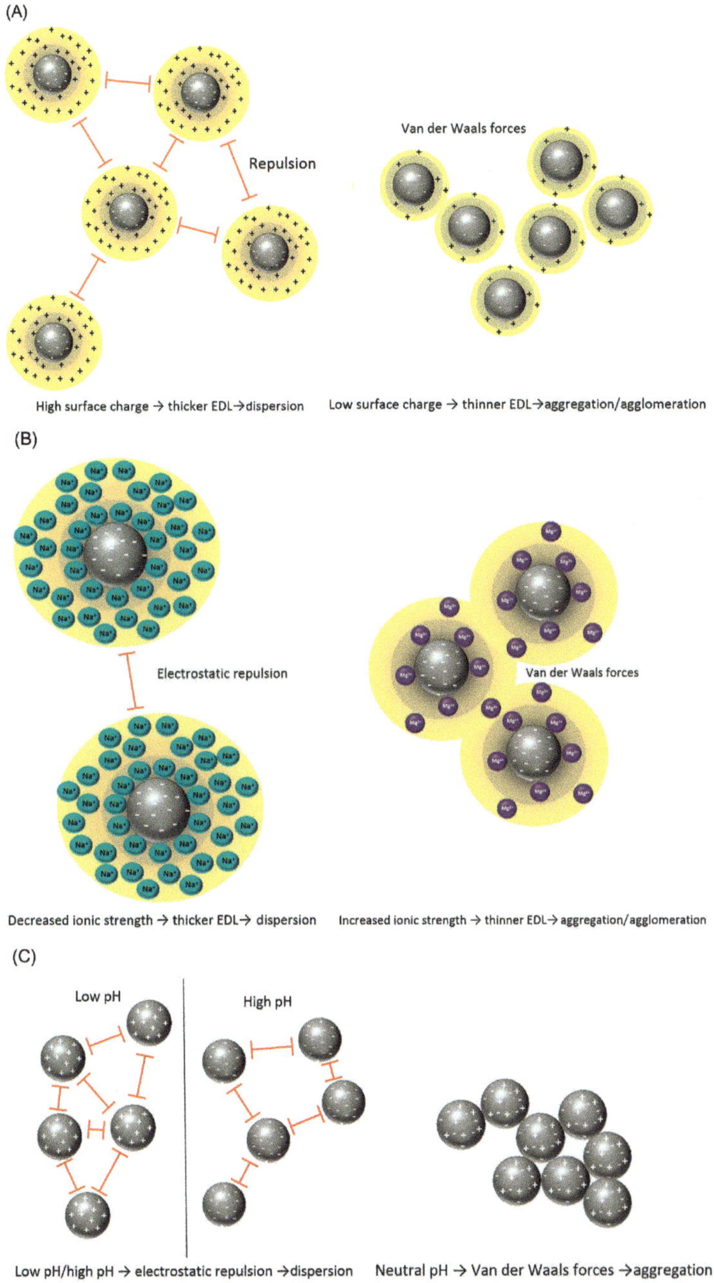

nanoparticle. Thus, the electrical double layer of the nanoparticle and their repulsive forces are small and they are forced to aggregate. (C) In a solution with extremely high or low pH values, the nanoparticles will be charged either positive or negative. Then the particles provide high repulsion and they keep on to be dispersed. In neutral pH ranges, these particles have a thin electrical double layer and thus tend to agglomerate.

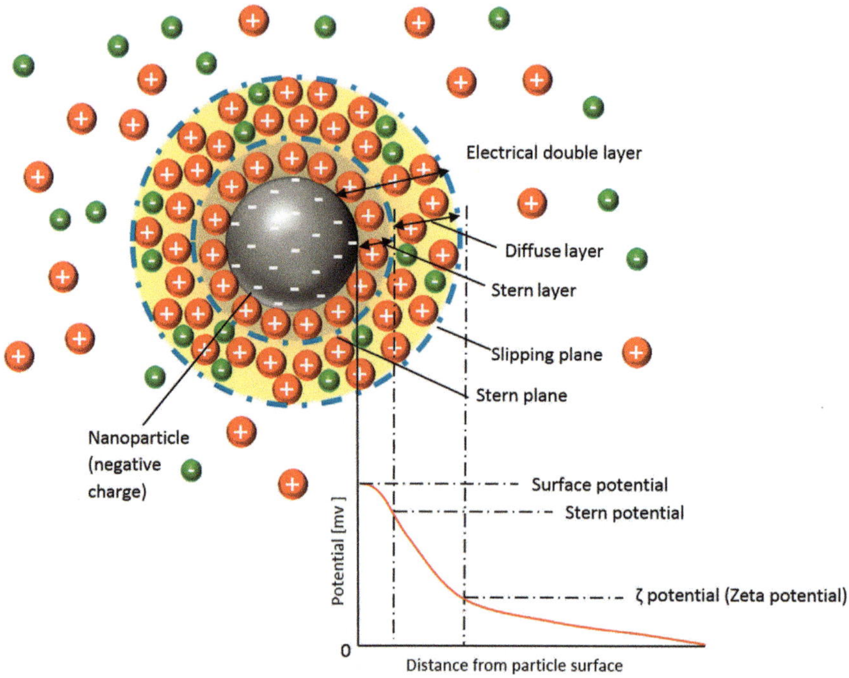

Figure 13.2 Model of a nanoparticle in aqueous solution. The nanoparticle has a negative charge in aqueous solutions. For neutralization, positive ions attach to the particle surface and create the "Stern layer." This first ion layer cannot completely neutralize the charge of the nanoparticle. Therefore more ions attach to the Stern layer. The binding of these ions to the particle is weaker due to the larger distance of these ions to the particle's surface and thus these ions are more mobile. This ion habit provided the name "Diffuse layer." Both ion layers are forming the electric double layer. With increasing thickness of the electrical double layer, the repulsive forces increase and the dispersions gets more stable. Each layer has its own potential. The potential of the electrical double layer is called zeta-potential and correlates with the stability of the dispersion.

13.6 Health risks of nanobiomaterials

The quote of Louis Pasteur "The role of the infinitely small in nature is infinitely large" has been used in a different context, but is incredibly true for nanoparticles. Their diverse nature is providing almost unlimited possibilities of applications, for example, in cosmetic, medical, textile, automotive industry, food industry, and cleaning products. Besides the unique usability of nanoparticles, some nanoparticles carry a health risk of partly known origin. In this case the different physicochemical properties of the nanoparticles are important. The surface charge is not only important for aggregation and agglomeration, but also has hematolytic activity. Positively charged nanoparticles increase the hemolysis, while negatively charged particles have no such effect. Nanoparticles with a PEG coating have a "stealth effect" and can hide from the immune system. Thereby they have a higher chance to reach their anatomical destination and be effective locally. The extended stay of nanoparticles in the cardiovascular system promotes an increased interaction of the nanoparticles with blood proteins and coagulation factors. Several studies have demonstrated that nanoparticles interact with thrombocytes and promote thrombus formation [53,54]. Moreover, it has been shown that in cases of nanoparticle interaction the activation of the coagulation cascade differs from normal activation pathways. The formation of aggregates with erythrocytes and coagulation proteins enhances the phagocytosis by antigen-presenting cells and therefore enhances the elimination of particles from the cardiovascular system [54]. Recently, an in vitro study demonstrates the effect by inhibiting coagulation through a dose-dependent effect by silver nanoparticles which were covered by citrate (AgNP-CIT-20 nanoparticles). However, with increasing concentration of nanoparticles the inhibition of coagulation will be reduced [55]. The effect of the agglomerates on the environment is controversially discussed. Gliga et al. have conducted a series of in vivo experiments using silver nanoparticles. They have shown that the agglomeration of the particles play a minor role addressing the cytotoxicity of the particles compared to previous reports. The comparison of coated and non-coated silver nanoparticles of different sizes demonstrated that particles of smaller diameter release a significant higher amount of silver into the cell which determine their higher toxicity of those nanoparticles. The uptake rate and quantity of coated and noncoated particles was similar in that case. Thus, the toxic effect is not based on the agglomerates, but on the concentration of the initial "primary" nanoparticles [56]. Nanoparticles seem to provide a multifold influence on the immune system. The interaction of nanoparticles with immune cells is changing the expression of immune-modulating surface proteins, for example, pattern-recognition receptors (PRRs), enzymes, and cytokines. By studying the surface proteins immune cells revealed the modulating expression of toll-like receptors after the exposure to various nanoparticles. Depending on the material an enhanced or reduced expression has been observed. Toll-like receptors belong to the group of PRRs and are used for the recognition of various pathogens. An enhanced expression of toll-like receptors can result in hyperbolic immune reactions and can induce autoreactivity. While a reduced expression of toll-like receptors could result in neglected pathogens and an absent immune response. In addition to modulations in PRRs, changes in the expression of MMP-2, AP-1, PTK, MHC-II, Arginase-1 as well as cytokines and transcription factors have been observed [57]. Also in late (adaptive) phase of the immune response to nanoparticles some variations from normal reactions have been observed. For example, Dark Agouti rats show during a normal immune response without nanoparticles the appearance of TH1 cells, DCs, and macrophages, while after exposure to nanoparticles the dominant cells are natural killer (NK) cells, NKt cells, and DCs [57]. Specific nanoparticles seem to have a toxic effect on lymphocytes. In a series of in vivo experiments it was shown that silver nanoparticles coated with PVP or citrate (CIT) reduce the proliferation and viability of lymphocytes [55].

Thus, nanobiomaterials are carrying a significant health risk which needs to be relialbly controlled before uncovering their therapeutic use.

References

[1] Potocnik J. Commission recommendation of 18 October 2011 on the definition of nanomaterial. Official J Eur Union 2011.

[2] Pool R. Clusters: strange morsels of matter: when metals or semiconductors are shrunk down to clumps only 10 or 100 atoms in size, they become a "totally new class of materials" with potentially valuable applications. Science 1990;248(4960):1186–8.

[3] Riedel E, Janiak C. Anorganische chemie. Walter de Gruyter GmbH & Co KG, Berlin; 2015.

[4] Barua S, Mitragotri S. Challenges associated with penetration of nanoparticles across cell and tissue barriers: a review of current status and future prospects. Nano Today 2014;9(2):223–43.

[5] Gao KP, Jiang XG. Influence of particle size on transport of methotrexate across blood brain barrier by polysorbate 80-coated polybutylcyanoacrylate nanoparticles. Int J Pharm 2006;310(1-2):213–9.

[6] Kuhn DA, et al. Different endocytotic uptake mechanisms for nanoparticles in epithelial cells and macrophages. Beilstein J Nanotechnol 2014;5:1625–36.

[7] Rabinovitch M. Professional and non-professional phagocytes: an introduction. Trends Cell Biol 1995;5(3):85–7.

[8] Kann B, et al. Raman microscopy for cellular investigations – from single cell imaging to drug carrier uptake visualization. Adv Drug Deliv Rev 2015;89:71–90.

[9] Hillaireau H, Couvreur P. Nanocarriers' entry into the cell: relevance to drug delivery. Cell Mol Life Sci 2009;66(17):2873–96.

[10] Mayor S, Pagano RE. Pathways of clathrin-independent endocytosis. Nat Rev Mol Cell Biol 2007;8(8):603–12.

[11] Cedervall T, et al. Detailed identification of plasma proteins adsorbed on copolymer nanoparticles. Angew Chem-Int Ed 2007;46(30):5754–6.

[12] Cedervall T, et al. Understanding the nanoparticle–protein corona using methods to quantify exchange rates and affinities of proteins for nanoparticles. Proc Natl Acad Sci USA 2007;104(7):2050–5.

[13] Lynch I, et al. The nanoparticle–protein complex as a biological entity; a complex fluids and surface science challenge for the 21st century. Adv Colloid Interface Sci 2007;134–135:167–74.

[14] Elsaesser A, Howard CV. Toxicology of nanoparticles. Adv Drug Deliv Rev 2012;64(2):129–37.

[15] Bertholon I, et al. Complement activation by core-shell poly(isobutylcyanoacrylate)-polysaccharide nanoparticles: influences of surface morphology, length, and type of polysaccharide. Pharm Res 2006;23(6):1313–23.

[16] Lundqvist M, et al. Nanoparticle size and surface properties determine the protein corona with possible implications for biological impacts. Proc Natl Acad Sci USA 2008;105(38):14265–70.

[17] Hu WJ, et al. Molecular basis of biomaterial-mediated foreign body reactions. Blood 2001;98(4):1231–8.

[18] Israelachvili J. Solvation forces and liquid structure, as probed by direct force measurements. Acc Chem Res 1987;20(11):415–21.

[19] Saptarshi SR, et al. Interaction of nanoparticles with proteins: relation to bio-reactivity of the nanoparticle. J Nanobiotechnol 2013;11.

[20] Zeinabad HA, et al. Thermodynamic and conformational changes of protein toward interaction with nanoparticles: a spectroscopic overview. Rsc Adv 2016;6(107):105903–105919.

[21] Lundqvist M, et al. Protein adsorption onto silica nanoparticles: conformational changes depend on the particles' curvature and the protein stability. Langmuir 2004;20(24):10639–47.
[22] Satzer P, et al. Protein adsorption onto nanoparticles induces conformational changes: particle size dependency, kinetics, and mechanisms. Eng Life Sci 2016;16(3):238–46.
[23] Wangoo N, et al. Interaction of gold nanoparticles with protein: a spectroscopic study to monitor protein conformational changes. Appl Phys Lett 2008;92:13.
[24] Nandiyanto ABD, et al. Synthesis of spherical mesoporous silica nanoparticles with nanometer-size controllable pores and outer diameters. Microporous Mesoporous Mater 2009;120(3):447–53.
[25] Natarajan SK, Selvaraj S. Mesoporous silica nanoparticles: importance of surface modifications and its role in drug delivery. Rsc Adv 2014;4(28):14328–34.
[26] Mudshinge SR, et al. Nanoparticles: emerging carriers for drug delivery. Saudi Pharm J 2011;19(3):129–41.
[27] Li LL, Wang H. Enzyme-coated mesoporous silica nanoparticles as efficient antibacterial agents in vivo. Adv Healthcare Mater 2013;2(10):1351–60.
[28] Almer G, et al. Interleukin 10-coated nanoparticle systems compared for molecular imaging of atherosclerotic lesions. Int J Nanomed 2014;9:4211–22.
[29] Ryman-Rasmussen JP, et al. Surface coatings determine cytotoxicity and irritation potential of quantum dot nanoparticles in epidermal keratinocytes. J Investig Dermatol 2007;127(1):143–53.
[30] Kedmi R, et al. The systemic toxicity of positively charged lipid nanoparticles and the role of toll-like receptor 4 in immune activation. Biomaterials 2010;31(26):6867–75.
[31] Moyano DF, et al. Modulation of immune response using engineered nanoparticle surfaces. Small 2016;12(1):76–82.
[32] Gamucci O, et al. Biomedical nanoparticles: overview of their surface immune-compatibility. Coatings 2014;4(1):139–59.
[33] Szebeni J, et al. Animal models of complement-mediated hypersensitivity reactions to liposomes and other lipid-based nanoparticles. J Liposome Res 2007;17(2):107–17.
[34] Hak S, et al. The effect of nanoparticle polyethylene glycol surface density on ligand-directed tumor targeting studied in vivo by dual modality imaging. Acs Nano 2012;6(6):5648–58.
[35] Schottler S, et al. Protein adsorption is required for stealth effect of poly(ethylene glycol)- and poly(phosphoester)-coated nanocarriers. Nat Nanotechnol 2016;11(4):372–7.
[36] Rodriguez PL, et al. Minimal "self" peptides that inhibit phagocytic clearance and enhance delivery of nanoparticles. Science 2013;339(6122):971–5.
[37] Parodi A, et al. Synthetic nanoparticles functionalized with biomimetic leukocyte membranes possess cell-like functions. Nat Nanotechnol 2013;8(1):61–8.
[38] Hu CMJ, et al. Erythrocyte membrane-camouflaged polymeric nanoparticles as a biomimetic delivery platform. Proc Natl Acad Sci USA 2011;108(27):10980–5.
[39] Blanco E, et al. Principles of nanoparticle design for overcoming biological barriers to drug delivery. Nat Biotechnol 2015;33(9):941–51.
[40] Oldenborg PA. CD47: a cell surface glycoprotein which regulates multiple functions of hematopoietic cells in health and disease. ISRN Hematol 2013;2013:614619.
[41] Singh L, et al. Intracellular localization of gold nanoparticles with targeted delivery in MT-4 lymphocytes. Adv Nat Sci—Nanosci Nanotechnol 2016;7:4.
[42] Bruinink A, et al. Effect of particle agglomeration in nanotoxicology. Arch Toxicol 2015;89(5):659–75.

[43] Allouni ZE, et al. Agglomeration and sedimentation of TiO_2 nanoparticles in cell culture medium. Colloids Surf B—Biointerfaces 2009;68(1):83–7.
[44] Markus AA, et al. Modeling aggregation and sedimentation of nanoparticles in the aquatic environment. Sci Total Environ 2015;506:323–9.
[45] Cho EC, et al. The effect of sedimentation and diffusion on cellular uptake of gold nanoparticles. Nat Nanotechnol 2011;6(6):385–91.
[46] Mahlalela LC, et al. Characterization and stability of TiO_2 nanoparticles in industrial dye stuff effluent. J Dispers Sci Technol 2017;38(4):584–93.
[47] French RA, et al. Influence of ionic strength, pH, and cation valence on aggregation kinetics of titanium dioxide nanoparticles. Environ Sci Technol 2009;43(5):1354–9.
[48] Romanello MB, de Cortalezzi MMF. An experimental study on the aggregation of TiO_2 nanoparticles under environmentally relevant conditions. Water Res 2013;47(12):3887–98.
[49] Jiang JK, et al. Characterization of size, surface charge, and agglomeration state of nanoparticle dispersions for toxicological studies. J Nanopart Res 2009;11(1):77–89.
[50] Xu RL. Progress in nanoparticles characterization: sizing and zeta potential measurement. Particuology 2008;6(2):112–5.
[51] Kirby BJ. Micro- and nanoscale fluid mechanics: transport in microfluidic devices. Cambridge University Press, New York; 2013.
[52] Obrien RW, et al. Electroacoustic studies of moderately concentrated colloidal suspensions. Farad Discuss 1990;90:301–12.
[53] Radomski A, et al. Nanoparticle-induced platelet aggregation and vascular thrombosis. Br J Pharmacol 2005;146(6):882–93.
[54] Dobrovolskaia MA, et al. Preclinical studies to understand nanoparticle interaction with the immune system and its potential effects on nanoparticle biodistribution. Mol Pharm 2008;5(4):487–95.
[55] Huang H, et al. An evaluation of blood compatibility of silver nanoparticles. Sci Rep 2016;6.
[56] Gliga AR, et al. Size-dependent cytotoxicity of silver nanoparticles in human lung cells: the role of cellular uptake, agglomeration and Ag release. Part Fibre Toxicol 2014;11.
[57] Hussain S, et al. Interactions of nanomaterials with the immune system. Wiley Interdiscip Rev—Nanomed Nanobiotechnol 2012;4(2):169–83.

Further Reading

EPA, 2017. EPA Chemical substances when manufactured or processed as nanoscale materials; TSCA reporting and recordkeeping requirements. United States Environmental Protection Agency (EPA) 2017.

Safety, regulatory issues, long-term biotoxicity, and the processing environment

14

Mehdi Razavi[1] *and Amirsalar Khandan*[2]
[1]Stanford University, Palo Alto, CA, United States
[2]Islamic Azad University, Isfahan, Iran

14.1 Introduction

In recent decades, there has been an explosion of great interest in nanoscale and microscale systems in order to initiate a better understanding of suitable and better carriers of drug delivery system as well as facilitate the immigration and transportation of cells and genes within the tissues, with as little side effect and destruction as possible [1–3]. In the world market today, the nanoparticles (NPs) have been developed and greatly advertised. The world market announced, in recent decades, that the cost of shopping for NPs globally has risen to over $10 billion [1]. With an increase in industrial demands and production capacity, a better understanding of how to safely develop and use these engineered nanomaterials are of huge concern to researchers [1–3]. The work done by Lacerda et al. [1] indicates that carbon nanotube (CNT) has the potential to be a viable component in drug delivery system within biomaterials engineering. This was further verified by their work in the translocation of single-walled carbon nanotubes (SWCNTs) and multiwalled carbon nanotubes (MWCNTs), when loaded with peptides, proteins, nucleic acids, and drugs into the mammalian cells [4–8]. CNTs are therefore a group of materials whose useful exploitable properties prompt an increase in production and utilization within the circle of diverse applications; this is to ensure that their safety is of vital importance [9]. Several researchers have worked on different metals and NPs with the potential for human health risk assessment for different NPs, including carbon fullerenes, titanium dioxide (TiO_2) [10,11]. These NPs are able to be used in the human body due to their excellent mechanical and biological properties such as large surface-to-volume ratio or proper bioactivity and biocompatibility of nonmetallic NPs [10]. The dialogue between the surgeons and materials engineers has led to a faster solution to clinical problems. The major issue that arises due to the implantation of NPs is the toxicity of NPs and this depends on the characteristics of biomaterials [12–16]. A large number of man-made medical devices such as hip joints, heart valves, dental roots, intraocular lens, and so on, are implanted into human bodies every year [17,18]. In this study, our objective is to build a uniform protocol and standard for the biological behavior of common NPs used in biomaterials field.

Nanobiomaterials Science, Development and Evaluation. DOI: http://dx.doi.org/10.1016/B978-0-08-100963-5.00014-8

14.2 Safety factors

There is a need for a highly sensitive system for evaluating the potential hazards that are brought by biomaterials because the innate properties of these materials, most often, do not permit an increased dosage to take place [19]. Moreover, a huge implausibility takes place when we extrapolate from one test system to another; a good example of this is from animals to human beings [12,13,19]. However, in order for this to be feasible, toxicologists take into account the idea of safety factors; with this, the toxicologists are able to scientifically outline the inter- and intraspecies variations that exist. In other words, there is a need to exaggerate the human clinical dosage that is foreseen within the nonhuman system test. When considering the toxicity model that is native to animals, there is an avenue for lowering down the dosage of the target cells by diffusion, distribution, variations in the amounts of cells exposed, that is due to the inflammatory response, and metabolism [12,19]. However, when considering the cell culture models, where the variables associated with distribution, metabolism, and absorption are reduced, the cell dosage is increased to give out an excellent test system that is highly sensitive.

14.3 Nanoparticle biomaterials safety

The NPs employed in the manufacture of human cosmetics such as the famous sunscreen is made from zinc dioxide [14,15] and TiO_2 [20] as a result of the ultraviolet radiation manipulation. Oral NP as well as intravenous administrations are more efficient in rapidly diluting into the blood stream when compared to the convention transdermal administration and so, once this has fully circulated into the blood stream, it has to go through the first-pass metabolism that is present in the liver; as a result, it can get stored up or spread through the vasculature to vital organs such as the cardiovascular, brain, skin, and so on. Now, even with its heavily guarded blood–brain–barrier (BBB) [21,22] against threats such as external chemicals, nanoparticulate matter can still break through the barrier and squeeze through tight junctions and so, this opens the brain to potential particulate toxicity [21]. Therefore, there is a need for concrete data on NP toxicity to be safe against adverse effects that are dangerous to the human anatomy. On the other hand, NPs acting as gene delivery system as well as a drug, have huge potential in the medical field; also, it can be applied in contrast agents [23,24], and for fluorescent labeling. The size range for meeting up with the standard of a true "NP" is from 1–100 nm; this must be a least one of the dimensions of the materials. NP as a carrier mechanism for chemotherapeutic drugs has been incredibly popular due to its efficiency in spotting cells that are cancerous and also, its ability to limit toxicity concentration [21]. An example of one of the clinically approved metal oxides is superparamagnetic iron oxide nanoparticles (SPIONs) and this has outstanding applications in the field of biomedicine such as the magnetic resonance imaging (MRI) [25], hyperthermic destruction of tumor tissue [26], and gene delivery [27].

14.4 Targets of drug deliver targets and hazard assessment

CNTs toxicity and toxicokinetics was crucially and carefully analyzed by Johnston et al. (2010) with primary concentration on the physiochemical characteristics that causes CNT toxicity [9]. In this section, more information that has surfaced recently will be discussed since Johnston et al. (2010) publication [9]; the focus will be on extracting and describing data that is required for assessing risk in a structure that is comparable to the regulatory assessment of the risk as shown in Fig. 14.1.

14.4.1 Liver targets

Now being the locality for the first-pass mechanism, there is a particular vulnerability the liver is open to when exposed to NPs toxicity and consistently, it has been seen to accumulate substances that have been administered; this is even after a long exposure. As a result, a thorough assessment of the NPs hepatocellular toxicity is still vital [28,29].

14.4.2 Dermal targets

From scientific evidence, it has been proven that the skin is one of the largest organs of the body and it is incredibly important because it provides the first line of barrier

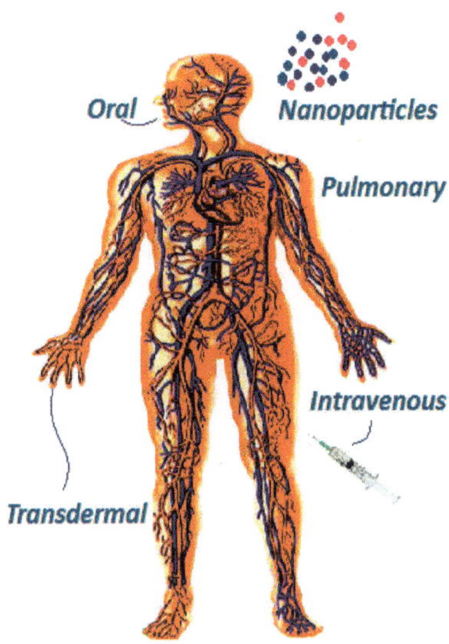

Figure 14.1 Routes of administration of nanoparticles and their advantages and disadvantages.
Source: Reproduced from Yildirimer, L., Thanh, N.T., Loizidou, M., & Seifalian, A.M. (2011). Toxicology and clinical potential of nanoparticles. Nano Today, 6(6), 585-607.

between the external environment and the internal organs [9]. Owing to this, the skin is an easy target for an array of environmental threats that reside within the atmosphere as well as toxic substances within cosmetic products, clothing, spray [21], and so on. Moreover, NPs that are topically applied have the ability to penetrate the skin and gain entry into the blood stream; also, this leads to more hostile effects in the human body at a systemic scale [9,21].

14.4.3 Lung targets

The lung presents an open target for delivery of drugs; this is as a result of the lung's large surface area, noninvasive nature of inhalation therapy, avoidance of the first-pass metabolism, and localization/accumulation of drugs within the pulmonary tissue; this results in a reduction in the systemic side effects [30–32]. In the past, a lot of authors have conducted research on the mechanism of operation of the CNT pulmonary toxicity with respect to the in vitro and have been able to prove that the CNTs were cytotoxic to various lung epithelial cell lines [9,21,28,29]. CNTs were shown to contain an outstanding high concentration of metals as impurities, that is about 30%, which played a role in its toxicity. On the other hand, however, CNTs that have been sanitized without the presence of biometals were shown to reduce the native oxidative stress development [30]; this suggests that just like the fullerenes, the reactive oxygen species (ROS) might be embedded via radical addition to the surface of the CNTs and this is due to their high electron affinity [33]. Researchers are strongly certain that the CNT presence caused the formation of granuloma; however, they pointed out that the SWCNT that houses the nickel (Ni), gave out a mortality rating that was incredibly higher [21].

14.4.4 Brain targets

Now unlike the liver, the brain has a very low regenerative ability and so, must be safeguarded against foreign threats. This is achieved, as stated previously by the BBB, which helps in stopping blood-borne pathogens from entering and damaging the brain permanently [21,22]. Nevertheless, bypassing the BBB might not be a bad option in some cases but rather it might be potentially lifesaving and advantageous in providing a solution to acute illnesses such as cerebral meningitis and also chronic conditions such as Parkinson's diseases [34,35]. A smaller amount of drugs is administered through the use of targeted drug delivery and so, it lowers the amount of systemic hostile effects. Targeted drug delivery allows the use of smaller drug doses and hence reduces systemic adverse effects [36].

14.5 Reaction of nanoparticles for clinical applications

14.5.1 Polymeric nanoparticles reaction

Polymeric NPs have the property of being surface modified, biocompatible, and are quite capable of maintaining a sustained drug discharge [21]. Researchers have been able to highlight its outstanding potential in the treatment of pulmonary diseases of different varieties such as chronic obstructive pulmonary disease (COPD) [21], asthma, lung cancer, and tuberculosis as well as the dreaded diabetes [37–41]. Currently, a multitude of organic nanopolymers exists, which includes the gelatine, Iranian Gum Tragacanth polymer [21,42], collagen, chitosan, bovine serum albumin (BSA), and the alginate [21]. Moreover, within the last 30 years, there has been an increase in the development of polymers that are synthetic such as the poly(lactic-co-glycolic acid) (PLGA), which is biodegradable and biocompatible and are employed in devices intended for drug carriage [30,43,44]. Now although nanoconfiguration of the loaded drug showcases a promising substitute for conventional cancer treatment, the level of its cytotoxicity needs to be carefully analyzed [3]. PLGA NP has been shown to improve the outcome of therapeutic as well as reduce the hostile effects via a targeted and sustained drug delivery process. According to Romero et al.'s findings, the cytotoxicity levels within the PLGA NPs can be lowered by stabilizing it with BSA [3,21].

14.5.2 Silica (SiO_2) nanoparticles reaction

Already, there has been a widespread usage of silica (SiO_2) NPs within the nonmedical arena; it has been used as an additive to chemical products such as cosmetics, varnishes, and polish, [21,45,46]. The study has shown that SiO_2 NPs are safer in moderate dosage, that is below 20 μg/mL, when compared to their crystalline counterparts that are classified as class-one carcinogens [46–48]. Now apart from the dependence on concentration, SiO_2 NPs were shown to have particle size-dependent cellular toxicity with a minute diameter, which resulted in greater harm when compared to its bigger counterparts as depicted in Napierska et al. [49]. Also, there are several factors or reasons that may be responsible for inconsistent results, that is the absence or presence or type of the specified coating play a major role in piecing together the interactions that NPs and the physiological environment will have, as well as the size of the particle [21]. Nevertheless, results have surfaced that contradict the theory of size-dependent toxicity and so, this requires further investigation to pinpoint the role of various routes of the administration of the particles. Most often, SiO_2 NPs have been employed in drug additives as well as cosmetics and are most often used as the nanovehicles for delivery of drugs [42,50–55].

14.5.3 Silver nanoparticles reaction

In terms of toxicity assessment, silver (Ag) is one of the most reviewed and studied metals. But there is a major setback in terms of its high cost and this is due to the fact that the AgNP has an inherent antimicrobial effect, which has been deployed in several products that range from clothing to wound dressings [21,42]. The concentration level is responsible for the toxicity assessment and it varies with respect to the coating at the surface. According to Samberg et al., there has been reports generated that a substantial amount of toxicity resides in AgNP that is uncoated with the human epidermal keratinocytes; this is in contrast to the particles that are coated with carbon [21,56]. Now aside, Au, AgNP has been proven to have neurodegenerative effects [57,58]. Recently, research that focuses on AgNP and BBB interaction has shown that the BBB undergoes functional disruption and subsequently, causes brain edema formation [22,57]. Furthermore, parameters that are responsible for affecting the toxicity level include its shape [59], size [60], particle concentration [61], and the ability to deplete cells of antioxidants [62].

14.5.4 Gold nanoparticles reaction

Gold (Au) NPs, that is AuNP, owing to its high potential for biofunctionalization and simplistic ability to be synthesized, there has been a range of research undertaken to find out about its applications clinically as well as its use in dermal drug delivery [63]. According to researchers, the Au compounds have generally been tagged safe and been routinely used clinically for several years, that is for treating ailments such as rheumatoid arthritis [64]. Nevertheless, once it has been shrunk to the nanoscale, there is a profound change that the particles undergo, which is with respect to its biochemical properties; this necessitates carrying out investigations into the profile of its cytotoxicity. Now, irrespective of the wealth of toxicity studies that have been carried out on AuNP, inconsistent findings are still the major drawbacks that truncate its transition into the clinical environment. A lot of research has demonstrated that the cellular uptake of Au NPs is a function of its particle size, time, and concentration. In a recent research conducted by Mironava et al. [65], the human dermal fibroblasts have exposed the Au NPs for a period of about 6 days [65,66]. About three sets of NP concentrations were uncovered for each of the two size variations. Also, the same group consider platinum folate NP toxicity in two various cell types (cancer and normal cells) [67].

14.5.5 Superparamagnetic nanoparticles reaction

Superparamagnetic NPs, also known as SPIONs, are made up of iron oxide core and a variable coating of carbohydrate that is responsible for governing the cellular uptake and half-life of its biology [19,21]. Now, of profound importance is the level of its surface coverage, which has been postulated to be the major parameter in its cellular uptake because incomplete coverage at the surface was demonstrated to promote rapid endocytosis as well as opsonization; however, SPION that is coated fully doesn't get opsonized and as a result, half-life of its plasma is lengthened (constant agents: ferumoxide, ferumoxtran, ferumoxsil) [23,24,68]. Another research suggests that particle size is actually the major factor that dictates the uptake of the macrophages [69]. Now, regardless of the SPION routine usage, the neurotoxicity level, as well as its long-term effect, hasn't been evaluated extensively. SPION in particular is incredibly valuable for novel therapeutic and diagnostic applications. Moreover, the reduction in its dimension may induce cytotoxicity and therefore, interfere with the functionality of the cell as well as its components [70,71]. Also, studies have shown a correlation between the types of surface coating, magnetic properties, particle size, concentration, products breakdown, the degree of opsonization and cytotoxicity in cultured cells, and concentration [72–77]. Nowadays, orthoferrite ceramics, $RFeO_3$ (R = rare earth metals), have been the target of attention of researchers owing to their useful properties in various applications ranging from solid oxide fuel cells [75–78], sensors [79], environmental catalysts [80] to magnetic materials [81], and biomagnetite properties function in hyperthermia treatment [82,83]. Besides, high domain-wall velocity as well as the existence of Bloch lines making them applicable in magneto-optical data storage devices [77].

14.5.6 Zirconia nanoparticles reaction

The osteoconductivity, biocompatibility, and osseointegration characteristics of zirconia (ZrO_2) have been discussed in various studies [14,15, and 84]. Moreover, there is a high flexural strength that is inherent to ZrO_2 as well as its fracture toughness. And so, a coating that has been prepared is a combination of these two properties, that is the novel natural hydroxyapatite (NHA)/zircon [14]. As a matter of fact, this coating with respect to its bioactivity speeds up the osseointegration. But however, this needs to be verified by future animal studies as well as the culturing of cells. Possible improvement of the interface that links the implants with the bone can increase the roughness level, which will in effect speed up its quality and osseointegration [84]. According to a consensus conducted in 2009, the report showed that rough surfaces or moderately rough surfaces provided an enhanced bone amalgamation when compared to conventionally using a minimal and smooth rough surface [85].

14.5.7 Titanium dioxide nanoparticles reaction

There are several properties that are inherent to TiO_2 NPs that make it a valuable asset in active ingredients for the production of cosmetics and commercial sunscreens. Moreover, these NPs demonstrate better chemical stability, UV-light-blocking properties, and as a result give out better transparency and aesthetics to creams [20,21]. Cell-type-dependent TiO_2 toxicity with respect to in vitro research affects the normal cell's functionality, which includes differentiation, cell proliferation, apoptosis, and mobility [86,87]. Effects such as this can also replicate itself in vivo. To be able to gauge its capacity to penetrate, research studies on dermal infiltration has been carried out on human volunteers by utilizing various investigative methodology. A research conducted by Lademan et al. [88], on the penetrative effect of repeated administration of the TiO_2 that had an element of sunscreen, was applied to the volunteers' skin [21,88]. From these facts, it can be seen that varying grades of toxicity and permeation with respect to the functionalization of the TiO_2 NP and surface coating as well as the follicle pore's number at the surface of the skin facilitate the uptake of the particle. Mavon et al. [89] showed near total recovery of sunscreen after 15 tape strippings with no TiO_2 deposition in hair follicles or skin layers.

14.5.8 Core–shell nanoparticles reaction

An outstanding coating required for magnetic as well as various particles to be functions of targeted drug delivery is Au. Iron oxides (Fe_2O_3 and Fe_3O_4), and Au are both incredibly biocompatible and are suitable for human usage. Another key advantage of this metal is that it is very easy to track within the human body and it can be a function of bioorganic and organic molecules; this includes enzymes and proteins [82]. Furthermore, iron and its oxides' NPs, have an inherent magnetic characteristic that can be administered to tissues, organs, or cancer tumors by making use of an outer magnetic field [21,82].

14.5.9 Calcium orthophosphate bioceramics reaction

Two independent postulations were made by Kuboki et al. [90] and Ripamonti [91] that the geometric configuration of the calcium orthophosphate bioceramic was indeed a key parameter when the issue of bone induction arose [92]. There have also been speculations that the rough surface of the nanostructure or a given surface charge of the implants might be responsible for the asymmetric division of the stem cells into osteoblasts [93]. However, in in vivo experiments, an observation of an inflammation occurred after the calcium orthophosphate bioceramics was implanted [94–96]; as a general conclusion, utilizing calcium orthophosphate with Ca/P ionic ratio, that is within the range of 1.0–1.7, is that all available implants aren't only nontoxic in property but produce zero foreign reactions and inflammation to the human body. One reason that inflammation occurs is as a result of highly porous HA bioceramics, which could be due to sharp implant edges [95]. Another factor causing this is the micro movements of implants [92].

14.5.10 Magnesium reaction

Based on a study conducted by Razavi et al. [55], the rapid degradation of magnesium could be controlled by having the surface of the magnesium implants modified by utilizing the fluoridated hydroxyapatite (FHA) through the combination of an electrophoretic deposition (EPD) [18] and microarc oxidation (MAO) [12]. A coated AZ91 magnesium alloy was examined for its biocompatibility when implanted into the greater trochanter area of rabbits. According to the results uncovered from in vivo test on the animal, there was a substantial improvement in the FHA/MAO-coated implant's biocompatibility when compared to the ones that were uncoated. Furthermore, when the AZ91 implants were coated with FHA/MAO, the magnesium ion that was released into the blood plasma was reduced and the weight problem was also significantly reduced.

14.5.11 Carbon nanotubes reaction

CNTs are commonly utilized for in vivo inhalation; CNTs can be divided into MWCNTs and SWCNTs, where the former represents the one with a higher cytotoxicity level. Now, what makes the toxicity level vary is as a result of the larger surface area of the SWCNTs unlike the multilayered alternative [97]. Moreover, CNTs shows true promise in biomedicine in fields such as photodynamic therapy (PDT) [98], drug delivery, and as tissue engineering scaffolds [9,28,29].

14.6 Characterization for different exposure routes

14.6.1 Cardiovascular effects

According to a research study in vitro and in vivo, an exposure to CNTs with respect to the cardiovascular system could have a detrimental effect on the human body and this could result in complications such as prothrombic responses [99], vascular damage, sites distal to the exposure site having oxidative responses or inflammatory problems [100,101], as well as an increased risk of cardiovascular disease that affects the normality of the electrophysiology [102].

14.6.2 Irritation/Corrosivity

An experiment was carried out by Lange and Huczko in 2001, whereby the rabbits' eyes were modified by drenching it with a high concentration carbon of SWCNTs; from the results, it was shown that no eye irritation occurred [103]. Also, this same carbon didn't irritate the skin in patch test conducted within a phase of 96h, which was done on 40 volunteers that gave a report of various irritation and allergies. One test conducted by Kishore et al. in 2009 was in two varying sizes of MWCNTs on the potential of the eye and dermal irritability in vitro and in vivo [104]. A 0.5mg dosage of MWCNTs, which was applied every 4h on the clipped area of the rabbits' skin didn't prompt any dermal responses such as edema and erythema until about 72h of postexposure. According to an experiment conducted in the in vitro, it showed that about 10mg of MWCNTs didn't result in any irritation [28].

14.6.3 Oral exposure

With respect to SWCNTs, only one acute oral toxicity research was carried out [28]. A single dose of 1000mg/kg bodyweight of about three various types of SWCNTs was administered to a mice by Kolosnjaj-Tabi et al. [105]. The result showed that despite the large dosage administered to the mouse, no changes occurred in the body weight and also, no abnormalities sprang up during the duration of 14 days of pathological examination.

14.6.4 Inhalation/Pulmonary exposure

A lot of studies or researches have been conducted that investigated the pulmonary effects due to exposure by aspiration, instillation, and inhalation. Now, when it comes to the human anatomy, the intratracheal instillations as well as pharyngeal aspirations aren't conventional exposure entry sites; however, these medium have been used on animals such as rats and mice to conduct an experiment on the systematic and potential pulmonary toxicity of high levels of the CNTs [106,107].

14.6.5 Oxidative stress

The oxidative stress is defined by the imbalance taking place between the antioxidants and the production of oxidants defences. Now with regard to the oxidants, it has been postulated to be a major mechanism that suppresses the biological effects of the CNTs. Malone dialdehyde (MDA) content or the lungs protein thiols, that are biomarkers of oxidative stress, increases after undergoing an initial exposure to CNT for 24h [108,109].

14.6.6 Inflammation

From experiments conducted, the pulmonary exposure to CNT resulted in an inflammatory response induction. Moreover, this so-called induction is a preliminary phase that occurs as early as 6-24h after the exposure occurs initially with the enrolment of neutrophils in the bronchoalveolar lavage fluid (BALF) [30,48]. Now within 15 days after the preliminary exposure, neutrophil-driven infiltration is usually resolved and transient.

14.6.7 Pharmacological activity

With respect to the economic, regulatory, and political bodies, there could be massive consequences, when the demarcation of medical devices and medicinal products takes place.

In this section, the discussion is focused only on the demarcation that takes place between the biomaterial and the pharmaceutical product, that is of the biological active constituency. Theoretically, however, there arise some exceptions; this could be for the purpose of promoting biological activity within the body such as regeneration of bone, and undesirable activity of blood cloth or infections.

14.6.8 Gene therapy

Gene therapy shows true promise in providing a solution to certain diseases by altering, replacing, or perhaps supplementing the genes that aren't available or are abnormal, which are severe conditions that are responsible for various ailments. Now the question is how exactly do the desired genes get targeted to the cells in question in an effective and safe manner? Also, there must be clarity on the similarities in the precise delivery of highly potent drugs.

14.7 Legal aspects of biomaterials

Any reasonable student in the field of biomaterials engineering knows that no products, regardless of how much precision was put into its manufacture can last forever; also, medical implants usually have undesired side effects or repercussions to the body. In our world today, some of these factors can influence the patients and manufacturer's perspective and most often, induce worries in both parties as to the integrity and safety of these medical devices. When it comes to the law, there are product liability laws that impose some sort of legal responsibility on the manufacturers of products, that is car manufacturers, computer manufacturers, and so on, as well as other companies that are connected to the stream of commerce, which includes divisions such as distributors, wholesalers, retailers, and so on, when customers get injured or, worse, killed. As a matter of fact, there are three theories that are normally postulated by products liability plaintiffs: in the first theory, they claim that the manufacturers were careless, that is they failed in making sure that their products are safe for human usage. Secondly, they claim that the manufacturers breached the legally enforceable promises, which is also generally known as warranties, that is when the products don't perform optimally as expected or meet the quality standard by the regulatory bodies [19]. Finally, the legal actions are taken on manufacturers, that is under strict liability, the plaintiff sues the company and so the manufacturer is held accountable for the hazardous product, irrespective of the care and promises made by the manufacturers. In order to avoid such problems hovering around these legal theories, the medical devices must be manufactured with safety as its number one priority before it is sold to the public. Also, clear instructions must be highlighted on the manual to disclose to the physicians or sometimes the patients, the risk involved in using this product. Products liability usually falls within the arena of civil laws known as *torts*. Torts are just wrongful acts that are committed that give an avenue for a lawsuit to be executed.

14.8 Long-term testing in vivo

When considering long-term testing of tissues, there are two aspects to take into consideration. One involves the response of the tissue to the material concerned while the other involves the response of the material, that is degradation, to implantation. Now when talking about the long-term implantation of test material within the bones and muscles of rabbits, rats, and dogs, there are two species that are highly recommended, that is, the rabbits and the dogs. Now when considering the rabbits' implants, the standards usually call for about four healthy rabbits per period of sacrifice with usually one control and then the two test materials are introduced into paravertebral muscles of the spine at each side. When considering bone implants, the standard is usually using three implants for every femur. However, no standards are put in place for testing of devices on a long term. But when a device is required for a definite application, it is completely and absolutely important to conduct a credible device test [19]. When considering fixation fracture plates, it is recommended to use plates that are attached to the femoral osteotomies within dogs' bodies. In this research, the effects of implants on the tissue will be analyzed and also, the effect it has on the device in question will be reviewed, that is the material degradation. As stated earlier, the standard for long-term testing of implants hasn't been established by the American Society for Testing Materials (ASTM) yet; however, F1439, that is the Standard Guide for Performance of Lifetime Bioassay for the Tumorigenic Potential of Implant Materials, gives us some guidelines as to the type of testing to carry out.

14.9 Global regulatory strategy and intended use

For drug delivery system, the incorporation of biomaterial is essential and it is used as carriers, that is within packages for biologics and then integrated into components of key importance within the medical devices for various applications such as syringes and disposable tubing to implantable devices in order to sustain life or revive and restore limb as well as organ functionality. Now with respect to all these various applications, the biomaterials are regulated indirectly by the intended usage of the final product. And so, the regulation is correlated with the risk associated with its intended usage. Notwithstanding the numerous applications in other fields, a majority of its application has been in the field of biomedicine and so this chapter will concentrate on the regulatory limitations put on the development of the products using biomaterials [19].

14.10 Biological and environment reaction

The implant's surface is torched by bacteria and as a result, this leads to hydrogen corrosion as well as leaves a destructive imprint. Also, there are some reports that point toward corrosive activity taking place in the presence of cell and protein in order to destroy the metallic implants. Some vital or important factors such as cells and protein causing destruction without taking into account some factors such as the polarization reactions as well as the electrode potential was uncovered by some researchers. Some of the observations indicated that the proteins get attracted to the surface of the metal at outstanding amounts. Moreover, Jacobs et al. record their book chapter in [19,110], showed or highlighted that these proteins can bind with the ions of the metal and get transported to other parts of the body. In other words, protein plays a crucial role in influencing the corrosion rate of the metallic implant in terms of its dentistry and orthopedic prosthesis without deploying any kind of the distinctive mechanism.

14.11 Conclusions and future trends

There is a range of clinical applications that NPs presents, but there is a drawback in its application due to safety and toxicity consideration. And until these issues are dealt with thoroughly and fully understood, there will always be a limitation in its usage. Research has shown that the factors that are responsible for NPs toxicity include diameter, length, and purity, functionalization, and production methodology. And when these factors are altered or shaped, NPs can now become safe for human usage. In vivo studies have been remarkably informative in demonstrating that various methodology of administration can have different pathological results. While when considering the in vitro studies, these studies are useful for triangulating and identifying the causes of NP toxicity; however, drawing a decisive conclusion from a given literature can be complicated due to the inconsistencies among research. And so, this is a true depiction of the growing number of opinions that the conventional cytotoxicity aren't suitable enough for conducting nanotoxicity experiments due to the fact that NPs all have unique properties and so, might bring about inconsistencies in results. There is, therefore, an urgent need for a reputable standard in this field as well as a consensus for measuring accurately the nanotoxicity level. However, based on the research undertaken by us and countless others, specific types of functionalization can greatly limit the amount of toxicity level leaked into the body; and so far, there has been promising progress as to its clinical application in the future. Irrespective of the differences in terms of their wall number, metal contamination source, and particle dimensions, it has been demonstrated by a good number of investigators that several types of CNTs are capable of eliciting similar underlying toxicity, but with varying potencies. According to the research, one of the most important target organs with respect to inhalation is the lungs; however, the skin is also prone to inflammation. As a result, in order for risk assessment to be thoroughly executed, CNTs have been assumed to induce toxic effects with a degree of the threshold. On the other hand, more investigation of systemic effects, that is cardiovascular and immunological, and then, sustainability and reversibility effects, which follows the repeated exposure to inhalation as well as the trigger mechanism for systemic effects via the release of mediators and also, postexposure periods, that is within several months, should be greatly considered.

References

[1] Lacerda L, Bianco A, Prato M, Kostarelos K. Carbon nanotubes as nanomedicines: from toxicology to pharmacology. Advanced drug delivery reviews 2006;58(14):1460–70.

[2] Cheng J, Chan CM, Veca LM, Poon WL, Chan PK, Qu L, et al. Acute and long-term effects after single loading of functionalized multi-walled carbon nanotubes into zebrafish (Danio rerio). Toxicology and applied pharmacology 2009;235(2):216–25.

[3] Burugapalli K, Razavi M, Zhou L, Huang Y. In Vitro Cytocompatibility Study of a Medical β-Type Ti-35.5 Nb-5.7 Ta Titanium Alloy. Journal of Biomaterials and Tissue Engineering 2016;6(2):141–8.

[4] Pantarotto D, Singh R, McCarthy D, Erhardt M, Briand JP, Prato M, et al. Functionalized carbon nanotubes for plasmid DNA gene delivery. Angewandte Chemie 2004;116(39):5354–8.

[5] Pantarotto D, Briand JP, Prato M, Bianco A. Translocation of bioactive peptides across cell membranes by carbon nanotubes. Chemical Communications 2004;1:16–17.

[6] Kam NWS, Dai H. Carbon nanotubes as intracellular protein transporters: generality and biological functionality. Journal of the American Chemical Society 2005;127(16):6021–6.

[7] Wu W, Wieckowski S, Pastorin G, Benincasa M, Klumpp C, Briand JP, et al. Targeted delivery of amphotericin B to cells by using functionalized carbon nanotubes. Angewandte Chemie International Edition 2005;44(39):6358–62.

[8] Lu Q, Moore JM, Huang G, Mount AS, Rao AM, Larcom LL, et al. RNA polymer translocation with single-walled carbon nanotubes. Nano Letters 2004;4(12):2473–7.

[9] Johnston HJ, Hutchison GR, Christensen FM, Peters S, Hankin S, Aschberger K, et al. A critical review of the biological mechanisms underlying the in vivo and in vitro toxicity of

carbon nanotubes: The contribution of physico-chemical characteristics. Nanotoxicology 2010;4(2):207–46.
[10] Jeng HA, Swanson J. Toxicity of metal oxide nanoparticles in mammalian cells. Journal of Environmental Science and Health Part A 2006;41(12):2699–711.
[11] Tsuji JS, Maynard AD, Howard PC, James JT, Lam CW, Warheit DB, et al. Research strategies for safety evaluation of nanomaterials, part IV: risk assessment of nanoparticles. Toxicological sciences 2006;89(1):42–50.
[12] Razavi M, Fathi M, Savabi O, Vashaee D, Tayebi L. In vivo assessments of bioabsorbable AZ91 magnesium implants coated with nanostructured fluoridated hydroxyapatite by MAO/EPD technique for biomedical applications. Materials Science and Engineering: C 2015;48:21–7.
[13] Razavi M, Fathi MH, Savabi O, Vashaee D, Tayebi L. Biodegradation, bioactivity and in vivo biocompatibility analysis of plasma electrolytic oxidized (PEO) biodegradable Mg implants. Physical Science International Journal 2014;4(5):708.
[14] Karamian E, Motamedi MRK, Khandan A, Soltani P, Maghsoudi S. An in vitro evaluation of novel NHA/zircon plasma coating on 316L stainless steel dental implant. Progress in Natural Science: Materials International 2014;24(2):150–6.
[15] Karamian E, Khandan A, Kalantar Motamedi MR, Mirmohammadi H. Surface characteristics and bioactivity of a novel natural HA/zircon nanocomposite coated on dental implants. BioMed research international 2014:2014.
[16] Khandan A, Abdellahi M, Ozada N, Ghayour H. Study of the bioactivity, wettability and hardness behaviour of the bovine hydroxyapatite-diopside bio-nanocomposite coating. Journal of the Taiwan Institute of Chemical Engineers 2016;60:538–46.
[17] Cui FZ, Li DJ. A review of investigations on biocompatibility of diamond-like carbon and carbon nitride films. Surface and Coatings Technology 2000;131(1):481–7.
[18] Khandan A, Abdellahi M, Barenji RV, Ozada N, Karamian E. Introducing natural hydroxyapatite-diopside (NHA-Di) nano-bioceramic coating. Ceramics International 2015;41(9):12355–63.
[19] Ratner BD, Hoffman AS, Schoen FJ, Lemons JE. Biomaterials science: an introduction to materials in medicine. Academic press; 2004.
[20] Karamian E, Abdellahi M, Khandan A, Abdellah S. Introducing the fluorine doped natural hydroxyapatite-titania nanobiocomposite ceramic. Journal of Alloys and Compounds 2016;679:375–83.
[21] Yildirimer L, Thanh NT, Loizidou M, Seifalian AM. Toxicology and clinical potential of nanoparticles. Nano today 2011;6(6):585–607.
[22] Franke H, Galla HJ, Beuckmann CT. Primary cultures of brain microvessel endothelial cells: a valid and flexible model to study drug transport through the blood–brain barrier in vitro. Brain Research Protocols 2000;5(3):248–56.
[23] Cheng R, Feng F, Meng F, Deng C, Feijen J, Zhong Z. Glutathione-responsive nanovehicles as a promising platform for targeted intracellular drug and gene delivery. Journal of controlled release 2011;152(1):2–12.
[24] Benson JD, Chen YNP, Cornell-Kennon SA, Dorsch M, Kim S, Leszczyniecka M, et al. Validating cancer drug targets. Nature 2006;441(7092):451–6.
[25] Ito A, Shinkai M, Honda H, Kobayashi T. Medical application of functionalized magnetic nanoparticles. Journal of bioscience and bioengineering 2005;100(1):1–11.
[26] Gupta AK, Gupta M. Synthesis and surface engineering of iron oxide nanoparticles for biomedical applications. Biomaterials 2005;26(18):3995–4021.
[27] Veiseh O, Gunn JW, Kievit FM, Sun C, Fang C, Lee JS, et al. Inhibition of tumor-cell invasion with chlorotoxin-bound superparamagnetic 2009.

[28] Aschberger K, Johnston HJ, Stone V, Aitken RJ, Hankin SM, Peters SA, et al. Review of carbon nanotubes toxicity and exposure—Appraisal of human health risk assessment based on open literature. Critical reviews in toxicology 2010;40(9):759–90.
[29] Schipper ML, Nakayama-Ratchford N, Davis CR, Kam NWS, Chu P, Liu Z, et al. A pilot toxicology study of single-walled carbon nanotubes in a small sample of mice. Nature nanotechnology 2008;3(4):216–21.
[30] Crouzier D, Follot S, Gentilhomme E, Flahaut E, Arnaud R, Dabouis V, et al. Carbon nanotubes induce inflammation but decrease the production of reactive oxygen species in lung. Toxicology 2010;272(1):39–45.
[31] Yang W, Peters JI, Williams RO. Inhaled nanoparticles—a current review. International Journal of Pharmaceutics 2008;356(1):239–47.
[32] Patton JS, Byron PR. Inhaling medicines: delivering drugs to the body through the lungs. Nature Reviews Drug Discovery 2007;6(1):67–74.
[33] Ryter SW, Kim HP, Hoetzel A, Park JW, Nakahira K, Wang X, et al. Mechanisms of cell death in oxidative stress. Antioxidants & redox signaling 2007;9(1):49–89.
[34] Selkoe DJ. Cell biology of protein misfolding: the examples of Alzheimer's and Parkinson's diseases. Nature cell biology 2004;6(11):1054–61.
[35] Hu K, Shi Y, Jiang W, Han J, Huang S, Jiang X. Lactoferrin conjugated PEG-PLGA nanoparticles for brain delivery: preparation, characterization and efficacy in Parkinson's disease. International journal of pharmaceutics 2011;415(1):273–83.
[36] Brigger I, Dubernet C, Couvreur P. Nanoparticles in cancer therapy and diagnosis. Advanced drug delivery reviews 2002;54(5):631–51.
[37] Matsuo Y, Ishihara T, Ishizaki J, Miyamoto KI, Higaki M, Yamashita N. Effect of betamethasone phosphate loaded polymeric nanoparticles on a murine asthma model. Cellular immunology 2009;260(1):33–8.
[38] Pison U, Welte T, Giersig M, Groneberg DA. Nanomedicine for respiratory diseases. European Journal of Pharmacology 2006;533(1):341–50.
[39] Sosnik A, Carcaboso ÁM, Glisoni RJ, Moretton MA, Chiappetta DA. New old challenges in tuberculosis: potentially effective nanotechnologies in drug delivery. Advanced drug delivery reviews 2010;62(4):547–59.
[40] Sarfati G, Dvir T, Elkabets M, Apte RN, Cohen S. Targeting of polymeric nanoparticles to lung metastases by surface-attachment of YIGSR peptide from laminin. Biomaterials 2011;32(1):152–61.
[41] Rink JS, McMahon KM, Chen X, Mirkin CA, Thaxton CS, Kaufman DB. Transfection of pancreatic islets using polyvalent DNA-functionalized gold nanoparticles. Surgery 2010;148(2):335–45.
[42] Heydary HA, Karamian E, Poorazizi E, Heydaripour J, Khandan A. Electrospun of polymer/bioceramic nanocomposite as a new soft tissue for biomedical applications. Journal of Asian Ceramic Societies 2015;3(4):417–25.
[43] Yang R, Yang SG, Shim WS, Cui F, Cheng G, Kim IW, et al. Lung-specific delivery of paclitaxel by chitosan-modified PLGA nanoparticles via transient formation of microaggregates. Journal of pharmaceutical sciences 2009;98(3):970–84.
[44] Tian F, Cui D, Schwarz H, Estrada GG, Kobayashi H. Cytotoxicity of single-wall carbon nanotubes on human fibroblasts. Toxicology in vitro 2006;20(7):1202–12.
[45] Lin W, Huang YW, Zhou XD, Ma Y. In vitro toxicity of silica nanoparticles in human lung cancer cells. Toxicology and applied pharmacology 2006;217(3):252–9.
[46] Akhtar MJ, Ahamed M, Kumar S, Siddiqui H, Patil G, Ashquin M, et al. Nanotoxicity of pure silica mediated through oxidant generation rather than glutathione depletion in human lung epithelial cells. Toxicology 2010;276(2):95–102.

[47] Yang H, Liu C, Yang D, Zhang H, Xi Z. Comparative study of cytotoxicity, oxidative stress and genotoxicity induced by four typical nanomaterials: the role of particle size, shape and composition. Journal of applied Toxicology 2009;29(1):69–78.
[48] Lu S, Duffin R, Poland C, Daly P, Murphy F, Drost E, et al. Efficacy of simple short-term in vitro assays for predicting the potential of metal oxide nanoparticles to cause pulmonary inflammation. Environmental health perspectives 2009;117(2):241.
[49] Napierska D, Thomassen LC, Rabolli V, Lison D, Gonzalez L, Kirsch-Volders M, et al. Size-Dependent Cytotoxicity of Monodisperse Silica Nanoparticles in Human Endothelial Cells. Small 2009;5(7):846–53.
[50] Meng H, Liong M, Xia T, Li Z, Ji Z, Zink JI, et al. Engineered design of mesoporous silica nanoparticles to deliver doxorubicin and P-glycoprotein siRNA to overcome drug resistance in a cancer cell line. ACS nano 2010;4(8):4539–50.
[51] Shi X, Wang Y, Varshney RR, Ren L, Zhang F, Wang DA. In-vitro osteogenesis of synovium stem cells induced by controlled release of bisphosphate additives from microspherical mesoporous silica composite. Biomaterials 2009;30(23):3996–4005.
[52] Kazemi A, Abdellahi M, Khajeh-Sharafabadi A, Khandan A, Ozada N. Study of in vitro bioactivity and mechanical properties of diopside nano-bioceramic synthesized by a facile method using eggshell as raw material. Materials Science and Engineering: C 2016.
[53] Najafinezhad A, Abdellahi M, Ghayour H, Soheily A, Chami A, Khandan A. A comparative study on the synthesis mechanism, bioactivity and mechanical properties of three silicate bioceramics. Materials Science and Engineering: C 2017;72:259–67.
[54] Sharafabadi AK, Abdellahi M, Kazemi A, Khandan A, Ozada N. A novel and economical route for synthesizing akermanite ($Ca_2 MgSi_2 O_7$) nano-bioceramic. Materials Science and Engineering: C 2016.
[55] Yazdimamaghani M, Razavi M, Vashaee D, Moharamzadeh K, Boccaccini AR, Tayebi L. Porous magnesium-based scaffold tissue engineering. Materials Science and Engineering: C 2016.
[56] Samberg ME, Oldenburg SJ, Monteiro-Riviere NA. Evaluation of silver nanoparticle toxicity in skin in vivo and keratinocytes in vitro. Environmental health perspectives 2010;118(3):407.
[57] Sharma HS, Hussain S, Schlager J, Ali SF, Sharma A. Influence of nanoparticles on blood–brain barrier permeability and brain edema formation in rats Brain edema XIV. Vienna: Springer; 2010. p. 359–64.
[58] Tang J, Xiong L, Wang S, Wang J, Liu L, Li J, et al. Distribution, translocation and accumulation of silver nanoparticles in rats. Journal of nanoscience and nanotechnology 2009;9(8):4924–32.
[59] Arora S, Jain J, Rajwade JM, Paknikar KM. Cellular responses induced by silver nanoparticles: in vitro studies. Toxicology letters 2008;179(2):93–100.
[60] Lankveld DPK, Oomen AG, Krystek P, Neigh A, Troost–de Jong A, Noorlander CW, et al. The kinetics of the tissue distribution of silver nanoparticles of different sizes. Biomaterials 2010;31(32):8350–61.
[61] Kim S, Choi JE, Choi J, Chung KH, Park K, Yi J, et al. Oxidative stress-dependent toxicity of silver nanoparticles in human hepatoma cells. Toxicology in vitro 2009;23(6):1076–84.
[62] Teodoro JS, Simões AM, Duarte FV, Rolo AP, Murdoch RC, Hussain SM, et al. Assessment of the toxicity of silver nanoparticles in vitro: a mitochondrial perspective. Toxicology in Vitro 2011;25(3):664–70.
[63] Pornpattananangkul D, Olson S, Aryal S, Sartor M, Huang CM, Vecchio K, et al. Stimuli-responsive liposome fusion mediated by gold nanoparticles. ACS nano 2010;4(4):1935–42.

[64] Murphy CJ, Gole AM, Stone JW, Sisco PN, Alkilany AM, Goldsmith EC, et al. Gold nanoparticles in biology: beyond toxicity to cellular imaging. Accounts of chemical research 2008;41(12):1721–30.
[65] Mironava T, Hadjiargyrou M, Simon M, Rafailovich MH. Gold nanoparticles cellular toxicity and recovery: Adipose Derived Stromal cells. Nanotoxicology 2014;8(2):189–201.
[66] Mironava T, Hadjiargyrou M, Simon M, Jurukovski V, Rafailovich MH. Gold nanoparticles cellular toxicity and recovery: effect of size, concentration and exposure time. Nanotoxicology 2010;4(1):120–37.
[67] Mironava T, Simon M, Rafailovich MH, Rigas B. Platinum folate nanoparticles toxicity: cancer vs. normal cells. Toxicology in Vitro 2013;27(2):882–9.
[68] Jung CW, Jacobs P. Physical and chemical properties of superparamagnetic iron oxide MR contrast agents: ferumoxides, ferumoxtran, ferumoxsil. Magnetic resonance imaging 1995;13(5):661–74.
[69] Raynal I, Prigent P, Peyramaure S, Najid A, Rebuzzi C, Corot C. Macrophage endocytosis of superparamagnetic iron oxide nanoparticles: mechanisms and comparison of ferumoxides and ferumoxtran-10. Investigative radiology 2004;39(1):56–63.
[70] Brunner TJ, Wick P, Manser P, Spohn P, Grass RN, Limbach LK, et al. In vitro cytotoxicity of oxide nanoparticles: comparison to asbestos, silica, and the effect of particle solubility. Environmental science & technology 2006;40(14):4374–81.
[71] Oberdörster G, Stone V, Donaldson K. Toxicology of nanoparticles: a historical perspective. Nanotoxicology 2007;1(1):2–25.
[72] Berry CC, Wells S, Charles S, Curtis AS. Dextran and albumin derivatised iron oxide nanoparticles: influence on fibroblasts in vitro. Biomaterials 2003;24(25):4551–7.
[73] Berry CC, Wells S, Charles S, Aitchison G, Curtis AS. Cell response to dextran-derivatised iron oxide nanoparticles post internalisation. Biomaterials 2004;25(23):5405–13.
[74] Mahmoudi M, Simchi A, Imani M, Shokrgozar MA, Milani AS, Häfeli UO, et al. A new approach for the in vitro identification of the cytotoxicity of superparamagnetic iron oxide nanoparticles. Colloids and Surfaces B: Biointerfaces 2010;75(1):300–9.
[75] Saeedi M, Abdellahi M, Rahimi A, Khandan A. Preparation and characterization of nanocrystalline barium ferrite ceramic. Functional Materials Letters 2016;9(05):1650068.
[76] Ghayour H, Abdellahi M, Bahmanpour M, Khandan A. Simulation of dielectric behavior in RFeO_ {3} orthoferrite ceramics (R = rare earth metals). Journal of Computational Electronics 2016;15(4):1275–83.
[77] Jabbarzare S, Abdellahi M, Ghayour H, Arpanahi A, Khandan A. A study on the synthesis and magnetic properties of the cerium ferrite ceramic. Journal of Alloys and Compounds 2017;694:800–7.
[78] Zhang TS, Ma J, Kong LB, Chan SH, Kilner JA. Aging behavior and ionic conductivity of ceria-based ceramics: a comparative study. Solid State Ionics 2004;170(3):209–17.
[79] Wu A, Shen H, Xu J, Wang Z, Jiang L, Luo L, et al. Crystal growth and magnetic property of YFeO 3 crystal. Bulletin of Materials Science 2012;35(2):259–63.
[80] Ameta J, Kumar A, Ameta R, Sharma VK, Ameta SC. Synthesis and characterization of CeFeO3 photocatalyst used in photocatalytic bleaching of gentian violet. Journal of the Iranian Chemical Society 2009;6(2):293–9.
[81] Abbad A, Benstaali W, Bentounes HA, Bentata S, Benmalem Y. Search for half-metallic ferromagnetism in orthorhombic Ce (Fe/Cr) O3 perovskites. Solid State Communications 2016;228:36–42.
[82] Liu X, Novosad V, Rozhkova EA, Chen H, Yefremenko V, Pearson J, et al. Surface functionalized biocompatible magnetic nanospheres for cancer hyperthermia. IEEE transactions on magnetics 2007;43(6):2462–4.

[83] Jordan A, Scholz R, Wust P, Schirra H, Schiestel T, Schmidt H, et al. Endocytosis of dextran and silan-coated magnetite nanoparticles and the effect of intracellular hyperthermia on human mammary carcinoma cells in vitro. Journal of Magnetism and Magnetic Materials 1999;194(1):185–96.
[84] Ehrenfest DMD, Coelho PG, Kang BS, Sul YT, Albrektsson T. Classification of osseointegrated implant surfaces: materials, chemistry and topography. Trends in biotechnology 2010;28(4):198–206.
[85] Lang NP, Jepsen S. Implant surfaces and design (Working Group 4). Clinical Oral Implants Research 2009;20(s4):228–31.
[86] Kiss B, Bíró T, Czifra G, Tóth BI, Kertész Z, Szikszai Z, et al. Investigation of micronized titanium dioxide penetration in human skin xenografts and its effect on cellular functions of human skin-derived cells. Experimental dermatology 2008;17(8):659–67.
[87] Pan Z, Lee W, Slutsky L, Clark RA, Pernodet N, Rafailovich MH. Adverse effects of titanium dioxide nanoparticles on human dermal fibroblasts and how to protect cells. Small 2009; 5(4):511–20.
[88] Lademann J, Weigmann HJ, Rickmeyer C, Barthelmes H, Schaefer H, Mueller G, et al. Penetration of titanium dioxide microparticles in a sunscreen formulation into the horny layer and the follicular orifice. Skin Pharmacology and Physiology 1999; 12(5):247–56.
[89] Mavon A, Miquel C, Lejeune O, Payre B, Moretto P. In vitro percutaneous absorption and in vivo stratum corneum distribution of an organic and a mineral sunscreen. Skin pharmacology and physiology 2006;20(1):10–20.
[90] Kuboki Y, Takita H, Kobayashi D, Tsuruga E, Inoue M, Murata M, et al. BMP-induced osteogenesis on the surface of hydroxyapatite with geometrically feasible and nonfeasible structures: topology of osteogenesis. Journal of biomedical materials research 1998;39(2):190–9.
[91] Ripamonti U. The morphogenesis of bone in replicas of porous hydroxyapatite obtained from conversion of calcium carbonate exoskeletons of coral. J Bone Joint Surg Am 1991;73(5):692–703.
[92] Dorozhkin SV. Bioceramics of calcium orthophosphates. Biomaterials 2010;31(7):1465–85.
[93] Habibovic P, Yuan H, van der Valk CM, Meijer G, van Blitterswijk CA, de Groot K. 3D microenvironment as essential element for osteoinduction by biomaterials. Biomaterials 2005;26(17):3565–75.
[94] Nagase M, Baker DG, Schumacher Jr HR. Prolonged inflammatory reactions induced by artificial ceramics in the rat air pouch model. The Journal of rheumatology 1988;15(9):1334–8.
[95] Rooney T, Berman S, Indresano AT. Evaluation of porous block hydroxylapatite for augmentation of alveolar ridges. Journal of Oral and Maxillofacial Surgery 1988;46(1):15–18.
[96] Prudhommeaux F, Schiltz C, Lioté F, Hina A, Champy R, Bucki B, et al. Variation in the inflammatory properties of basic calcium phosphate crystals according to crystal type. Arthritis & Rheumatism 1996;39(8):1319–26.
[97] Dresselhaus MS, Dresselhaus G, Saito R. Physics of carbon nanotubes. Carbon 1995;33(7):883–91.
[98] Dougherty TJ, Gomer CJ, Henderson BW, Jori G, Kessel D, Korbelik M, et al. Photodynamic therapy. Journal of the National Cancer Institute 1998;90(12):889–905.
[99] Radomski A, Jurasz P, Alonso-Escolano D, Drews M, Morandi M, Malinski T, et al. Nanoparticle-induced platelet aggregation and vascular thrombosis. British journal of pharmacology 2005;146(6):882–93.

[100] Yang ST, Wang X, Jia G, Gu Y, Wang T, Nie H, et al. Long-term accumulation and low toxicity of single-walled carbon nanotubes in intravenously exposed mice. Toxicology letters 2008;181(3):182–9.

[101] Li Z, Hulderman T, Salmen R, Chapman R, Leonard SS, Young SH, et al. Cardiovascular effects of pulmonary exposure to single-wall carbon nanotubes. Environmental health perspectives 2007:377–82.

[102] Helfenstein M, Miragoli M, Rohr S, Müller L, Wick P, Mohr M, et al. Effects of combustion-derived ultrafine particles and manufactured nanoparticles on heart cells in vitro. Toxicology 2008;253(1):70–8.

[103] Huczko A, Lange H. Carbon nanotubes: experimental evidence for a null risk of skin irritation and allergy. Fullerene Science and Technology 2001;9(2):247–50.

[104] Kishore AS, Surekha P, Murthy PB. Assessment of the dermal and ocular irritation potential of multi-walled carbon nanotubes by using in vitro and in vivo methods. Toxicology letters 2009;191(2):268–74.

[105] Kolosnjaj-Tabi J, Hartman KB, Boudjemaa S, Ananta JS, Morgant G, Szwarc H, et al. In vivo behavior of large doses of ultrashort and full-length single-walled carbon nanotubes after oral and intraperitoneal administration to Swiss mice. Acs Nano 2010;4(3):1481–92.

[106] Maynard AD, Baron PA, Foley M, Shvedova AA, Kisin ER, Castranova V. Exposure to carbon nanotube material: aerosol release during the handling of unrefined single-walled carbon nanotube material. Journal of Toxicology and Environmental Health, Part A 2004;67(1):87–107.

[107] Methner M, Hodson L, Dames A, Geraci C. Nanoparticle emission assessment technique (NEAT) for the identification and measurement of potential inhalation exposure to engineered nanomaterials—Part B: Results from 12 field studies. Journal of occupational and environmental hygiene 2010;7(3):163–76.

[108] Folkmann JK, Risom L, Jacobsen NR, Wallin H, Loft S, Møller P. Oxidatively Damaged DNA in Rats Exposed by Oral Gavage to C_{60} Fullerenes and Single-Walled Carbon Nanotubes. Environmental health perspectives 2009;117(5):703.

[109] Migliore L, Saracino D, Bonelli A, Colognato R, D'Errico MR, Magrini A, et al. Carbon nanotubes induce oxidative DNA damage in RAW 264.7 cells. Environmental and molecular mutagenesis 2010;51(4):294–303.

[110] Jacobs H, Okano T, Lin JY, Kim SW. PGE1—Heparin conjugate releasing polymers. Journal of Controlled Release 1985;2:313–9.

Practical aspects

15

Serda Kecel-Gunduz, Sefa Celik and Aysen E. Ozel
Istanbul University, Istanbul, Turkey

15.1 Introduction

Nanotechnology is about the functional design and production of structures from atoms and molecules, at scales of 1–100 nm, and the examination of those structures and their effective utilization [1]. The size and distribution of the particles is the most important characteristic for studies at nanoscales: namely nanoscience [2–3]. In addition to basic research in physics, chemistry, and biological sciences, nanotechnology and nanoscience is widely used in many areas. These areas include nanoelectronics and computer technologies (fiber optic communication networks), aviation and space research, environment and energy, agriculture, chemical engineering and the defense industry, and especially biomedical and medical fields due to the nanoscales possible. The most important development in these fields was the invention of the scanning tunneling microscope in 1981 by Binning and Rohrer, who won a Nobel Prize for their invention [4]. That study made it possible to examine the surface of biological materials at nanoscales. Another development was the discovery of fullerene particles, which are the building blocks for synthetic carbon nanostructures, by Kroto et al. in 1985 [5]. Fullerene particles are C60 allotropes that form carbon nanotube arrays.

Nanotechnology can be explained in two ways, using a "top-down" approach or a "bottom-up" approach, that can be summarized as follows:

Bottom-up: (From atoms to molecules, from molecules to materials)
This is an approach from the small scale to the big scale. It is about creating molecules by aligning atoms, the most fundamental building blocks of matter.
Top-down: (From materials to molecules, from molecules to atoms)
This is an approach from the big scale to the small scale. It is about decomposing materials into its atoms via mechanical or chemical processes and rearranging them. Owing to technological advances, this method is the more commonly performed (Fig. 15.1).

Nanotechnological products occur in our daily lives in so many areas and make our lives easier by replacing the materials we use with smarter, long-lasting ones. There are many examples of the application of nanotechnology, from self-cleaning paints to drip-dry and dirt-repellent fabrics; from elastic but more solid concrete to diamond-hard coatings; from killing cancer cells without harming the body to nanotechnological drug-carrying systems, creams with effects that last for days, antibacterial and odor-free socks, and antimicrobial fridges.

Nanobiomaterials Science, Development and Evaluation. DOI: http://dx.doi.org/10.1016/B978-0-08-100963-5.00015-X

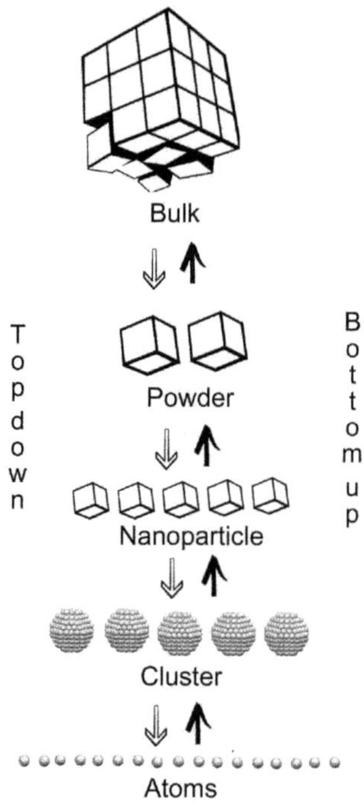

Figure 15.1 Schematic representation of the top-down and bottom-up synthesis processes of nanomaterials.

15.2 Part I: Nanomaterials and their types

15.2.1 Nanotechnological drug-carrying systems

Nanotechnology has developed new drug-carrying systems for the delivery of active molecules to the target tissue or cells in the body. The idea of using carrying systems for drugs was initially proposed by Paul Ehrlich in the form of magic bullets, which are now widely used in medicine [6].

Nanocarriers provide useful, enhanced systems for diagnosis and treatment by quickly solving the problems encountered when dealing with the absorption of the drugs and their delivery to the correct parts of the body. Especially in cancer treatments, the nanocarriers are crucial in avoiding the unwanted side effects of the drugs released into the body by directly targeting the cancer cells. Nanocarriers are solid, colloidal particles at submicron-scales, generally with radii of 10–1000 nm. They are prepared from polymers with specific physicochemical properties and are used as carrying systems after being loaded with drugs. Drug-carrying nanoparticle systems can be classified as nanocapsules, nanospheres, nanotubes, nanocrystals, or nanoemulsions.

Nanoparticles: These are solid, matrix-type structures with a circular form having particle sizes between 100 nm and 200 nm. They are usually obtained from natural or synthetic polymers. The drug is dissolved in the polymer matrix where it is trapped and encapsulated by being chemically bound or adsorbed. Inside the body, nanoparticles allow the release of various drugs, vaccines, and hydrophobic and hydrophilic biological macromolecules. Additionally, studies show that nanoparticles allow controlled drug release to specific organs and cells [7]. The nanoparticles either encapsulate the drug molecules or carry those using covalent bonds when delivering them to the tumorous tissue. Nanoparticles fix the stability, solubility, and permeability of the drug by reducing its decay under physiological conditions. They decrease the drug concentration within healthy tissues and the toxic side effects associated with this by passive and active targeting methods to increase the drug concentration within the tumorous tissues and—through the active targeting method and surface modification method—provide the specific delivery of the drug, enabling penetration of the tumor.

Nanotubes: Peptide nanotubes are highly organized materials that are formed by noncovalent hydrogen bond interactions and van der Waals interactions [8]. Owing to the conformations and functional varieties of proteins and peptides, peptide nanotubes are versatile molecules for the development of nanometer scale devices [9–12], and they are used in many different fields such as biochemistry, chemistry, biology, and medicine [13]. Depending on the specific interactions between the peptide nanotubes and the biomolecules, they are used in molecular-recognition procedures and as medicine-recognition docks. Peptide nanotubes are classified into two groups as either cyclic or linear nanotubes. Studies have been carried out on cyclic peptide nanotubes since 1974, and they have become an important research topic in ion or small molecule delivery. The structure, the dynamic characteristics, and the carrying properties of cyclic peptides have been examined through experimental and theoretical studies [14–18]. One of the reasons behind the use of cyclic peptide structures is that they are easy to synthesize, have pores with varying radii, have a changing surface chemistry, and they act as a new type of antibiotics against bacterial pathogens [19].

Ghadiri et al. have become the pioneers in the design of cyclic peptide nanotubes [20]. Cyclic peptides have characteristic structural properties [21–22]. The structure of the nanotube depends on the D- and L-α-amino acids in an alternating order. Cyclic D- and L-α-peptides have structural properties that peptide antibiotics and their derivatives do not [23]. Cyclic nanotubes that have D- and L-α-peptide arrangements are antibacterial and have an important place in applications as drug-carrying agents [24]. Zang et al. demonstrated the nanotube formation using unpaired linear peptide monomers. Those peptides have two different surfaces: hydrophilic and hydrophobic [25].

Amino acid chains that make up the linear peptide combine to form nanotube structures by themselves. The best example of these are the nanotubes with radii varying between 20 nm and 50 nm that are obtained from α-lactalbumin. The formation of this nanotube depends on the structure of α-lactalbumin and can be used for protection of the drugs [26]. Linear peptides are a member of the bolaamphiphile peptide class. The structures of bolaamphiphile peptide-based nanotubes can be investigated using X-ray and Raman spectroscopy. In a study in 2000, it was observed that metal-covered nanowires could be produced from bolaamphiphile peptide nanotubes

[27]. In that study, researchers used glycylglycine bolaamphiphile crystals. Ordered nanofibers, formed by ionic peptides (a peptide subcategory), were used in tissue engineering for cell renewal. In 2005, Hidenori Yokoi et al. did important studies on the three-dimensional (3D) cell culture, tissue repair, and cell renewal using the nanofiber structure of the RADARADARADARADA (RADA16-I) ionic peptide [28]. The first applications of peptide nanotubes have been in antibiotic agents interacting with bacterial membranes. It was found by some studies that peptide nanotubes are an effective carrier allowing membrane trespassing (hence an antibiotic agent) for ions and molecules such as water or glucose [29–30]. Many peptides are being used safely on living organisms (in vivo) or in the laboratory (in vitro); nevertheless, short- and long-term side effects are still a matter of concern. In a study by Westermark et al. in 2009, it was observed that amyloid remnants were found in rats that had been given peptides including RADA16-I and silver nitrate [31]. Amyloid is a harmful peptide sequence that breaks the communication between the cells and makes the tissue (or the organ) dysfunctional by increasing cell death [32]. It became possible to diagnose many diseases early on, such as cancer or oriental sore, with the use of modified electrodes [33]. In another study by Katerina A. Drouvalakis et al. in 2008, nanotube-based immunosensors were used for the first time for direct identification of antibodies related to the diseases in human serum [34]. In 2013, studies were done for the detection of cancer cells using folic acid peptide nanotubes applied to modified graphene electrodes. Phe–Phe dipeptide and its derivatives, which already have an important role in cancer treatments and drug-carrying systems, will continue to have a significant part in future studies, as reported by Silvia et al. [35]. The structure of linear peptides are being studied in both theoretical and experimental works [36–40].

Nanospheres: Nanospheres, found in amorphous or crystalline structures in nature, have the ability to protect the drug against enzymatic and chemical decay. Biocompatible and recyclable polymeric materials are used in the preparation of nanospheres as drug carriers. Nanospheres can be categorized as immune nanospheres and magnetic nanospheres. Immunomagnetic nanospheres that are prepared from a combination of the two types improve the targeting considerably. Since these carrying systems are nanosize, they can pass through the smallest blood vessels and penetrate the target cells or tissues. Nowadays, nanospheres are used in many applications using polypeptides, proteins, amino acids, and genes. Further studies are being done to improve nanosphere drug-carrying systems in terms of parameters such as drug release rate, surface modification, and drug-carrying capacity [41–43].

Nanocrystals: Colloidal nanocrystals comprise an important class of materials with a potentially high number of different applications ranging from medicine to electronics and optoelectronic devices [44]. Within recent years, nanocrystal formulations have become important as carriers for oral, parenteral, and other drug applications with low solubility [45]. Drugs in the form of nanocrystals—solid particles at nanosizes—do not require any solvents and/or encapsulation chemicals in their application. Since there is no need for encapsulation, and their formulation is easy, nanocrystals can be produced in large amounts. The key property of drug nanocrystals with nanometer size is that their content is 100% drug, like the polymeric nanoparticles, but with no carrier material. Since there are no solid dissolution agents in their formulations, nanocrystals are expected to have a low toxicity and a high anticancer effect [46]. They are obtained via milling, precipitation, or homogenization, or by a combination of those three methods. All of the industrial methods aim to obtain smaller sizes from a drug powder.

Nanocapsules: Nanocapsules are a subcategory of nanoparticles that are vesicular systems consisting of an inner core of colloidal size, encircled by a polymeric protector [47–49]. They have become interesting for biomedical research because they can protect enzymes, proteins, and other alien cells and focus the drugs onto their targets and control their release [50–52]. Some of those systems are liposomes, nanoparticles, active matter polymer conjugates, polymeric micelles, dendrimers, hydrogels, and solid lipid particles. The use of polymeric materials, especially as the encapsulating material, is very common.

Polymers that are used in medical applications—such as polyethylene (PE), polyurethane (PU), polytetrafluoroethylene (PTFE), polyacetal (PA), polymethylmethacrylate (PMMA), polyethylene teraphthalate (PET), silicon rubber (SR), polysulfone (PS), polylactic acid (PLA), and polyglycolic acid (PGA)—can be produced in various compositions and shapes (fiber, film, gel, bead, nanoparticles) and therefore have a broad spectrum of use as biomaterials [53].

Polymeric nanoparticles—poly(alkyl cyanoacrylates) (PACA), chitosan-PLA, poly(lactic-co-glycolic acid) (PLGA) nanoparticles—are micelle-based systems, dendrimers, phospholipid, and lipid-based systems. It is seen that chitosan-coated polycaprolactone has the biopotential to provide drug release for the treatment of bladder cancer, whereas pemetrexed loaded magnetic O-carboxmethyl chitosan nanoparticles have that ability for lung cancer and golden nanoparticle-drug conjugates for a variety of cancers [54].

Proteins comprise a class of natural molecules that has functionality and potential applications in biology. Nanomaterials produced from proteins are recyclable, antigenic, and can be easily bonded to the surfaces of drugs and ligands. Interest in polymeric nanoparticles has increased gradually throughout past years. Nowadays, active research is focused on the preparation of nanoparticles using proteins such as albumin and gelatin. The delivery of treating molecules via polymeric nanoparticles is an important application for cancer treatment [55].

Nanoemulsions: Nanoemulsions are colloidal particle systems with sizes between 10 nm and 1000 nm, and are used as carriers for drug molecules. These carriers are solid spheres and their surfaces are negatively charged, amorphous, and lipophilic. Nanoemulsions, whose basic content is lipid and aqueous phases, can easily penetrate the cells of microorganisms such as bacteria or fungi and terminate them, thus minimizing the toxic reaction. They protect the drug and increase its bioactivity [56–58], and are therefore widely used in drug-carrying systems. In 2003, it was seen that nanoemulsions with no side effects on the mucosa membrane showed biological activity against harmful viruses via a study on rats and other animals [59]. More research and development on nanoemulsions is expected [60] (Fig. 15.2).

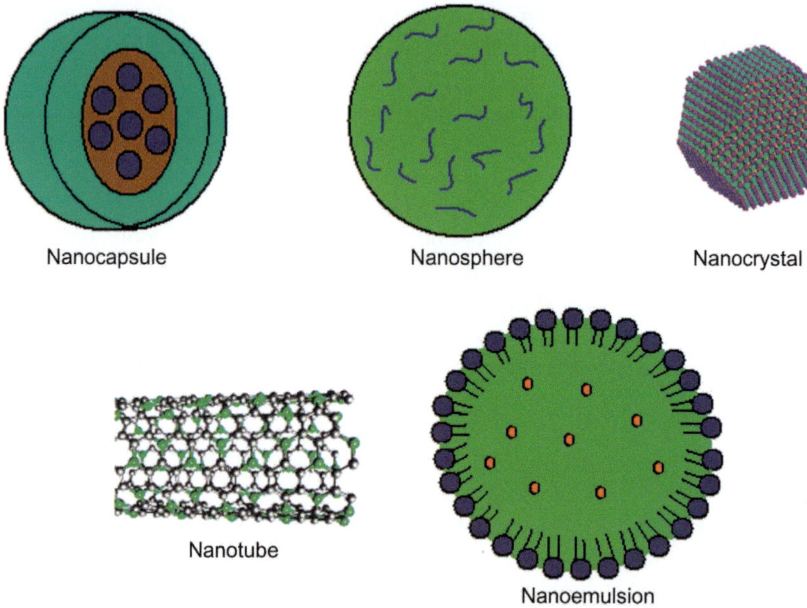

Figure 15.2 Schematic representation of the nanocapsule, nanosphere, nanocrystal, nanotube, and nanoemulsion.

15.3 Part II: The uses of nanomaterials

15.3.1 Nanotechnology in cancer diagnosis and treatment

The use of nanotechnology in the detection, diagnosis, and treatment of diseases is one of the biggest innovations in the medical field. Responding to cancer cells at the early stages of the mutation can stop the evolution of cancer [61]. Currently, the growth or changes in the organs can be monitored via classical methods, but the cancer diagnosis can be made only with a biopsy if there is any doubt. With nanostructures, a single tumor cell can be penetrated, and with the developments in related imaging technologies, tumors can be diagnosed at an earlier stage compared to classical methods. The diagnosis of breast cancer via mammography requires one million tumor cells to be present; however, it is possible to make a diagnosis with fewer than 100 cells using nanotechnological structures [62]. Iron oxide nanoparticles are being used as contrast agents in magnetic resonance imaging of cancer cells. Iron oxide nanoparticles have low toxicity, can adhere in the blood for a long time and can be broken down biologically [63,64]. Semiconducting quantum dots (QDs) are particles at nanometer size with optical and electronic features, enhanced signal intensity, and stability. With QDs emitting radiation at different wavelengths, it is possible to image and monitor more than one tumor indicator at the same time. This increases the sensitivity for detection of cancerous cells.

Sathe et al. have performed studies on imaging of cancerous cells using nanocrystals with iron oxide and QDs. From these studies, it has been determined that the combination of nanocrystals with iron oxide and QDs can be used to get the best image quality [65].

It is shown that QD nanoparticles that are actively targeted at the MUC1 mucin protein can be used in imaging ovarian cancer [66], whereas QDs targeted at HER2 receptors can be used in imaging breast tumor cells [67], and QDs targeted at tumor-related glycoprotein 72 (TAG-72) can be used in imaging gastric cancer cells [68].

The primary methods in cancer treatment are radiotherapy, chemotherapy, and surgery. Radiotherapy relies on the destruction of cancer cells with radiation at specific frequencies. The disadvantages of this method are the exposure of healthy cells to radiation and the loss of functionality in the tissue, and the inability to distribute radiation to the cancer cells equally. The most important aim in chemotherapy is to annihilate the mechanisms sustaining the division of cancerous cells. For this purpose, drugs with toxic effects are used to kill cancerous cells. However, the drugs are not targeted within the body and they affect the healthy cells as well as the cancerous ones. Surgical methods involving the removal of cancerous tissues also has disadvantages, such as the possible loss of an organ, risk of recurrence of the disease, and the inability to perform it on all types of cancer.

Important innovations have been made in nanooncology to increase the concentration of the treatment drugs within the cancerous cells and to minimize the toxic effects on the healthy cells [69].

Aptamers are DNA or RNA oligonucleotides used in targeted therapy that adhere to the target molecules. Owing to their small size, they do not interact with the whole surface of the molecule and stay stable in the circulatory system without losing their activity for a long time [70].

P-glycoprotein is a protein that enables drugs to be transported within the body. Any change in its activity may reduce the curative effects of the drug and increase its toxic effects. With targeted therapy using nanotechnological methods, the release of P-glycoprotein can be controlled.

Since peptides with amino acid sequences typical to cancer cells are smaller than antibodies, and are chemically durable, their use in targeted cancer treatment is increasing. Various studies show that they can be combined with various drugs or drug-carrying systems and be selectively targeted at cancerous cells [33].

15.3.2 Nanotechnology in tissue engineering and dental treatment

Nanotechnology, together with nanomaterials, nanorobots, and related biotechnologies, is being used in dentistry, tissue engineering, implantology, and restorative dental treatments [71,72]. Resin-based composites is one of the most important nanotechnological developments in dental treatment. The main reason behind the use of nanofillings—and hence nanotechnology—in dentistry and dental treatments are that nanocomposites can be used in all teeth. They have good polishing and adherence qualities, a wide range of colors, and good mechanical properties [73]. With the use of noninjection nanorobotic painkillers in dental treatments, analgesic activity can be controlled, the process will be speeded up and the side effects minimized. Thus, patient concerns and fears will be resolved resulting in increased comfort. Technological studies are being carried on the identification and destruction of plaque within the oral cavity and of pathogenic bacteria elsewhere by nanorobots [74]. Nanohydroxyapatite is a highly biocompatible and bioactive material that is used in dentistry for osteogenesis and remineralization. In various studies, it has been shown that toothpastes containing nanohydroxyapatite are more effective in avoiding caries compared to other toothpastes [75,76]. Nanofibers produced from biopolymers have an important place in biomedical sciences due to their properties. They are used as wound dressings since they do not contain toxic materials, they stop fungus reproduction, and they are hemostatic, antiallergic, and breathable. As reported in research material, antibacterial nanofiber wound dressings produced from biopolymers containing silver ions can sustain an effective defense against various bacteria [77,78]. Replacing dead tissue with artificial tissue produced for the human body using steady, resistant, and durable nanomaterials will be one of the most important contributions of nanotechnology to tissue engineering.

15.3.3 Nanotechnology in the treatment of eye diseases

PMMA, PACA, polycaprolactone, albumin, gelatin, PLA, chitosan, and Eudgarid are nanoparticles that are used in drug delivery to the eye due to their drug-loading capacity, drug release rate, and biocompatibility of the polymers used. Chitosan is the most preferable nanoparticle for drug delivery to the eye for the treatment of many diseases such as glaucoma, ocular infections, and ocular inflammations, due to its biodegradability, biocompatibility, and stability [79–81].

15.3.4 Nanotechnology in the treatment of cardiovascular diseases

Nanocarriers are also preferred in the field of cardiology, because their small sizes allow them to travel inside the blood vessels, they are biodegradable, biocompatible, and have low toxicity. Magnetic nanoparticles with super-paramagnetic properties, coated with carbohydrate or polymers containing an iron oxide core, are very important for the imaging of cardiovascular diseases. Nanostents developed using nanotechnology help the healing process for cardiac patients and prohibit blood coagulation [82].

15.3.5 Nanotechnology in the treatment of neurological diseases

The blood brain barrier (BBB) is a defense mechanism developed by the brain against pathogens and toxins. This barrier acts as a filter that stops many water-soluble active substances such as antibiotics, neuropeptides, and other oligo- and macro-molecules from trespassing to the central nervous system. Various carrying strategies have been developed for the delivery of water-soluble active substances. Nanoparticles and nanovesicles are used as drug-carrying systems. Additionally, the local application of convection-enhanced delivery (CED) liposome is a method that is used in diagnosis and treatment. Apart from brain tumors, this method can also be used for the diagnosis and treatment of neurodegenerative diseases such as Alzheimer's or Parkinson's disease [83,84].

15.3.6 Nanotechnology in the cosmetics industry and its applications

Nanotechnology has many application areas in cosmetics, ranging from suntan creams to moisturizers, and from perfumes to hair conditioners. Nanotitanium dioxide (TiO_2) and zinc oxide (ZnO) particles are widely used for protection in suntan creams. The particles block ultraviolet (UV) rays, spread more evenly on the skin, are more transparent, less scented, and leave no residuals [85,86]. In vitro studies showed that nano-TiO_2 and ZnO particles penetrate the stratum corneum layer of the skin and accumulate there [86,87]. There are also products being developed containing nanoiron molecules instead of nano-TiO_2 or ZnO to protect against UV rays [87]. In the production of dyes for hair, eyelashes, eyebrows, and nails, nanocelluloses are used. Nanocelluloses are categorized into three groups according to their features: microfiber cellulose, nanocrystal cellulose, and bacterial nanocellulose. Bacterial nanocellulose has a high water-holding capacity (99% water), and therefore it is used in the production of moisturizing creams and face masks [88]. Nanosilver particles are used in many cosmetic products such as soap, lotions, acne products, antiseptic sprays, and creams because they are antibacterial, antiviral, antifungal, and antimicrobial. Additionally, deodorants with nanosilver particles eliminate the odor resulting from the combination of bacteria due to their antibacterial features [89]. Another nanomaterial that is found in foundations, eyeliners, eye shadows, mascaras, and nail polishes is carbon black, a coloring agent in make-up products. However, this material was identified as a possible carcinogenic for humans by the International Agency for Research on Cancer (IARC) [90].

15.4 Part III: Common nanoparticles and their harmful effects

Owing to their unique chemical and physical properties, nanomaterials have a wide range of applications. With smaller sizes, the physical properties of nanotechnological materials can change: (electrical, magnetic, optical, stiffness, robustness, conductivity, melting point, etc.). For example, metals have become stronger, lighter, and more conducting, whereas ceramics have become more elastic, and plastics have become more conductive. Nanomaterials consist of nanoparticles of sizes between 0.1 nm and 100 nm. The physical, chemical, and mechanical properties of nanoparticles differ dramatically from macroscopic solids of the same kind. For example, silicon is a semiconductor macroscopically, but at nanosizes it behaves as a conductor. The physicochemical properties, size-range quantum effects, size-dependence of the electronic structure, unique properties of the surface atoms, and high surface-to-volume ratio can all make a nanoparticle desirable. In the fields of computation, construction, cosmetics, energy, environment, food, medical packaging, dyes, coating, sports, entertainment, textile, clothing, and transportation, the most preferred nanoparticles are Ag, Fe, Pt, Sn, Al, Cu, Zr, Se, Ca, Mg, TiO_2, ZnO, CeO_2, SiO_2, Al_2O_3, carbon black, fullerene, nanoclay, ceramics, QDs, and many more. Nanoparticles with bigger surface areas increase the performance of batteries and fuel cells and are important for the efficiency of structures such as electrodes [91].

Silver nanoparticles are used mainly in cosmetics (soap, lotion, antiseptic creams) and textiles (socks, shirts, antiallergic cloths, masks, gloves, antibacterial carpets, antibacterial polymeric floor liners, and wallpaper) because of their antimicrobial and antibacterial properties [92,93]. These particles also increase the sensitivity and performance of metal oxide sensors.

Golden nanoparticles are commonly used in health (cardiac patients, diagnosis of cancer, and infection agents) and as catalyzers for fuel cells and in the production of nanodevices [94–97].

Iron nanoparticles can be used in cleaning pollutants such as uranium from soil and water. They can also be used as drug carriers, magnetic storage devices, sensors, and electrode materials [92–98].

Copper nanoparticles, which have good conductivity, are used in print technology and in cleansing underground waters of heavy metals [99]. Copper oxide nanoparticles are used in dyes and in the production of electronic devices [100].

Zinc oxide (ZnO) nanoparticles are used as antimicrobial agents, especially in foot protection creams, since they stop mold and fungus growth [101–102]. Additionally, they have a wide range of use in electronics, optics, and optoelectronics as varistors and catalyzers [103]. Zinc oxide doped with manganese, cobalt, and silver sees changes in its structural, optical, photocatalytic, and antibacterial properties [104].

Titanium dioxide nanoparticles are especially used in self-cleaning glasses and paints due to their photocatalytic and hydrophilic properties [105–106], in coatings and air cleaning due to their antibacterial properties, in cosmetics due to their biocompatibility, and also in solar batteries [107]. To favor their antibacterial properties, they are doped with silver to produce silver titanium dioxide metal/metal oxide nanoparticles. These nanoparticles are mainly used in antibacterial plastic, coatings, and medical applications [108].

Nickel oxide nanoparticles are used as cathodic material for batteries in addition to applications in sensors [103–109].

Aluminum oxide, iron oxide, and tin oxide nanoparticles are used in polishing jewelry, and cerium oxide nanoparticles are used in polishing optical and fiber optic materials. Lead oxide nanoparticles are used in battery applications due to their reliability and low cost, and indium oxide nanoparticles are mainly preferred in gas sensors and optoelectronic devices.

Commonly used nanoparticles can easily penetrate the body in different ways: via respiration, nutrition, or through the skin, and therefore, they can cause various diseases by affecting different organs.

The risks and uncertainties of the effects on living tissue and the environment caused by nanoparticles should not be ignored when developing new application fields for nanotechnology.

Potential health risks related to exposure to these particles must be identified and precautions against them must be developed. Depending on their shape, size, and ions, these particles can be toxic. Nanoparticles, especially those with cytotoxic and genotoxic effects, are shown in Table 15.1 along with their areas of use and their harmful effects on humans.

Table 15.1 **Properties, areas of use, and harmful effects of nanoparticles [110,111]**

NP	Properties	Areas of use	Harmful effects
TiO_2	Biocompatibility, photocatalytic, optical and electrical properties, corrosion resistance, mechanical strength, bleaching, opaqueness.	Cosmetics, food, toothpaste, sun cream, printing ink, dyes, polish, plastic, paper, industrial materials, rubber, cleaning supplies, photocatalytic applications, solar cells for refinement of organic matter in waste water and catalyzers [112,113].	Carcinogenic when inhaled [112,113]. Accumulated at different sites in brain and causes change in neural structure [114]. When exposed to TiO_2, changes in the sodium, potassium, magnesium, calcium, iron, and zinc levels in the brain were observed [114,115]. TiO_2 nanoparticles can be genetically inherited from mothers, therefore diseases regarding the brain development and nervous system of the newborn are possible [116,117].
ZnO	Antibacterial	Sun creams, biosensors, food additives, cement, tires, ceramic materials, pigments, plastics, catalyzers, and electronic materials.	Dissolved Zn^{+2} ions cause toxicity. Inflammatory effects related to ZnO toxicity [118]. Neurotoxicity of ZnO nanoparticles at different sizes was observed for neural stem cells of rats. When taken orally by mammals, ZnO nanoparticles increase the blood viscosity and pathological regions in the stomach, liver, kidneys, pancreas, and spleen [119].
Ag	Shiny, silvery white, soft metal. Antibacterial and antifungal.	In medical devices, textile, personal care products, food services, construction materials, and in washing machines as an antibacterial agent; in the production of ethylene oxide as a catalyzer; conductors, mirrors, and photographic applications; air-fresheners, wall paints, and laundry detergent [120–122].	Penetrates the body easily and accumulates in the organs: kidneys, liver, testicles, lungs, or brain. Toxicity was observed in the cells from the liver, skin, vascular system, lungs, and reproductive systems. Can cause oxidative stress and cell death in human skin carcinoma and fibrosarcoma cells [123]. Produces damage in DNA [124]. Neurotoxic effects detected by in vitro and in vivo studies [125].

(Continued)

Table 15.1 (Continued)

NP	Properties	Areas of use	Harmful effects
Iron oxide (FeO, Fe_2O_3, Fe_3O_4)	Supermagnetic	Industrial and biomedical applications; biomedical imaging (magnetic resonance imaging, positron emission tomography, or ultrasound), gene and drug delivery, tissue renewal, cancer treatment; brain imaging and targeted drug delivery to the brain.	Increase of use of Fe_3O_4 nanoparticles in industry and biomedical sciences can trigger fibrillation in polluted air. Increasing fibrillation encourages neurodegenerative diseases such as Alzheimer's or Parkinson's [126–127]. When intranasal exposure to Fe_2O_3 nanoparticles occur, neurons are damaged and oxidative stress increases [128].
Copper and copper oxide	Responsible for the production of neurotransmitters such as epinephrine and norepinephrine that can be found in the brain at high levels.	Ink, oiler, coatings, semiconductors, heat transfer fluids, antimicrobial preparates, and intrauterine devices [129].	CuO nanoparticles are extremely toxic in comparison with other metal oxide nanoparticles [130].
Aluminum oxide (alumina, Al_2O_3)	Good electrical and anticorrosive properties.	Coatings resistant to scratching, alloys and sensors, motor vehicles, electronic materials or isolators, exterior linings, and personal care products [131].	Neurotoxicological effects that cause mitochondrial weakening [132].

15.5 Conclusions and future directions

This chapter has offered a detailed guide to nanomaterials (nanoparticles, nanotubes, nanospheres, nanocrystals, nanoemulsions, and nanocapsules) and their application areas (cancer diagnosis and treatment, low-toxicity drug carriers [133], treatment of eye diseases, treatment of cardiovascular diseases, treatment of neurological diseases, and tissue engineering, textile, cosmetics, electronics, computers, food, and agriculture). In addition to the application areas and successes of nanotechnological materials, their harmful effects have also been detailed in tabular form. Since the full environmental effects of nanoparticle pollution created by nanotechnology are as yet unknown, there are increasing concerns that nanoparticles will affect human health in a harmful way. There is a large body of research on nanoparticles that are commonly used and their harmful effects. Research done on humans and animals show that some nanoparticles can penetrate the body and the organs via vascular and lymphatic systems, and yet their use in medical science for diagnosis [134] and treatment [135–136] is very important and cannot be neglected. The importance of nanotechnology in industry increases day by day. However, it is also very important that the developments in nanotechnology must be pursued safely and cautiously considering the effects on the environment and human health.

References

[1] Thrall JH. Nanotechnology and medicine 1. Radiology 2004;230(2):315–8.

[2] Jahanshahi M. ISBN: 964-2571-10-2 Molecular nanotechnology & nanobiotechnology. Academic University (Mazandaran) Publications; 2007.

[3] Jahanshahi M, Babaei Z. Protein nanoparticle: a unique system as drug delivery vehicles. Afr J Biotechnol 2008;7(25):4926–34.

[4] Baro AM, Miranda R, Alaman J, et al. Determination of surface topography of topography of biological specimens at high resolutuion by scanning tunnelling microscopy. Nature 1985;315:253–4.

[5] Curl RF, Smalley RE, Kroto HW, O'Brien S, Heath JR. How the news that we were not the first to conceive of soccer ball C60 got to us. J Mol Graph Model 2001;19:185–6.

[6] Ribatti D. Protagonists of medicine. Dordrecht: Springer Science+Business Media B.V.; 2010.

[7] Ravi Kumar MNV. A review of chitin and chitosan applications. React Funct Polym 2000;46(1):1–27.

[8] Zhou Y. Patenting activity in synthesis of lipid nanotubes and peptide nanotubes. Recent Pat Nanotechnol 2007;1(1):21–8.

[9] Adler-Abramovich L, Reches M, Sedman VL, Allen S, Tendler SJ, Gazit E. Thermal and chemical stability of diphenylalanine peptide nanotubes: implications for nanotechnological applications. Langmuir 2006;22(3):1313–20.

[10] Zhao X, Pan F, Lu JR. Recent development of peptide self-assembly. Prog Nat Sci 2008;18(6):653–60.

[11] Banerjee IA, Yu L, Matsui H. Location-specific biological functionalization on nanotubes: attachment of proteins at the ends of nanotubes using Au nanocrystal masks. Nano Lett 2003;3(3):283–7.

[12] Scanlon S, Aggeli A. Self-assembling peptide nanotubes. Nano Today 2008;3(3):22–30.
[13] Pignataro B. ISBN: 3527630546, 9783527630547 Ideas in chemistry and molecular sciences: advances in nanotechnology, materials and devices, Vol. 3. John Wiley & Sons; 2010.
[14] Lewis JP, Pawley NH, Sankey OF. Theoretical investigation of the cyclic peptide system cyclo[(D-Ala-Glu-D-Ala-Gln)m=1-4]. J Phys Chem B 1997;101(49):10576–83.
[15] Çelik S, Özel A, Akyüz S. Comparative study of antitumor active cyclo(Gly-Leu) dipeptide: a computational and molecular modeling study. Vib Spectrosc 2016;83:57–69.
[16] Çelik S, Özel A, Kecel S, Akyüz S. Structural and IR and Raman spectral analysis of cyclo(His-Phe) dipeptide. Vib Spectrosc 2012;61:54–65.
[17] Çelik S, Özel A, Akyüz S, Kecel S, Agaeva G. Conformational preferences, experimental and theoretical vibrational spectra of cyclo(Gly-Val) dipeptide. J Mol Struct 2011;993:341–8.
[18] Chen GJ, Su SJ, Liu RZ. Theoretical studies of monomer and dimer of cyclo[(-L-Phe1-D-Ala2-)n] and cyclo[(-L-Phe1-D-MeN-Ala2-)n] (n) (3-6). J Phys Chem B 2002;106(7):1570–5.
[19] Jain KK. The handbook of nanomedicine. Springer Science & Business Media: Humana Press; 2012.
[20] Ghadiri MR, et al. Self-assembling organic nanotubes based on a cyclic peptide architecture. Nature 1993;366(6453):324–7.
[21] Knoll Wolfgang. Handbook of biofunctional surfaces. Pan Stanford: CRC Press; 2013.
[22] Mandal D, Shirazi AN, Parang K. Self-assembly of peptides to nanostructures. Org Biomol Chem 2014;12(22):3544–61.
[23] Fernandez-Lopez S, Kim HS, Choi EC, Delgado M, Granja JR, Khasanov A, et al. Antibacterial agents based on the cyclic D, L-α-peptide architecture. Nature 2001;412(6845):452–5.
[24] Khurana E, Nielsen SO, Ensing B, Klein ML. Self-assembling cyclic peptides: molecular dynamics studies of dimers in polar and nonpolar solvents. J Phys Chem B 2006;110(38):18965–72.
[25] Jason C, Luc B, Jonathan H. Amino acids, peptides and proteins. Royal Society of Chemistry; 2012.
[26] Gülfem Ü. Süt Proteinlerinin Gıda Endüstrisinde Nanoteknolojik Olarak Uygulama Alanları. Gıda 2012;37(3):181–8.
[27] Matsui H, Pan S, Gologan B, Jonas SH. Bolaamphiphile nanotube-templated metallized wires. J Phys Chem B 2000;104(41):9576–9.
[28] Yokoi H, Kinoshita T, Zhang S. Dynamic reassembly of peptide RADA16 nanofiber scaffold. Proc Natl Acad Sci U S A 2005;102(24):8414–9.
[29] Engels M, Bashford D, Ghadiri MR. Structure and dynamics of self-assembling peptide nanotubes and the channel-mediated water organization and self-diffusion. A molecular dynamics study. J Am Chem Soc 1995;117(36):9151–8.
[30] Granja JR, Ghadiri MR. Channel-mediated transport of glucose across lipid bilayers. J Am Chem Soc 1994;116(23):10785–6.
[31] Westermark P, Lundmark K, Westermark GT. Fibrils from designed non-amyloid-related synthetic peptides induce AA-amyloidosis during inflammation in an animal model. PLoS One 2009;4(6):e6041.
[32] Chaudhuri TK, Paul S. Protein-misfolding diseases and chaperone-based therapeutic approaches. FEBS J 2006;273:1331–49.
[33] Castillo JJ, Svendsen WE, Rozlosnik N, Escobar P, Martinez F, Castillo-Leon J. Detection of cancer cells using a peptide nanotube–folic acid modified graphene electrode. Analyst 2013;138(4):1026–31.

[34] Drouvalakis KA, Bangsaruntip S, Hueber W, Kozar LG, Utz PJ, Dai H. Peptide-coated nanotube-based biosensor for the detection of disease-specific autoantibodies in human serum. Biosens Bioelectron 2008;23(10):1413–21.
[35] Marchesan S, Vargiu AV, Styan KE. The Phe-Phe motif for peptide self-assembly in nanomedicine. Molecules 2015;20(11):19775–88.
[36] Kecel S, Özel A, Akyüz S, Çelik S, Agaeva G. Conformational analysis and vibrational spectroscopic investigation of L-proline-tyrosine (L-Pro-Tyr) dipeptide. J Mol Struct 2011;993:349–56.
[37] Kecel S, Özel A, Akyüz S, Çelik S. Conformational analysis and vibrational spectroscopic investigation of L-alanyl-L-glutamine dipeptide. Spectrosc Int J 2010;3–4:219–32.
[38] Chahkandi B, Hosseini BS. Investigation of various conformations of HCO-Gly-L-Val-Gly-NH_2 tripeptide in elastin: Ab initio and DFT calculations (No. 5) Bulucea CA, Mladenov V, Pop E, Leba M, Mastorakis N, editors. WSEAS international conference. Proceedings. Recent advances in biology and biomedicine. WSEAS; 2009.
[39] Guisasola EEB, Masman MF, Enriz RD, Rodriguez AM. Structure of isolated tyrosyl-glycyl-glycine tripeptide. A comparative conformational study with peptides containing an aromatic ring. Cent Eur J Chem 2010;8(3):566–75.
[40] Kecel Gündüz S, Çelik S, Özel A, Akyüz S. The conformational and vibrational behavior of the inhibitory neuropeptide derived from beta-endorphin (Article in press). J Biomol Struct Dyn 2016;26:1–20.
[41] Singh A, Garg G, Sharma PK. Nanospheres: a novel approach for targeted drug delivery system. Int J Pharm Sci Rev Res 2010;5(3):84–8.
[42] Fulekar MH. Nanotechnology: importance and applications. IK International Pvt Ltd.; 2010.
[43] Fanun M. Colloids in drug delivery, Vol. 150. CRC Press; 2010.
[44] Kovalenko MV, Manna L, Cabot A, Hens Z, Talapin DV, Kagan CR, et al. Prospects of nanoscience with nanocrystals. ACS Nano 2015;9(2):1012–57.
[45] Shegokar R, Müller RH. Nanocrystals: industrially feasible multifunctional formulation technology for poorly soluble actives. Int J Pharm 2010;399:129–39.
[46] Christin PH. Nanocrystals of chemotherapeutic agents for cancer theranostics: development and in vitro and in vivo evaluation. Theses and Dissertations—Pharmacy; 2012.
[47] Benita S. Microparticulate drug delivery systems: release kinetic models. Microspheres, Microcapsules Liposomes 1998;2:155–81.
[48] Microspheres AR. Microcapsules and liposomes: general concepts and criteria. MML Series 1999;1:11.
[49] Kothamasu P, Kanumur H, Ravur N, Maddu C, Parasuramrajam R, Thangavel S. Nanocapsules: the weapons for novel drug delivery systems. Bioimpacts 2012;2:71–81.
[50] Diaspro A, Krol S, Cavalleri O, Silvano D, Gliozzi A. Microscopical characterization of nanocapsules templated on ionic crystals and biological cells toward biomedical applications. IEEE Trans Nanobioscience 2002;1(3):110–5.
[51] Zhang Y, Hsu BYW, Ren C, Li X, Wang J. Silica-based nanocapsules: synthesis, structure control and biomedical applications. Chem Soc Rev 2015;44(1):315–35.
[52] Kontermann R. Therapeutic proteins: strategies to modulate their plasma half-lives (Vol. 48). John Wiley & Sons; 2012.
[53] Lee HB, Khang G, Lee JH. Polymeric biomaterials, the biomedical engineering handbook, 2nd ed. CRC Press LLC; 2000.
[54] Bilensoy E, Erdo⊠ar N, Mungan NA. Role of nanoparticles in the treatment of noninvasive bladder cancer. Bull Urooncol 2015;14:61–6.

[55] Borislav A. Study of structure and properties of polymeric nanoparticles for biomedical applications. Theses and Dissertations, http://www.imc.cas.cz/en/umch/an210Angel.htm.
[56] Gasco MR, Gallarate M, Pattarino F. In vitro permeation of azelaic acid from viscosized microemulsions. Int J Pharm 1991;69:193–6.
[57] Kriwet K, Muller-Goymann C. Diclofenac release from phospholipid drug systems and permeation through excised human stratum corneum. Int J Pharm 1995;125:231–42.
[58] Trotta M. Influence of phase transformation on indomethacin release from microemulsions. J Control Release 1999;60:399–405.
[59] Myc A, Kukowska-Latallo JF, Bielinska AU, Cao P, Myc PP, Janczak K, et al. Development of immune response that protects mice from viral pneumonitis after a single intranasal immunization with influenza A virus and nanoemulsion. Vaccine 2003;21(25):3801–14.
[60] Jaiswal M, Dudhe R, Sharma PK. Nanoemulsion: an advanced mode of drug delivery system. 3 Biotech 2015;5(2):123–7.
[61] Auyang YS. Cancer causes and cancer research on many levels of complexity; 2006 http://www.creatingtechnology.org/biomed/cancer.pdf.
[62] Singh KK. Nanotechnology in cancer detection and treatment. Technol Cancer Res Treat 2005;4:583–4.
[63] Tan YF, Chandrasekharan P, Maity D, Yong CX, Chuang KH, Zhao Y, et al. Multimodal tumor imaging by iron oxides and quantum dots formulated in poly (lactic acid)-d-alpha-tocopheryl polyethylene glycol 1000 succinate nanoparticles. Biomaterials 2011;32:2969–78.
[64] Fan C, Gao W, Chen Z, Fan H, Li M, Deng F, et al. Tumor selectivity of stealth multi-functionalized superparamagnetic iron oxide nanoparticles. Int J Pharm 2011;404:180–90.
[65] Sathe TR, Agrawal A, Nie S. Mesoporous silica beads embedded with semiconductor quantum dots and iron oxide nanocrystals: dual – function microcarriers for optical encoding and magnetic seperation. Anal Chem 2006;78:5627–32.
[66] Savla R, Taratula O, Garbuzenko O, Minko T. Tumor targeted quantum dot-mucin 1 aptamerdoxorubicin conjugate for imaging and treatment of cancer. J Control Release 2011;153:16–22.
[67] Balalaeva IV, Zdobnova TA, Krutova IV, Brilkina AA, Lebedenko EN, Deyev SM. Passive and active targeting of quantum dots for whole-body fluorescence imaging of breast cancer xenografts. J Biophotonics 2012;5:860–7.
[68] Zhang YP, Sun P, Zhang XR, Yang WL. In vitro gastric cancer cell imaging using near-infrared quantum dot-conjugated CC49. Oncol Lett 2012;4:996–1002.
[69] Kumar B, Yadav PR, Goel HC, Moshahid M, Rizvi A. Recent developments in cancer therapy by use of nanotechnology. Digest J Nanomater Biostr 2009;4(1):1–12.
[70] Farokhzad OC, Cheng J, Teply BA, et al. Nanoparticle – aptamer bioconjugates result in significant tumor reduction in vivo. Proc Natl Acad Sci U S A 2006;103(6):6315–20.
[71] Freitas RJ. Nanodentistry. J Am Dent Assoc 2000;131:1559–65.
[72] Ozak ST, Ozkan P. Nanotechnology and dentistry. Eur J Dent 2013;7:145–51.
[73] Craig BD, Mitra SB, Kobussen GA, Doruff MC, Lechuga HL, Atkinson MR. Polish retention comparison of experimental and commercial restorative composite materials. J Dent Res 2009;88:1506.
[74] Patil M, Mehta DS, Guvva S. Future impact of nanotecnology on medicine and dentistry. J Indian Soc Periodontol 2008;12:34–40.
[75] Hanning M, Hanning C. Nanomaterials in preventive dentistry. Nat Nanotechnol 2010;5:565–9.
[76] Comar LP, Souza BM, Gracindo LF, Buzalaf MA, Magalhaes AC. Impact of experimental nano-HAP pastes on bovine enamel and dentin submitted to a pH cycling model. Braz Dent J 2013;24:273–8.

[77] Choi JS, Leong KW, Yoo HS. In vivo wound healing of diabetic ulcers using electrospun nanofibers immobilized with human epidermal growth factor (EGF). Biomaterials 2008;29:587–96.
[78] Rujitanaroj P, Pimpha N, Supaphol P. Wound-dressing materials with antibacterial activity from electrospun gelatin fiber mats containing silver nanoparticles. Polymer (Guildf) 2008;49:4723–32.
[79] Baldrick P. The safety of chitosan as a pharmaceutical excipient. Regul Toxicol Pharmacol 2010;56:290–9.
[80] De La Fuente M, Ravina M, Paolicelli P, Sanchez A. Chitosan-based nanostructures: a delivery platform for ocular therapeutics. Adv Drug Deliv Rev 2010;62:100–17.
[81] De Campos A, Sanchez A, Alonso M. Chitosan nanoparticles: a new vehicle for the improvement of the delivery of drugs to the ocular surface. Application to cyclosporin A. Int J Pharm 2001;224:159–68.
[82] Gupta AK, Gupta M. Synthesis and surface engineering of iron oxide nanoparticles for biomedical applications. Biomaterials 2005;26(18):3995–4021.
[83] Sengel-Türk CT, Hasçelik C, Gönül N. Nanoparticulate drug delivery systems for targeting the drugs to the brain. J Neurol Sci 2007;24:254–63.
[84] Re F, Gregori M, Masserini M. Nanotechnology for neurodegenerative disorders. Nanomedicine 2012;8:S51–8.
[85] DeLouise LA. Applications of nanotechnology in dermatology. J Invest Dermatol 2012;132:964–75.
[86] Contri RV, Fiel LA, Pohlmann AR, Guterres SS, Beck RC. Transport of substances and nanoparticles across the skin and in vitro models to evaluate skin permeation and/or penetration Nanocosmetics and nanomedicines. Heidelberg: Springer Berlin; 2011.
[87] Schilling K, Bradford B, Castelli D, Dufour E, Nash JF, Pape W, et al. Human safety review of “nano” tita- nium dioxide and zinc oxide. Photochem Photobiol Sci 2010;9(4):495–509.
[88] Klemm D, Schumann D, Kramer F, Heßler N, Hornung M, Schmauder HP, et al. Nanocelluloses as innovative polymers in research and application Polysaccharides II. Heidelberg: Springer Berlin; 2006.
[89] Das R, Nath SS, Chakdar D, Gope G, Bhattacharjee R. Preparation of silver nanoparticles and their characterization. J Nanotechnol 2009;5:1–6.
[90] Baan R, Straif K, Grosse Y, et al. Carcinogenicity of carbon black, titanium dioxide, and talc. Lancet Oncol 2006;7:295–6.
[91] Holister P, Weener JW, Vas CR, Harper T. Nanoparticles; Technology White Papers nr. 3. Cientifica; 2003.
[92] Brar SK, Verma M, Tyagi RD, Surampalli RY. Engineered nanoparticles in wastewater and wastewater sludge–evidence and impacts. Waste Manage 2010;30(3):504–20.
[93] Chou K, Ren C. Synthesis of nanosized silver particles by chemical reduction method. Mater Chem Phys 2000;64:241–6.
[94] Paciotti GF, Myer L, Weinreich D, Goia D, Pavel N, McLaughlin RE, et al. Colloidal gold: a novel nanoparticle vector for tumor directed drug delivery. Drug Deliv 2004;11(3):169–83.
[95] Cheng Y, Samia AC, Meyers JD, Panagopoulos I, Fei B, Burda C. Highly efficient drug delivery with gold nanoparticle vectors for in vivo photodynamic therapy of cancer. J Am Chem Soc 2008;130(32):10643–7.
[96] Solanki PR, Kaushik A, Agrawal VV, Malhotra BD. Nanostructured metal oxide-based biosensors. NPG Asia Mater 2011;3(1):17–24.
[97] Li Y, Schluesener HJ, Xu S. Gold nanoparticle-based biosensors. Gold Bull 2010;43(1):29–41.

[98] Dickinson M, Scott T. The application of zero-valent iron nanoparticles for the remediation of a uranium-contaminated waste effluent. J Hazard Mater 2010;178:171–9.
[99] Huang C, Shang-Lien Lo, Lien HL. Zero-valent copper nanoparticles for effective dechlorination of dichloromethane using sodium borohydride as a reductant. Chem Eng J 2012;203:95–100.
[100] Gencer Ö. Bakır ve Bakır Oksit Nanopartiküllerinin Ultrasonik Sprey Piroliz (USP) Yöntemi İle Üretimi. Theses and Dissertations; 2009.
[101] Kandavelu V, Kastien H, Ravindranathan-Thampi K. Photocatalytic degradation of isothiazolin-3-ones in water and emulsion of paints containing nanocrystalline TiO_2 and ZnO catalysts. Appl Catal B 2004;48:101–11.
[102] Liu G, Wang D, Wang J, Mendoza C. Effect of ZnO particles on activated sludge: role of particle dissolution. Sci Total Environ 2011;409:2852–7.
[103] Masoomi MY, Morsali A. Applications of metal–organic coordination polymers as precursors for preparation of nano-materials. Coord Chem Rev 2012;256(23):2921–43.
[104] Rekha K, Nirmala M, Nair MG, Anukaliani A. Structural, optical, photocatalytic and antibacterial activity of zinc oxide and manganese doped zinc oxide nanoparticles. Phys B 2010;405(15):3180–5.
[105] Meyer DE, Wood K, Bachas LG, Bhattacharyya D. Degradation of chlorinated organics by membrane-immobilized nanosized metals. Environ Prog 2004;23:232–42.
[106] Mann S. Nanotechnology and construction. Nanoforum report. Stirling: Institute of Nanotechnology; 2006.
[107] Othman SH, Rashid SA, Ghazi TIM, Abdullah N. Dispersion and stabilization of photocatalytic TiO_2 nanoparticles in aqueous suspension for coatings applications. J Nanomater 2012;2012:2.
[108] Cheng Q, et al. Surface-modified antibacterial TiO_2/Ag^+ nanoparticles: preparation and properties. Appl Surf Sci 2006;252(12):4154–60.
[109] Kiani MA, Mousavi MF, Ghasemi S. Size effect investigation on battery performance: comparison between micro-and nano-particles of β-$Ni(OH)_2$ as nickel battery cathode material. J Power Sources 2010;195(17):5794–800.
[110] Karmakar A, Zhang Q, Zhang Y. Neurotoxicity of nanoscale materials. J Food Drug Anal 2014;22(1):147–60.
[111] Bystrzejewska-Piotrowska G, Golimowski J, Urban PL. Nanoparticles: their potential toxicity, waste and environmental management. Waste Manage 2009;29(9):2587–95.
[112] Chen J, Dong X, Zhao J, Tang G. In vivo acute toxicity of titanium dioxide nanoparticles to mice after intraperitioneal injection. J Appl Toxicol 2009;29(4):330–7.
[113] National Institute for Occupational Safety and Health. Occupational exposure to titanium dioxide. Publication No. 2011-160 Cincinnati. US Department of Health and Human Services, Public Health Service, Centers for Disease Control, National Institute of Occupational Safety and Health, DHHS (NIOSH); 2011.
[114] Wang J, Chen C, Liu Y, Jiao F, Li W, Lao F, et al. Potential neurological lesion after nasal instillation of TiO_2 nanoparticles in the anatase and rutile crystal phases. Toxicol Lett 2008;183(1):72–80.
[115] Wang JX, et al. Influence of intranasal instilled titanium dioxide nanoparticles on monoaminergic neurotransmitters of female mice at different exposure time. Zhonghua Yu Fang Yi Xue Za Zhi 2007;41(2):91–5.
[116] Ma L, Liu J, Li N, et al. Oxidative stress in the brain of mice caused by translocated nanoparticulate TiO2 delivered to the abdominal cavity. Biomaterials 2010;31:99–105.
[117] Shimizu M, et al. Maternal exposure to nanoparticulate titanium dioxide during the prenatal period alters gene expression related to brain development in the mouse. Part Fibre Toxicol 2009;6.1:1.

[118] Heng BC, Zhao X, Tan EC, et al. Evaluation of the cytotoxic and inflammatory potential of differentially shaped zinc oxide nanoparticles. Arch Toxicol 2011;85:1517–28.
[119] Wang J, Wang B, Wang TC, et al. Acute toxicological impact of nano- and submicro-scaled zinc oxide powder on healthy adult mice. J Nanopart Res 2008;10:263–76.
[120] Lee HY, Park HK, Lee YM, et al. A practical procedure for producing silver nanocoated fabric and its antibacterial evaluation for biomedical applications. Chem Commun (Camb) 2007;28:2959–61.
[121] Jain P, Pradeep T. Potential of silver nanoparticle-coated polyurethane foam as an anti-bacterial water filter. Biotechnol Bioeng 2005;90:59–63.
[122] Zhang YY, Sun J. A study on the bio-safety for nano-silver as anti-bacterial materials. Chin J Med Instrum 2007;31.1:36–8. 16.
[123] Arora S, Jain J, Rajwade JM, et al. Cellular responses induced by silver nanoparticles: in vitro studies. Toxicol Lett 2008;179:93–100.
[124] Soto K, Garza KM, Murr LE. Cytotoxic effects of aggregated nanomaterials. Acta Biomater 2007;3:351–8.
[125] Zhang Y, Ferguson SA, Watanabe F, et al. Silver nanoparticles decrease body weight and locomotor activity in adult male rats. Small 2013;9:1715–20.
[126] Kong SD, Lee J, Ramachandran S, et al. Magnetic targeting of nanoparticles across the intact bloodebrain barrier. J Control Release 2012;164:49–57.
[127] Calderon-Garciduenas L, Solt AC, Henriquez-Roldan C, et al. Long-term air pollution exposure is associated with neuroinflammation, an altered innate immune response, disruption of the blood-brain barrier, ultrafine particulate deposition, and accumulation of amyloid beta-42 and alpha-synuclein in children and young adults. Toxicol Pathol 2008;36:289–310.
[128] Wang B, Feng W, Zhu M, et al. Neurotoxicity of low-dose repeatedly intranasal instillation of nano- and submicronsized ferric oxide particles in mice. J Nanopart Res 2009;11:41–53.
[129] Aruoja V, Dubourguier HC, Kasemets K, et al. Toxicity of nanoparticles of CuO, ZnO and TiO_2 to microalgae Pseudokirchneriella subcapitata. Sci Total Environ 2009;407:1461–8.
[130] Karlsson HL, Cronholm P, Gustafsson J, et al. Copper oxide nanoparticles are highly toxic: a comparison between metal oxide nanoparticles and carbon nanotubes. Chem Res Toxicol 2008;21:1726–32.
[131] Darlington TK, Neigh AM, Spencer MT, et al. Nanoparticle characteristics affecting environmental fate and transport through soil. Environ Toxicol Chem 2009;28:1191–9.
[132] Zhang QL, et al. In vivo toxicity of nano-alumina on mice neurobehavioral profiles and the potential mechanisms. Int J Immunopathol Pharmacol 2010;24(1 Suppl):23S–9S.
[133] Topuzogullari Murat, et al. Conjugation, characterization and toxicity of lipophosphoglycan-polyacrylic acid conjugate for vaccination against leishmaniasis. J Biomed Sci 2013;20(1):35.
[134] Budama-Kılınc Y, Cakır-Koc R, Badur S. The development of a universally conserved M2e and hemagglutinin peptide-based ELISA method against Influenza A. J Clin Anal Med 2016. http://dx.doi.org/10.4328/JCAM.4883.
[135] Eroglu BI, Kilinc YB, Mustafaeva Z. Bioconjugation of Hepatitis B antigenic peptide with polymeric carriers through various carbodiimide chemistry. Turk J Biochem 2011;36:222–9.
[136] Kilinc Yasemin Budama, Akdeste Zeynep Mustafaeva, Koc Rabia Cakir, Bagirova Melahat, Allahverdiyev Adil. Synthesis and characterization of antigenic influenza A M2e protein peptide-poly(acrylic) acid bioconjugate and determination of toxicity in vitro. Bioengineered 2014;5(6):357–62.

Summary and future of nanomaterials in medicine/biomaterials

16

M. Miraftab
University of Bolton, Bolton, Lancashire, United Kingdom

16.1 What are nanomaterials and why are they important?

The concept of measurement in the form of meter, centimeter, and millimeter is well understood by all and regularly used to express size in a meaningful way. However, working with 1000 parts in a millimeter, otherwise known as micrometer (μm) is less familiar to most people and the thought of 1000,000 parts in 1 mm or more appropriately, nanometer (nm) is beyond most people's scope of perception. Hence materials described by nanometer scale are not only very small but are of significant importance when it comes to precision engineering and efficient functionality.

Distinction between nanoparticle and nanomaterials lies in the dimensional characteristics of these materials. The term *particle* refers to a substance of small dimension in all its axes for example, a fine powder. Therefore, nanoparticles are described as those with dimensions between 1 and 100 nm in size. Nanomaterials, on the other hand, are not necessarily the same as they need to have at least one dimension in nanoscale for example, nanofibers with possibly infinite length are in this category. In either scenario, the overall effect is a function of the material surface area and the consequences that has on the material behavior. To better illustrate the surface area perspective, the depictions below show two cylindrical objects of identical volumes; however, due to their different internal structures, their overall surface area are very different.

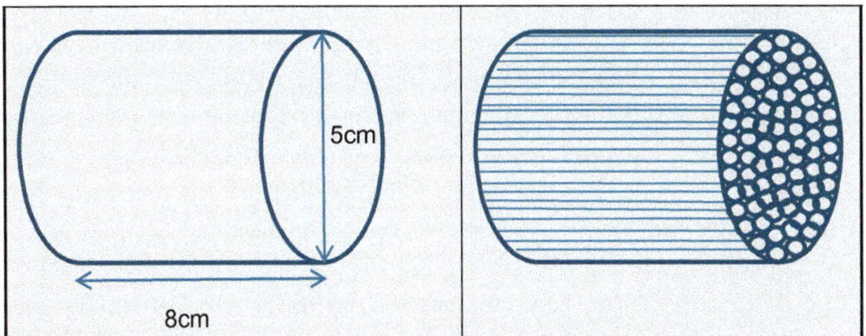

$ø = 5\,\text{cm}, l = 8\,\text{cm}, n = 1$ Surface area $= 2\pi rh + 2\pi r^2$ $= 2\pi \times 2.5 \times 8 + 2\pi \times 2.5^2$ $= 164.85\,\text{cm}^2$	$ø = 0.4\,\text{cm}, l = 8\,\text{cm}, n = 75$ Surface area $= 75\,(2\pi rh + 2\pi r^2)$ $= 75\,(2\pi 0.2 \times 8 + 2\pi \times 0.2^2)$ $= 772.44\,\text{cm}^2$

Nanobiomaterials Science, Development and Evaluation. DOI: http://dx.doi.org/10.1016/B978-0-08-100963-5.00016-1

The large difference in the surface area has a number of implications in terms of material behavior and functionality. For start, the greater surface area within a given volume allows greater absorption of liquids, dyes, or drugs and likewise a quicker or more efficient means of releasing or dispatching the loaded material. For a given material, the bulk object also has a much lower flexibility, tenacity, and resilience compared to its high surface area counterpart. Nanomaterials are often described as a bridge between bulk materials and atomic or molecular structures [1]. The change in physical properties at nanoscale is of immense interest and has opened up a whole new field of engineering, design, and application needs.

At this fine level, what is known as "quantum effects" governs the behavior and overall properties of nanomaterials [2]. Details of quantum effects is beyond the scope of this chapter; however, its presence at nanolevel is the source that leads to novel optical, thermal, electrical, and mechanical behaviors, which are distinctly different to those of bulk materials. Specific examples include melting temperature of gold nanoparticles at about 300°C as opposed to ~1065°C in bulk, or appearance of gold nanoparticles in shades of red or purple rather than the deep yellow color we are all familiar with in bulk gold [3,4]. Furthermore, materials such as ceramics that are brittle, hard, strong in compression but weak in shear, and tensile loading, at nanoscale behave as ductile materials when subjected to elevated temperatures [5]. Inclusion of nano-inorganic particles in composites could also alter their dielectric constant and hence influence their photonic band-gap structures [6,7].

Nanomaterials are found abundantly in natural habitat and to a searching eye are full of clues and instructions as to the nature of their complex behaviors and properties. Despite their existence, due to technological limitations and unavailability of right investigative tools, they have remained out of reach and therefore out of sight for a long time. With the advent of the electron microscopes in the 1930s and their full commercialization in the 1960s, a new horizon beyond what had been possible until then was unveiled and with it there came an explosion of opportunities and potentials for new forms of investigation at molecular or nanoscale domain [8]. The term *nanotechnology* was subsequently first used by Norio Taniguvhi in 1974 and since then the all-inclusive terminology has blossomed into an area of great interest around the globe [9]. This is largely due to man's desire to explore, investigate, and, where possible, control and manipulate matter at its lowest level of existence that is, atoms and molecules.

In nature, many biological species and inorganic objects are made from nanomaterials. However, our appreciation of their existence has only just begun. For instance, self-cleaning feature of lotus leaf is governed by its intricate surface nanostructure, which minimizes water droplet contacts and makes them roll away henceforth removing dirt [10], or the fact that Geckos can walk upside down on glass is purely down to their nanoscale spatulae feet structure that utilizes otherwise very weak Van der Waals forces to its advantage [11]. The skin, bones, hair, and nails have similar nanostructures with specific in-built functions without which they would not be able to operate.

This is also true with inorganic matter where nanostructures are developed through crystal growth in diverse chemical conditions of the earth's crust. Such examples include complex nanostructures of clay, hydrated amorphous form of silica known as opal and pyrogenic silica otherwise known as fumed silica [12].

Generally, nanomaterials can be classified based on three variables of origin, dimension, and structural configurations.

Origin: Natural nanomaterials originate from nature itself and includes a range of species such as viruses, protein molecules, minerals such as clays, colloids such as milk and blood, gelatine, or mineralized materials such as shells, corals, bones, insect wings, and so on. Artificial or manmade nanomaterials, however, are those that are produced through precision fabrication processes, which include carbon nanotubes, semiconductors such as quantum dots, and so forth.

Dimensions: Nanomaterials could be categorized into zero-, one-, two-, or three-dimensional materials. Zero-dimensional nanomaterials include gold and silver nanoparticles and semiconductors (quantum dots). They are often spherical in shape and their dimensions range between 1 nm and 50 nm. One-dimensional nanomaterials have one dimension outside the nanometer range, which include nanowires, nanorods, and nanotubes, mainly based on metals and their oxides. Two-dimensional nanomaterials have two dimensions outside the nanometer range. Nanofilms, nanosheets or nanowalls are some of these examples. Three-dimensional nanomaterials have all their three dimensions outside the nanoscale but they are composed of individual blocks that have nanometer scales [8,13].

Structural configurations: On this basis, nanomaterials are often classified into four categories:

- Carbon-based nanomaterials: For example, fullerenes consisting of spherical and ellipsoidal configurations or single- and multiwalled nanotubes.
- Metal-based nanomaterials: For example, nanogold/silver, metal oxides, and quantum dots.
- Dendrimers: These are branched macromolecules with distinct surface characteristics that could be functionalized.
- Composites: These are multiphase materials where any of their three dimensions could be in nanoscale, for example, colloids and gels.

Nanomaterials maybe produced by what is known as top-down technique or bottom-up technique [8,9,14].

Top-down technique basically starts off with a large piece of a material and it is gradually grinded down to nanomaterial size using high energy methods. These include milling, sputtering, etching, or laser ablations. Detailed insight into operational procedures of these techniques is beyond the scope of this chapter.

Bottom-up technique involves building from the lowest point that is, atoms and molecules upward. This may be achieved by various techniques including sol–gel processing, aerosol deposition, or atomic/molecular condensation and self-assembly. Again, details of these processing techniques are beyond the limit of this chapter, although further reference to one of these techniques; that is, self-assembly including electrospinning will be made later on in the chapter.

What needs to be borne in mind is, to manufacture nanodevices for different sectors, high purity materials/ceramics, polymers, and composite materials are required to achieve high performance. If this is not achievable, the packing becomes nonuniform and the irregularity in the physical shape of nanoparticles would cause differences in the packing density.

Nonuniformity can also be brought about by agglomeration that is beyond control. Because of this shortfall, the material may be subjected to permeability disorders and hence experience property change from plastic to brittle status.

Even if the uniformity is preserved during manufacturing, the material may be subjected to certain anomalies during the packing time. This will cause changes in the density of the material, and would be liable to increase during fusing or the sintering process.

Because of these likelihoods, it is best to process nanomaterial in such a way that distribution of components and permeability within them is physically uniform; hence the intricacy and the artful assembly of nanomaterials are maintained.

Carbon nanotubes (CNTs) are typical examples of such assemblies where depending on production technique impurities such as polydisperse mixtures that is, metallic and semiconducting single-wall nanotubes, can drastically influence product performance and undermine their potentials. Although the primary use of highly purified devices has been in electronics, there is growing interest in using them for a variety of biomedical applications including vehicles for targeted delivery of drugs to cancer cells with least side effects and excessive doses, or in functionalized CNTs where near-infrared light could be used to transfer the generated heat to the target cell and thus destroy it.

16.1.1 Characterization of biomaterials

The naked eye can see objects down to ~20 μm and no further. Optical microscopes push this resolution boundary down to ~0.2 μm and no more, limited by the wavelength of the visible light. Hence to view objects at nanoscales, electrons rather than light are used, which provide resolutions down to 0.001 μm or 1 nm scale. These specialized characterization tools include scanning electron microscope (SEM), transmission electron microscope (TEM), scanning tunneling microscope (STM), and atomic force microscope (AFM). Although the principles of all these techniques are different they all produce high-resolution images of material surfaces and bulks. For further in-depth details of each of these techniques, readers are referred to more specialized textbooks [15]. Raman spectroscopy could also be used to study rotational, vibrational, and other low-frequency modes in a given nanostructure. This technique essentially relies on Raman scattering of monochromatic laser light. The shift or variation in energy level gives information about the subject under examination [16]. Other characterization techniques include wide-angle X-ray diffraction and particle size analysis by various methods including dynamic light scattering or DLS [17]. Detail discussions on these techniques are again beyond the limit of this chapter and will not be pursued further.

16.2 What is their application in healthcare and medicine?

Universally useful behavior of nanomaterials makes them suitably viable in almost all conceivable forms of applications and allows all disciplines to benefit from these fundamental behaviors. Since their emergence in the 1980s, research and development in nanomaterials and nanotechnology has mushroomed and has in recent years matured into a commercial reality. To keep within the context of this section, references only to their use and application in general healthcare and specifically medicine are made here.

Generally, there are three distinctive areas within the healthcare that nanotechnology and nanomaterials have or could have long-lasting impact. These include:

- Diagnosis;
- Prevention; and
- Treatment.

Diagnosis is the first step in finding out what is wrong with a patient. A wrong diagnosis can have consequential implications that could lead to wasted efforts, trauma, and considerable costs both to the patients and the clinicians in charge. Hence, nanoparticles that could identify cancer cells and tumors by the release of the so-called biomarkers or detection of magnetic nanoparticles by nuclear magnetic resonance (NMR) [18] or using carbon nanotubes and gold nanoparticles in sensors that detect proteins in oral cancers and indeed antibody-coated nanofiber meshes that bind to individual cancer cells [19] are only few examples of the diagnostic techniques that have been developed or are currently under development.

Prevention rather than treatment is the best way of avoiding disease or ill health particularly if the consequences are likely to be permanent or irreversible. Hence nanotechnology and nanomaterials that can monitor environment, air, and health hazards such as pollutants, bacteria, and viruses could limit, if not completely stop, the devastating effect of such predators. Some of these preventative measures include the inclusion or coating of food containers with silver nanoparticles to kill bacteria and prolong shelf life [20] or the presence of gold nanoparticles in toothpastes, which helps to prevent plague formation, cavities, and gingivitis [21]. Other examples include the development of nanofilters where pathogenic microbes including viruses are captured and zapped by nanobased antimicrobials or ultraviolet (UV) lights [22].

Treatment is the inevitable action once damage is done and the way this is carried out could have much physical, psychological, and clinical impact on the patients as well as the physicians. Nanomedicine and nanomaterials are revolutionizing treatments of cancer by targeting affected cells, organs, or bone and teeth regeneration, and repairs like never before. Treating lung cancer by inhaling nanodrugs and localized treatments with minimal side effects are becoming increasingly routine treatment procedures [23].

To elaborate further on the scope of nanomaterials application with the healthcare, they may be broadly divided into four general categories.

16.2.1 Drug and gene deliveries

Traditionally, drugs have been taken orally because it is noninvasive and convenient; however, some drugs, particularly those carrying peptides or proteins, get damaged within harsh acidic conditions of the stomach and ultimately destroy or reduce their bioavailability where needed. This is indeed the reason why type I diabetics have to inject themselves with insulin [24]. Nanoencapsulation of insulin using biocompatible materials that can resist the severity of stomach environment is currently a subject of much research with promising results [25].

Nanoparticles as healing agents can be delivered to preidentified targets, including sites that cannot be easily accessed by standard drugs. For example, if the drug can be chemically fused to a nanoparticle, it can then be guided to the location of the disease or the infection by external electromagnetic signals. These nanodrugs could subsequently be released either because of the presence of certain molecules or be signaled into action by external stimuli such as radio waves or infrared heat. This strategy will not only offer a better and more effective treatment but could avoid potential harmful side effects at the expense of reduced dosages [26].

Delivery of drug to the brain is highly challenging due to the presence of the so-called blood–brain barrier. Nanoparticles as carriers of drugs could be used to carry out this task effectively, thus improving drug efficiency and reducing drug toxicity [27]. Another application of nanotechnology and nanoparticles is the delivery of antigens for vaccination and enhancement of immunizations [28].

Diseases such as cancer, hemophilia, hypercholesterolemia, and neurodegenerative malfunctions could benefit from gene therapy [29]. This effectively means introducing genes at the targeted sites where correction or elimination of the faulty genes can take place. For reasons beyond the scope of this chapter, genes are susceptible to damage and cannot be introduced into the body in their raw form. To overcome this issue, they may be encapsulated in carefully selected nanoparticles, some of which includes lipid-based, or polymer-based, or even inorganic nanoparticles. However, issues relating to biodegradation, biocompatibility, and aggregation in physiological fluids or nonspecific adsorption by undesired tissues are challenges that are still being tackled by many researchers around the world [29,30].

16.2.2 Nanobased medical devices

The function of implantable nanomedical devices are to continuously sense and monitor the environment so that they can perform a range of tasks including delivering drugs, sampling body fluids, maintaining normal blood flow in arteries, and even killing undesirable cells such as cancer cells [31]. Although these may be achieved, to a certain extent, by biological systems, their material properties and speeds at which they can be enacted are somewhat limited.

Implantable medical devices based on nanodevice electronics such as nanostructured electronics, actuators, sensors, and the like, are simply a revolution in the way diseases and malfunctioning organs can be detected at a very early stage and how the knowledge could be used to prompt action long before any damage is done. These could operate independently or be prompted into action by outside stimuli such as electromagnetic waves, heat, or sound waves [8,31]. Materials including nanotubes, nanowires, and other suitable nanoscale materials are the key components in self-assembly and/or precision production at this level [31].

Nanorobots are a natural progression of this technology whereby built-in intelligence at nanoscale would have specific tasks in detection, delivery, and dispensation of what is required in the human body. Manufacturing such devices is an ongoing challenge both in terms of size and costs as well as safety issues [32]. There are also ongoing work on biodegradable devices and robots that corrode and eventually discharge from the body once their task is complete, thus avoiding any unnecessary presence of materials in the body. The implication and overall consequences of such degradation products are currently under investigation [33].

16.2.3 Tissue engineering/scaffolds

Tissue engineering is now a well-established method of combining cells with materials to improve or replace biological functions. To achieve this, cells are grown on appropriately made scaffolds before they can be used. The scaffolding materials and their structure are crucial in allowing cell survival and proliferation. Scaffolds made from nanomaterials, particularly nanofibers, play this role quite effectively because of their huge surface area and superior strengths and their close resemblance to extracellular matrix (ECM). These can be produced by a number of techniques including direct drawing from solution, melt processing, phase separations, self-assemblies, and the so-called island in the sea process or electrospinning [34]. Electrospinning by far is the preferred method of nanofiber production, given the versatility of the technology and the relative ease of their production. The process uses electrostatic forces to draw fibers from a liquid polymer solution or melt, with the application of high voltage. In comparison to the conventional spinning techniques such as wet spinning, dry spinning, melt spinning, and gel spinning, which produce fiber having diameters in micrometer range, electrospinning is a process capable of producing polymer fibers having diameters ranging from a few microns to tens of nanometers. Owing to their enormous advantages, electrospun fibers have been successfully applied in various applications ranging from the field of biomedical such as tissue engineering scaffolds, controlled drug release systems, filtration, pharmaceutical, healthcare, biotechnology, to environmental engineering [35]. Figs. 16.1–16.3 are some examples of possible applications of this technology.

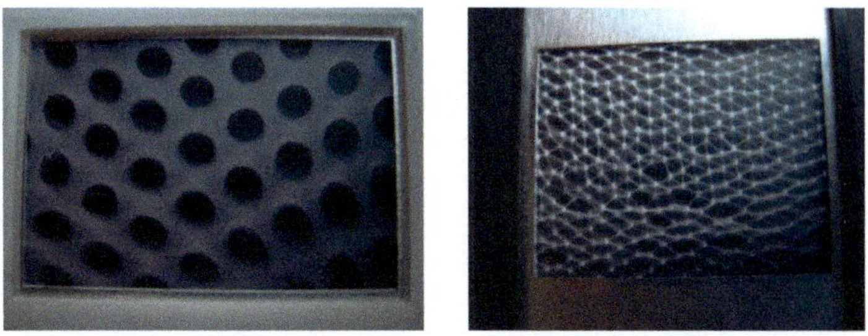

Figure 16.1 Example of possible electrospun membranes for fine filtration or as substrate for tissue engineering application.

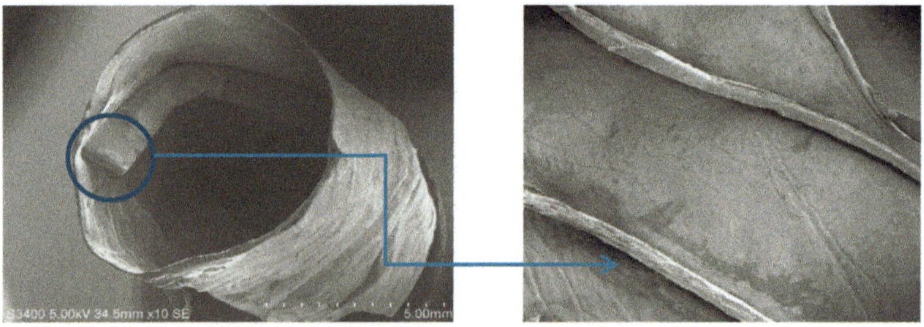

Figure 16.2 Example of electrospun narrow (<6 mm) vascular grafts with internal helices [36].

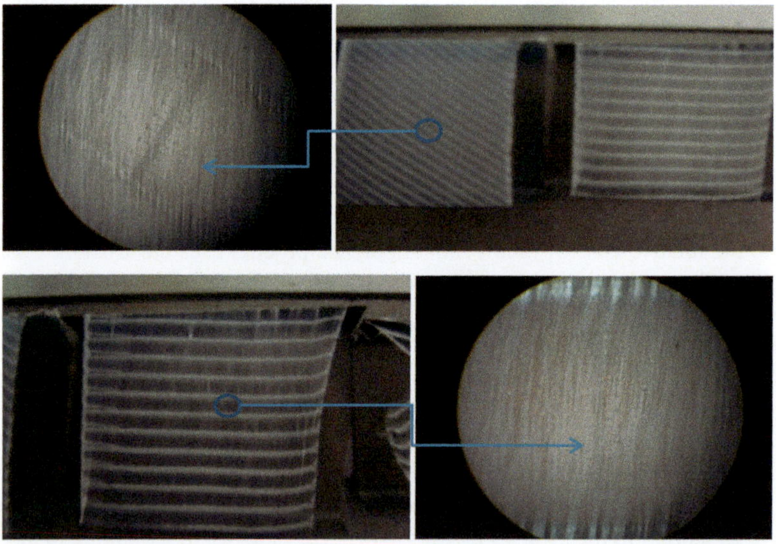

Figure 16.3 Example of continous production of electrospun membranes with preset nanofiber directional orientation illustrating the versatility of this production technique.

16.3 Modified implants

Hip and joint replacements have traditionally used titanium or stainless steel alloys, but despite being bioinert, their surface interaction with the nanostructure of bone often leads to lack of adhesion and ultimate seperation and loosening. This would then result in further trauma and possible second and third operations [37]. Nanocoating of such surfaces can closely emulate natural bone structures and hence promote and encourage osteoblast proliferation and integration, hence avoiding long-term problems and disassociations. These nanocoatings could be from a variety of materials including metals, polymers, ceramics, or carbon-based materials and composites made from them [38].

Other than the use of nanodrugs in treating teeth and gum problems, dental implant therapy has made huge advances in the recent times with respect to surface and interaction characteristics. Cell colonization, surface chemistry modifications, and improved wettability have all led to better results soley due to embracement and use of nanomaterials [39].

Quite a few cosmetic manufacturers nowadays regularly use nanomaterials in their products. For instance, nanoparticles of zinc and titanium oxides are regularly included in suntan lotions to provide better and more effective protection against UV light, or inclusion of protein-derived stem cells in creams are claimed to prevent aging, and so on [40].

16.4 What are their potentials and future prospects?

In the 21st-century, nanomaterials and nanotechnology in general will continue to dominate and lead research and development. In 2014, the global nanomaterial market reached $3.4 billion, and by 2020, depending on which estimates are to be believed, it can reach anything from $11.8 billion to $30 billion [41,42]. This market is largely dominated by the United States but Europe accounts for 30% of the total market share.

Huge investments made in the emerging economies of China, India, and some Southeast Asian countries are expected to be the fastest growing markets, given their rapid industrialization programs. It is generally believed that nanomaterials market in healthcare would surpass that of electrical and electronics market in not too distant future, based on the huge advancements being made in the biomedical field [41–43].

The key drivers of the nanomaterials' market are the ever-increasing range of applications. In healthcare, specifically, this is geared to increasing population of the elderly and life expectancy of most people across the world [40,41].

Nanotechnology has shown the potentials to revolutionize all aspects of science and engineering over and beyond what could have been imagined only 20 years ago and nowhere this is more evident than in the medical health and medical device arena. All this, without a doubt, is in the interest of all, particularly the new generation where preventative medicine, personal health management at will, and safety concerns at affordable costs will help them lead healthier lifestyle.

16.4.1 Safety of nanomaterials

Despite the advantages and ever-increasing practicality of nanomaterials, it must be noted that working at nanoscale is not an entirely safe and danger-free practice, ironically due to the very same reasons that make nanomaterials technically so attractive. Their potency may be divided into three means by which they can affect human health.

- Inhalation
- Ingestion
- Dermal penetration.

Inhalation is the first and foremost means by which nanoparticles could be transported into the body. Hence the respiratory tract leading to lungs is first affected. Depending on size, they may then enter the blood stream and therefore find access to other tissues and organs and even the brain and possibly the fetus of pregnant women [40,44]. Furthermore, depending on the active nature of the nanomaterial, a number of associated hazards may follow. For instance, when metal nanoparticles are used, they are prone to attack by the body environment and can undergo corrosion, transformation, and lose their integrity or, in the event of oxygen being present, they can become highly explosive due to their high surface area.

Ingestion can arise from manual handling of nanomaterials and hand-to-mouth transfer from contaminated surfaces or by taking in contaminated water or food. Through the stomach and the digestive system, they would eventually reach the blood stream, tissues, and various other organs [45]. More alarmingly however, increasingly, nanomaterials are deliberately put into food and dairy products to enhance color, flavor, and texture and to prolong shelf life. Examples of such nanoparticles include titanium dioxide, silicon oxide, and zinc oxide [46]. These could potentially damage DNA and proteins in cells with serious consequences. There currently exists very little study on long-term effects of such materials in the body and their safety remains an open question [42–45].

Dermal penetration, although unbroken skin is a reasonable barrier to nanoparticle entry, any incision or skin injury could allow free access to such particles through unintentional exposure or in the form of consumer products such as creams and other ointments [47]. However, there is a body of evidence that suggest that nanomaterials included in sunscreens and personal care products could potentially be toxic. Since nanomaterials can much more easily cross biological membranes than larger particles, their greater surface area increase production of reactive free radicals and oxygen species, which can result in oxidative stress, inflammation, and ultimately damage to DNA [48].

Despite these known facts, there is still knowledge deficiency in the available information regarding toxicity of nanomaterials, which makes risk assessments difficult without much hard evidence. It may therefore be years before full effects of nanomaterials on human health become apparent.

16.5 Conclusion

Nanotechnology, and nanomaterials in particular, in the context of medical and clinical healthcare applications, play an increasing crucial role in the 21st-century medicine where designing "bottom-up" has become the key in many diagnostic and preventative treatments. Nanoparticle loadings and functionalization of biomaterials has allowed localized administration of drugs and achievement of desired properties via various compound attachments. Having proved their viability, doctors and scientists are changing their classic views of treating disease and are increasingly drawn to methodologies that offer prevention of ill health prior to their manifestations in the traditional ways. Placing nanosensors in blood streams to alert risks of heart attacks, inclusion of graphene-based biosensors to detect biomolecules, proteins, and DNA, or indeed the development of 3D-printed nanobatteries to power nanorobots are only some of the new preventative developments taking place in the area. Just as much as nanoparticles and nanomaterials are becoming integral to everyday life, their possible toxicity and potential negative impact on the environment and health in general are becoming important and a subject of much-needed research.

References

[1] Farre M, Barcelo D. Analysis and Risk of Nanomaterials in Environmental and Food Samples, vol. 59. Elsevier Publication; 2012.
[2] Mohseni M, Omar Y, Plenio MB, Quantum Effects in Biology, ISBN: 9780511863189, 2014.
[3] Carabineiro SAC, Colloidal gold, colloids: classification, properties and applications, pp. 1–24, 2012.
[4] Uehara N, Ookubo K, Shimizu T. Colorimetric assay of glutathione based on the spontaneous disassembly of aggregated gold nanocomposites conjugated with water-soluble polymer. Langmuir 2010;26(9):6818–25.
[5] Pelleg J. The strength and strengthening of ceramics, mechanical properties of ceramics, Volume 213 of the series Solid Mechanics and Its Applications, pp. 351–415. 2014.
[6] Dastjerdi R, Montazer M. A review on the application of inorganic nano-structured materials in the modification of textiles: focus on anti-microbial properties. Colloids Surf B Biointerfaces 2010;79(1):5–18.
[7] Abdullah OG, Salman YAK, Saleem SA. Electrical conductivity and dielectric characteristics of in situ prepared PVA/HgS nanocomposite films. J Mater Sci Mater Electronics 2016;27(4):3591–8.
[8] D'Arrigo J, Chapter 1 Nanotechnology and nanomaterials, Studies in Interface Science, 23, 2006, 1–69, Elsevier, Amsterdam.
[9] Nimesh S, Gene Therapy, Potential Applications of Nanotechnology, Nanotechnology: an introduction, Woodhead Publishing, Cambridge, 2013, 1-12.
[10] McLauchlin ML, Yang D, Aella P, Hayes MA. Evaporative properties and pinning strength of laser-alblated, hydrophilic sites on Lotus-leaf-like, nanostructured surfaces. Langmur 2007;23(9):4871–7.
[11] Maynard J. Solved: Mystery how geckos use their feet to stick to walls and ceilings, Tech Times, 2014.
[12] Hyde EDER, Seyfaee A, Neville F, Moreno-Atanasio R. Colloidal Silica Particle Synthesis and Future Industrial Manufacturing Pathways: A Review, I & EC Industrial and Engineering Chemistry Research, 2016.
[13] Tiwaria JN, Tiwarib RN, Kima KS. Zero-dimensional, one-dimensional, two-dimensional and three-dimensional nanostructured materials for advanced electrochemical energy devices. Prog Mater Sci 2012;57(4):724–803.
[14] Sutariya VB, Pathak V, Groshev A, Chougule MB, Naik S, Patel D, et al., Introduction-biointeractions of nanomaterials: challenges and solutions, ISBN: 978-1-4665-8238-5, pp. 1–48.
[15] Russell P, Batchelor D, Thornton J. SEM and AFM: Complementary Techniques for High Resolution Surface Investigations, di Digital Instruments, Veeco Metrology Group.

[16] Cardell C, Guerra I. An overview of emerging hyphenated SEM-EDX and Raman spectroscopy systems: applications in life, environmental and materials sciences. TrAC - Trends Anal Chem 2016;77:156–66.
[17] Xu R. Light scattering: a review of particle characterization applications. Particuology February 2015;18:11–21.
[18] Brigger I, Dubernet C, Couvreur P. Nanoparticles in cancer therapy and diagnosis. Adv Drug Deliv Rev 2012;64(Supplement):24–36.
[19] Jacobs CB, Peairs MJ, Venton BJ. Review: carbon nanotube based electrochemical sensors for biomolecules. Anal Chim Acta 2010;662(2):105–27.
[20] Bastarrachea LJ, Denis-Rohr A, Goddard JM. Antimicrobial food equipment coatings: applications and challenges. Annu Rev Food Sci Technol 2015;6:97–118.
[21] Kishen A. ISBN: 978-3-319-13574-8 Nanotechnology in Endodontics - Current and Potential Clinical Applications. Springer; 1978.
[22] Heidarpour F, Wan Ab Karim Ghani WA, Fakhru'l-Razi A, Mozafari MR. Complete removal of pathogenic bacteria from drinking water using nano silver-coated cylindrical polypropylene filters. Clean Technol Environ Policy 2011;13(3):499–507.
[23] Lee W-H, Loo C-Y, Traini D, Young PM. Inhalation of nanoparticle-based drug for lung cancer treatment: advantages and challenges. Asian J Pharmaceut Sci 2015;10(6):481–9.
[24] Dourovic I, Poljak M, Posavčević M, Sršen F, Vidović T, Sertić M. Diabetes - The 21st century disease. Farm Glas 2014;70(6):383–97.
[25] Ramesan RM, Sharma CP. Challenges and advances in nanoparticle-based oral insulin delivery. Expert Rev Med Devices 2009;6(6):665–76.
[26] Savii C, Putz A-M, Recent advances in bioresponsive nanomaterials, carbon bonding and structures, Volume 5 of the series Carbon Materials: Chemistry and Physics pp 379–435, 2011.
[27] Li X, Tsibouklis J, Weng T, Zhang B, Yin G, Feng G, et al. Nano carriers for drug transport across the blood–brain barrier. J Drug Target 2016:1–12.
[28] Boraschi D, Italiani P. From antigen delivery system to adjuvanticy: the board application of nanoparticles in vaccinology. Vaccines 2015;3(4):930–9. http://dx.doi.org/10.3390/vaccines3040930.
[29] Kaufmann KB, Büning H, Galy A, Schambach A, Grez M, Gene therapy on the move, EMBO Molecular Medicine, 2013.
[30] Chen J, Guo Z, Tian H, Chen X, Production and clinical development of nanoparticles for gene delivery, Molecular Therapy-Methods & Clinical Development, Review Article, 2016.
[31] Fitzpatrick D, Implantable electronic medical devices, 1st Edition, ISBN: 978-124165779, 2014.
[32] Nikitin MP, Nanorobots for biomedical applications, Proceedings - 2016 International Conference Laser Optics, LO 2016, 23 August 2016, Article number 7549994, Page S227.
[33] Rus D, Tolley MT. Design, fabrication and control of soft robots. Nature 2015;521:467–75.
[34] Dragostin OM, Lupascu F, Dragan O, Apotrosoaei M, Velicescu C, Pieptu D, et al. Polymeric materials as nanofibres used in the treatment of burns. Pharmacy, Rev Med Chir Soc Med Nat, Iasi 2015;119(3).
[35] Teo WE, Ramakrishna S, A review on electrospinning design and nanofibre assemblies, Nanotechnology, Volume 17, Number 14.
[36] PhD thesis, University of Bolton.
[37] Agrawal CM, Ong JL, Appleford MR and Mani G., Introduction to Biomaterials.

[38] Zhang BGX, Myers DE, Wallace GG, Brandt M, Choong PFM. Bioactive coatings for orthopaedic implants—recent trends in development of implant coatings. Int J Mol Sci 2014;15(7):11878–921.
[39] Neel EAA, Bozec L, Perez RA, Kim H-W, Knowles JC. Nanotechnology in dentistry: prevention, diagnosis, and therapy. Int J Nanomedicine 2015;10:6371–94.
[40] Steinfeldt M, von Gleich A, Petschow U, Haum R. ISBN: 978-3-540-73882-4 Nanotechnologies, hazards and resource efficiency, a three-tiered approach to assessing the implications of nanotechnology and influencing its development. Springer; 2007.
[41] Global Nanomaterials Market - Segmented by Product Type, End-User Industry, and Geography - Trends and Forecasts (2015–2020), PRNwswire, 2015.
[42] Nanotechnology recent developments, risks and opportunities, RISKS, Lloyd's emerging risk team report 2007.
[43] Koo JH, Fundementals, properties, and applications of polymer nanocomposites, ISBN: 978-1-107-02996-5. 648-678.
[44] Oberdorster G. Safety assessment for nanotechnology and nanomedicine: concepts of nanotoxicology. J Intern Med 2010;267(1):89–105.
[45] Amoabediny G, Naderi A, Malakootikhah J, Rashedi H. Guidelines for safe handling, use and disposal of nanoparticles. J Phys Conf Ser 2009;170(1).
[46] Contado C. Nanomaterials in consumer products: a challenging analytical problem. Front Chem 2015;3.
[47] Crosera M, Bovenzi M, Maina G, Adami G, Zanette C, Florio C, et al. Nanoparticle dermal absorption and toxicity: a review of the literature. Int Arch Occup Environ Health 2009 Oct;82(9):1043–55.
[48] Iavicoli I, Fontana L, Nordberg G. The effects of nanoparticles on the renal system. Crit Rev Toxicol 2016;46(6):490–560.

Index

Note: Page numbers followed by "*f*" and "*t*" refer to figures and tables, respectively.

O

Q

R

S

X

Z

CPI Antony Rowe
Chippenham, UK
2017-06-08 17:59